Sexually Transmitted Diseases
SOURCEBOOK

Second Edition

Second Edition

Sexually Transmitted Diseases
SOURCEBOOK

*Basic Consumer Health Information about
Sexually Transmitted Diseases, Including
Information on the Diagnosis and Treatment of
Chlamydia, Gonorrhea, Hepatitis, Herpes, HIV,
Mononucleosis, Syphilis, and Others*

*Along with Information on Prevention, Such as
Condom Use, Vaccines, and STD Education; And
Featuring a Section on Issues Related to Youth
and Adolescents, a Glossary, and Resources for
Additional Help and Information*

Edited by
Dawn D. Matthews

Omnigraphics

615 Griswold Street • Detroit, MI 48226

Bibliographic Note

Because this page cannot legibly accommodate all the copyright notices, the Bibliographic Note portion of the Preface constitutes an extension of the copyright notice.

Each new volume of the *Health Reference Series* is individually titled and called a "First Edition." Subsequent updates will carry sequential edition numbers. To help avoid confusion and to provide maximum flexibility in our ability to respond to informational needs, the practice of consecutively numbering each volume will be discontinued.

Edited by Dawn D. Matthews

Health Reference Series

Karen Bellenir, *Series Editor*
Peter D. Dresser, *Managing Editor*
Maria Franklin, *Permissions Assistant*
Joan Margeson, *Research Associate*
Dawn Matthews, *Verification Assistant*
Jenifer Swanson, *Research Associate*

Omnigraphics, Inc.

Matthew P. Barbour, *Vice President, Operations*
Laurie Lanzen Harris, *Vice President, Editorial Director*
Kevin Hayes, *Production Coordinator*
Thomas J. Murphy, *Vice President, Finance and Comptroller*
Peter E. Ruffner, *Senior Vice President*
Jane J. Steele, *Marketing Coordinator*

Frederick G. Ruffner, Jr., Publisher

© 2001, Omnigraphics, Inc.

Library of Congress Cataloging-in-Publication Data

Sexually transmitted diseases sourcebook: basic consumer health information about sexually transmitted diseases, including information on the diagnosis and treatment of chlamydia, gonorrhea, hepatitis, herpes, HIV, mononucleosis, syphilis, and others; along with information on prevention, such as condom use, vaccines, and STD education; and featuring a section on issues related to youth and adolescents, a glossary, and resources for additional help and information / edited by Dawn D. Matthews.
    p. cm. -- (Health reference series)
  Includes bibliographical references and index.
  ISBN 0-7808-0249-7
    1. Sexually transmitted diseases--popular works. I. Matthews, Dawn D. II. Health reference series (Unnumbered)
RC200.2 .S387 2000
616.95'1--dc21

                                 00-047878

∞

This book is printed on acid-free paper meeting the ANSI Z39.48 Standard. The infinity symbol that appears above indicates that the paper in this book meets that standard.

Printed in the United States

Table of Contents

Part VI: Other Issues Related to Sexually Transmitted Diseases

Part VII: Additional Help and Information

Preface

About This Book

Sexually Transmitted Diseases (STDs) are among the most common infectious diseases in the United States today. More than 20 STDs have now been identified, and they affect more than 13 million men and women in this country each year. Men and women of all backgrounds are affected and nearly two-thirds of all STDs occur in people younger than 25 years of age. Understanding the basic facts about STDs—how they are spread, their symptoms, and how they are treated—is the first step toward prevention.

The *Sexually Transmitted Diseases Sourcebook, Second Edition* provides information about the symptoms, diagnosis, and treatment of most sexually transmitted diseases including chlamydia, gonorrhea, hepatitis, herpes, HIV, mononucleosis, syphilis, and others. It provides information on prevention issues, such as condom use, vaccines, and STD education, and a section on issues related to youth and adolescents. A glossary, and resources for additional help and information are also included.

How to Use This Book

This book is divided into parts and Chapters. Parts focus on broad areas of interest. Chapters are devoted to single topics within a part.

Part I: An Introduction to Sexually Transmitted Diseases offers information about the prevalence of sexually transmitted diseases among different populations, including statistics of STDs among youth and persons over age 50.

Part II: Types of Sexually Transmitted Diseases explains the different types of STDs, including chlamydia, gonorrhea, hepatitis, herpes, HIV, mononucleosis, syphilis, and others.

Part III: Risk and Prevention Issues gives informative advice on curbing STDs, including condom use and syringe exchange programs. It also addresses non-sexual transmission of STDs.

Part IV: Diagnosis and Treatment of Sexually Transmitted Diseases discusses the guidelines for the treatment of STDs, as well as addressing some testing and screening issues.

Part V: Issues Related to Youth and Adolescents contains information about topics of special concern to teens, the effectiveness of sex education, and vaccination recommendations for Hepatitis B.

Part VI: Other Issues Related to Sexually Transmitted Diseases discusses STDs and pregnancy, relationship of domestic violence to STDs, and occupational exposure to STDs.

Part VII: Additional Help and Resources includes a glossary of important terms and resources for further help and information.

Bibliographic Note

This volume contains documents and excerpts from publications issued by the following government agencies: Centers for Disease Control (CDC); National Institute of Allergy and Infectious Diseases (NAIAD); National Institute on Dental Research (NIDR); National Institutes of Health (NIH); United States Department of Health and Human Services (DHHS); United States Food and Drug Administration (FDA); United States Government Printing Office.

In addition, this volume contains copyrighted articles from American Academy of Family Physicians; American Health Consultants Inc.; American Medical Association; American Social Health Association; Charles W. Henderson; Cliggott Publishing Company; Clinical Reference Systems; Cortlandt Group; Crown Publishers Inc.; Lancet Ltd.; McGraw-Hill Inc.; Medical Economics Publishing; Sexuality Information and Education Council of the United States (SIECUS); Sigma Theta Tau International Honor Society of Nursing; Springhouse Corp.;

U.S. News and World Report Inc.; Washington Post/Newsweek Interactive Co.; Washington Times Corporation.

Full citation information is provided on the first page of each chapter. Every effort has been made to secure all necessary rights to reprint the copyrighted material. If any omissions have been made, please contact Omnigraphics to make corrections for future editions.

Acknowledgements

Thanks to Maria Franklin for her patience and to Bruce and Karen Bellenir for their help and support.

Note from the Editor

This book is part of Omnigraphics' *Health Reference Series*. The series provides basic information about a broad range of medical concerns. It is not intended to serve as a tool for diagnosing illness, in prescribing treatments, or as a substitute for the physician/patient relationship. All persons concerned about medical symptoms or the possibility of disease are encouraged to seek professional care from an appropriate health care provider.

Our Advisory Board

The *Health Reference Series* is reviewed by an Advisory Board comprised of librarians from public, academic, and medical libraries. We would like to thank the following board members for providing guidance to the development of this series:

Dr. Lynda Baker,
Associate Professor of Library and Information Science,
Wayne State University, Detroit, MI

Nancy Bulgarelli,
William Beaumont Hospital Library, Royal Oak, MI

Karen Imarasio,
Bloomfield Township Public Library, Bloomfield Township, MI

Karen Morgan,
Mardigian Library, University of Michigan-Dearborn,
Dearborn, MI

Rosemary Orlando,
St. Clair Shores Public Library, St. Clair Shores, MI

Health Reference Series *Update Policy*

The inaugural book in the *Health Reference Series* was the first edition of *Cancer Sourcebook* published in 1992. Since then, the *Series* has been enthusiastically received by librarians and in the medical community. In order to maintain the standard of providing high-quality health information for the lay person, the editorial staff at Omnigraphics felt it was necessary to implement a policy of updating volumes when warranted.

Medical researchers have been making tremendous strides, and it is the purpose of the *Health Reference Series* to stay current with the most recent advances. Each decision to update a volume will be made on an individual basis. Some of the considerations will include how much new information is available and the feedback we receive from people who use the books. If there is a topic you would like to see added to the update list, or an area of medical concern you feel has not been adequately addressed, please write to:

Editor
Health Reference Series
Omnigraphics, Inc.
615 Griswold Street
Detroit, MI 48226

The commitment to providing on-going coverage of important medical developments has also led to some format changes in the *Health Reference Series*. Each new volume on a topic is individually titled and called a "First Edition." Subsequent updates will carry sequential edition numbers. To help avoid confusion and to provide maximum flexibility in our ability to respond to informational needs, the practice of consecutively numbering each volume has been discontinued.

Part One

An Introduction to Sexually Transmitted Diseases

Chapter 1

An Overview of Sexually Transmitted Diseases (STDs)

Sexually transmitted diseases (STDs), once called venereal diseases, are among the most common infectious diseases in the United States today. More than 20 STDs have now been identified, and they affect more than 13 million men and women in this country each year. The annual comprehensive cost of STDs in the United States is estimated to be well in excess of $10 billion.

Understanding the basic facts about STDs—the ways in which they are spread, their common symptoms, and how they can be treated—is the first step toward prevention. The National Institute of Allergy and Infectious Diseases (NIAID), a part of the National Institutes of Health, has prepared a series of fact sheets about STDs to provide this important information. Research investigators supported by NIAID are looking for better methods of diagnosis and more effective treatments, as well as for vaccines and topical microbicides to prevent STDs. It is important to understand at least five key points about all STDs in this country today:

1. STDs affect men and women of all backgrounds and economic levels. They are most prevalent among teenagers and young adults. Nearly two-thirds of all STDs occur in people younger than 25 years of age.

2. The incidence of STDs is rising, in part because in the last few decades, young people have become sexually active earlier yet

National Institutes of Allergy and Infectious Diseases (NIAID), July 1999.

are marrying later. In addition, divorce is more common. The net result is that sexually active people today are more likely to have multiple sex partners during their lives and are potentially at risk for developing STDs.

3. Most of the time, STDs cause no symptoms, particularly in women. When and if symptoms develop, they may be confused with those of other diseases not transmitted through sexual contact. Even when an STD causes no symptoms, however, a person who is infected may be able to pass the disease on to a sex partner. That is why many doctors recommend periodic testing or screening for people who have more than one sex partner.

4. Health problems caused by STDs tend to be more severe and more frequent for women than for men, in part because the frequency of asymptomatic infection means that many women do not seek care until serious problems have developed.

    • Some STDs can spread into the uterus (womb) and fallopian tubes to cause pelvic inflammatory disease (PID), which in turn is a major cause of both infertility and ectopic (tubal) pregnancy. The latter can be fatal.

    • STDs in women also may be associated with cervical cancer. One STD, human papillomavirus infection (HPV), causes genital warts and cervical and other genital cancers.

    • STDs can be passed from a mother to her baby before, during, or immediately after birth; some of these infections of the newborn can be cured easily, but others may cause a baby to be permanently disabled or even die.

5. When diagnosed and treated early, many STDs can be treated effectively. Some infections have become resistant to the drugs used to treat them and now require newer types of antibiotics. Experts believe that having STDs other than AIDS increases one's risk for becoming infected with the AIDS virus.

HIV Infection and AIDS

AIDS (acquired immunodeficiency syndrome) was first reported in the United States in 1981. It is caused by the human immunodeficiency virus (HIV), a virus that destroys the body's ability to fight off infection. An estimated 900,000 people in the United States are currently infected with HIV. People who have AIDS are very susceptible to many life-threatening diseases, called opportunistic infections, and to certain forms of cancer. Transmission of the virus primarily occurs during sexual activity and by sharing needles used to inject intravenous drugs. If you have any questions about HIV infection or AIDS, you can call the AIDS Hotline confidential toll-free number: 1-800-342-AIDS.

Chlamydial Infection

This infection is now the most common of all bacterial STDs, with an estimated 4 to 8 million new cases occurring each year. In both men and women, chlamydial infection may cause an abnormal genital discharge and burning with urination. In women, untreated chlamydial infection may lead to pelvic inflammatory disease, one of the most common causes of ectopic pregnancy and infertility in women. Many people with chlamydial infection, however, have few or no symptoms of infection. Once diagnosed with chlamydial infection, a person can be treated with an antibiotic.

Genital Herpes

Genital herpes affects an estimated 60 million Americans. Approximately 500,000 new cases of this incurable viral infection develop annually. Herpes infections are caused by herpes simplex virus (HSV). The major symptoms of herpes infection are painful blisters or open sores in the genital area. These may be preceded by a tingling or burning sensation in the legs, buttocks, or genital region. The herpes sores usually disappear within two to three weeks, but the virus remains in the body for life and the lesions may recur from time to time. Severe or frequently recurrent genital herpes is treated with one of several antiviral drugs that are available by prescription. These drugs help control the symptoms but do not eliminate the herpes virus from the body. Suppressive antiviral therapy can be used to prevent occurrences and perhaps transmission. Women who acquire genital herpes during pregnancy can transmit the virus to their babies. Untreated HSV infection in newborns can result in mental retardation and death.

Genital Warts

Genital warts (also called venereal warts or condylomata acuminata) are caused by human papillomavirus, a virus related to the virus that causes common skin warts. Genital warts usually first appear as small, hard painless bumps in the vaginal area, on the penis, or around the anus. If untreated, they may grow and develop a fleshy, cauliflower-like appearance. Genital warts infect an estimated 1 million Americans each year. Genital warts can be injected with a type of interferon. If the warts are very large, they can be removed by surgery.

Gonorrhea

Approximately 400,000 cases of gonorrhea are reported to the U.S. Centers for Disease Control and Prevention (CDC) each year in this country. The most common symptoms of gonorrhea are a discharge from the vagina or penis and painful or difficult urination. The most common and serious complications occur in women and, as with chlamydial infection, these complications include PID, ectopic pregnancy, and infertility. Historically, penicillin has been used to treat gonorrhea, but in the last decade, four types of antibiotic resistance have emerged. New antibiotics or combinations of drugs must be used to treat these resistant strains.

Syphilis

The incidence of syphilis has increased and decreased dramatically in recent years, with more than 11,000 cases reported in 1996. The first symptoms of syphilis may go undetected because they are very mild and disappear spontaneously. The initial symptom is a chancre; it is usually a painless open sore that usually appears on the penis or around or in the vagina. It can also occur near the mouth, anus, or on the hands. If untreated, syphilis may go on to more advanced stages, including a transient rash and, eventually, serious involvement of the heart and central nervous system. The full course of the disease can take years. Penicillin remains the most effective drug to treat people with syphilis.

Other diseases that may be sexually transmitted include trichomoniasis, bacterial vaginosis, cytomegalovirus infections, scabies, and pubic lice.

STDs in pregnant women are associated with a number of adverse outcomes, including spontaneous abortion and infection in the newborn. Low birth weight and prematurity appear to be associated with STDs, including chlamydial infection and trichomoniasis. Congenital or perinatal infection (infection that occurs around the time of birth) occurs in 30 to 70 percent of infants born to infected mothers, and complications may include pneumonia, eye infections, and permanent neurologic damage.

What Can You Do to Prevent STDs?

The best way to prevent STDs is to avoid sexual contact with others. If you decide to be sexually active, there are things that you can do to reduce your risk of developing an STD.

- Have a mutually monogamous sexual relationship with an uninfected partner.

- Correctly and consistently use a male condom.

- Use clean needles if injecting intravenous drugs.

- Prevent and control other STDs to decrease susceptibility to HIV infection and to reduce your infectiousness if you are HIV-infected.

- Delay having sexual relations as long as possible. The younger people are when having sex for the first time, the more susceptible they become to developing an STD. The risk of acquiring an STD also increases with the number of partners over a lifetime.

Anyone who is sexually active should:

- Have regular checkups for STDs even in the absence of symptoms, and especially if having sex with a new partner. These tests can be done during a routine visit to the doctor's office.

- Learn the common symptoms of STDs. Seek medical help immediately if any suspicious symptoms develop, even if they are mild.

- Avoid having sex during menstruation. HIV-infected women are probably more infectious, and HIV-uninfected women are probably more susceptible to becoming infected during that time.

- Avoid anal intercourse, but if practiced, use a male condom.

- Avoid douching because it removes some of the normal protective bacteria in the vagina and increases the risk of getting some STDs.

Anyone diagnosed as having an STD should:

- Be treated to reduce the risk of transmitting an STD to an infant.

- Discuss with a doctor the possible risk of transmission in breast milk and whether commercial formula should be substituted.

- Notify all recent sex partners and urge them to get a checkup.

- Follow the doctor's orders and complete the full course of medication prescribed. A follow-up test to ensure that the infection has been cured is often an important step in treatment.

- Avoid all sexual activity while being treated for an STD.

Sometimes people are too embarrassed or frightened to ask for help or information. Most STDs are readily treated, and the earlier a person seeks treatment and warns sex partners about the disease, the less likely the disease will do irreparable physical damage, be spread to others or, in the case of a woman, be passed on to a newborn baby.

Private doctors, local health departments, and STD and family planning clinics have information about STDs. In addition, the American Social Health Association (ASHA) provides free information and keeps lists of clinics and private doctors who provide treatment for people with STDs. ASHA has a national toll-free telephone number, 1-800-230-6039. The phone number for the Herpes Hotline, also run by ASHA, is 919-361-8488. Callers can get information from the ASHA hotline without leaving their names.

Research

STDs cause physical and emotional suffering to millions and are costly to individuals and to society as a whole. NIAID conducts and supports many research projects designed to improve methods of prevention, and to find better ways to diagnose and treat these diseases. NIAID also supports several large university-based STD research centers.

Within the past few years, NIAID-supported research has resulted in new tests to diagnose some STDs faster and more accurately. New drug treatments for STDs are under investigation by NIAID researchers. This is especially important because some STDs are becoming resistant to the standard drugs. In addition, vaccines are being developed or tested for effectiveness in preventing several STDs, including AIDS, chlamydial infection, genital herpes, and gonorrhea.

It is up to each individual to learn more about STDs and then make choices about how to minimize the risk of acquiring these diseases and spreading them to others. Knowledge of STDs, as well as honesty and openness with sex partners and with one's doctor, can be very important in reducing the incidence and complications of sexually transmitted diseases.

Table 1.1. Sexually Transmitted Diseases and the Organisms Responsible

Disease	Organism(s)
Acquired Immunodeficiency Syndrome (AIDS)	Human immunodeficiency virus
Bacterial vaginosis	*Bacteroides* *Gardnerella vaginalis* *Mobiluncus spp.* *Mycoplasma hominis* *Ureaplasma urealyticum*
Chancroid	*Haemophilus ducreyi*
Chlamydial infections	*Chlamydia trachomatis*
Cytomegalovirus infections	Cytomegalovirus
Genital herpes	Herpes simplex virus
Genital (venereal) warts	Human papillomavirus
Gonorrhea	*Neisseria gonorrhoeae*
Granuloma inguinale (donovanosis)	*Calymmatobacterium granulomatis*
Leukemia-Lymphoma/Myelopathy	HTLV-I and II
Lymphogranuloma venereum	*Chlamydia trachomatis*
Molluscum contagiosum	Molluscum contagiosum virus
Pubic lice	*Phthirus pubis*
Scabies	*Sarcoptes scabiei*
Syphilis	*Treponema pallidum*
Trichomoniasis	*Trichomonas vaginalis*
Vaginal yeast infections	*Candida albicans*

Chapter 2

STDs: Are You Up-to-Date?

While many Americans believe STDs no longer present an urgent threat, these infections are alive and well in more people than you might guess. Here's the latest on what you need to know to help prevent and treat these common, potentially serious conditions.

Over the past four decades, vast progress has been made in this country toward the successful management and prevention of sexually transmitted diseases (STDs). The incidence of both syphilis and gonorrhea is the lowest ever in the United States, and about half of all current reported syphilis cases are concentrated in just 1% of US counties.[1] Syphilis rates are so low this year that the CDC is planning a campaign to eradicate that infection in this country.

Against this backdrop, national data indicate a significant resurgence of both primary and secondary syphilis in certain regions, particularly among minority members at lower socioeconomic levels, many of whom live in poverty, have limited access to health care, and use illegal drugs. This propagates congenital syphilis, which experts mistakenly believed would disappear after the advent of penicillin. Moreover, while gonorrhea rates have declined consistently since the 1970s, they remain dangerously high among teenagers, young adults, and African Americans.

Numerous studies also indicate that genital herpes simplex virus (HSV) infection continues to spread in many regions of the country.

Curative therapy remains unavailable, and the technologies that deliver the most effective care at this time are both expensive and fairly new. Human papillomavirus (HPV) infection appears to be increasing steadily among young people from middle and upper socioeconomic populations. In addition, chlamydial infections continue to be the most commonly reported bacterial STD.

Despite all the progress, STDs are still a substantial problem in the United States, which has the highest rates among industrialized nations. Each year, some 15 million Americans contract an STD. Approximately one third of these people are teenagers, some as young as 13. STDs on the Top 10 list include chlamydial infections, with about 4 million new cases yearly; trichomoniasis, with 3 million; and gonorrhea, with more than 1 million (see Table 2.1). The overall cost of STDs, about $17 billion annually, includes $6.7 billion associated with managing HIV infection and AIDS.[2] Almost all STDs dramatically increase the risk of both acquiring and spreading HIV.

Women sustain a disproportionate burden of complications directly related to STDs, including pelvic inflammatory disease (PID), infertility, potentially fatal ectopic pregnancies, and cancer of the reproductive tract. Infants infected during gestation or birth can suffer blindness, bone deformities, mental retardation, and even death. STDs remain a dire problem among teenagers, many of whom have multiple sex partners and engage in unprotected intercourse (see "STDs and US teens"). Studies indicate that a whole new generation of young people—especially young homosexuals—are participating in riskier sexual behavior than the preceding generation.

An extremely important advance has occurred in chlamydial screening with the licensing of a polymerase chain reaction test and a ligase chain reaction test, the latter developed to uncover both chlamydia and gonorrhea. While these tests have been on the market for several years, they have only just begun to receive the attention they deserve.

The Most Pressing Challenges

While only a few STDs are life-threatening—HIV infection, hepatitis B, and syphilis—the vast majority can lead to serious medical conditions for patients and their offspring. For example, when both the cervix and uterus are infected with HSV, the risk of cervical cancer is 8 times higher than in noninfected women.[1] Whether HSV actually causes the cancer remains unclear. What is known is that early initiation of intercourse and having multiple sex partners not only increase the chances of being infected with HSV but also of other STDs linked to cancer development.

Acute HSV Infection

This disease greatly increases a pregnant woman's chances of spontaneous abortion and premature labor. Women with this infection have a miscarriage rate more than 3 times that of uninfected women, and delivering an infant through an infected canal can expose a newborn to a virus that causes irreversible brain damage, if not death. Many experts believe, however, that patients infected with HSV-2 who have no active vaginal sores usually experience normal, safe deliveries.

HPV Infection

Currently the fastest-spreading STD in this country, HPV infection can linger throughout a lifetime. Patients with visible genital warts may be infected simultaneously with multiple HPV types, some of which have been associated with external genital squamous intraepithelial neoplasia such as squamous cell carcinoma in situ or Bowen's disease of the genitalia. These types also have been related to vaginal, anal, and cervical intraepithelial dysplasia and squamous cell carcinoma.

Bacterial Vaginosis (BV)

BV is no longer considered simply a bothersome illness that triggers a malodorous discharge. Experts now know it has the potential to increase the risk of upper tract infection following gynecologic surgery and, in certain patients, the risk of future premature births. Intra-amniotic infection and PID are also associated with BV.

Pelvic Inflammatory Disease

The serious consequences of PID almost exclusively affect sexually active women in their reproductive years. Delay in treatment increases the risk of infertility, ectopic pregnancy, chronic pelvic abscesses and pain, and the need for abdominal surgery. While acute PID may have a polymicrobial etiology, it remains the most common serious complication of chlamydial and gonococcal infections—the primary causes of PID in about 80% of cases involving women younger than 25.[3]

Asymptomatic Patients

Many cases of gonorrhea in women fail to produce recognizable symptoms until potentially serious complications such as PID have already occurred. Conversely, most male patients with gonorrhea present with urethritis and experience pain, difficulty urinating, and penile discharge, which usually prompt them to seek treatment soon enough to avoid serious sequelae. Asymptomatic chlamydial infection runs rampant among both men and women, and numerous cases of HSV are spread by patients who are completely unaware they harbor the infection or who are asymptomatic during transmission.

While syphilis and herpes infection can be asymptomatic in both sexes, men again are more likely to be diagnosed via a complaint such as penile lesions. Lesions in female patients are often found within the vagina and on the cervix, making them less evident.

Syphilis, which develops in stages, can be particularly difficult to diagnose and may be life-threatening if not detected expeditiously. The primary form often presents with painless chancres that, if left untreated, clear on their own. Patients with stage 2 syphilis present with systemic illness, including low-grade fever, hair loss, rash, and swollen lymph nodes—signs that often mimic mononucleosis. Because many patients mistake these signs for a less serious illness, medical evaluation is often delayed. In the meantime, *Treponema pallidum* can disseminate throughout the body, causing structural damage to the brain, liver, and aorta.

STDs that typically cause symptoms (such as trichomoniasis) can linger for a substantial time before signs or symptoms become apparent. In addition, most men infected with *Trichomonas vaginalis* have no symptoms, although a subgroup may have nongonococcal urethritis.

Risk Assessment

Preventing the spread of STDs requires that people at risk for transmitting or acquiring infection alter their sexual behavior. A logical first step is for physicians to incorporate sexual histories into their routine history taking. Many physicians worry about their ability to initiate such a conversation or about opening up "a can of worms" that might consume too much office time. A national survey found that primary care physicians assessed sexual behavior in less than half of all patients.[2]

The more sexual histories you take, the more comfortable you will become and the more adept at keeping them brief. Furthermore, surveys have shown that most patients actually welcome having their doctors show an interest in their sexual lives and don't object to succinct, nonjudgmental questions. The key to initiating a successful interview is to develop a standardized approach, keeping in mind that questions need to be tailored to individual patients. The recently widowed 72-year-old woman, for instance, requires a much different sexual history than the single woman in her 20s. Before broaching this topic, patients should be told why it is necessary to inquire about their sex lives. Otherwise, some may become suspicious of the sudden interest in this topic.

Among the questions to cover:

- Are you sexually active?
- Are you involved in a monogamous relationship, or do you have multiple sex partners?
- Are you involved with someone who has an STD or multiple sex partners?
- Have you ever had an STD or PID?
- Do you use protective barrier contraception during sex?
- Do you have sex with men, women, or both?
- Do you participate in vaginal, oral, and/or anal sex?

Remember that anal intercourse is the riskiest activity for sexual transmission of HIV infection. Age at first sexual experience is important. The longer a person has been having intercourse, the greater the chances of having been exposed to STDs. Ask if they engage in casual sex (for example, in bars or bathhouses). Transmission of some STDs is highly associated with this type of anonymous sexual activity. Some people tend to put themselves at high risk on weekends, during travel, and when they are intoxicated or feeling depressed. Determine, also, if any of your patients ever offered sex in exchange for food, money, drugs, or a place to sleep, or if they were ever forced into sexual activity.

Find out whether patients or their partners experience painful intercourse or urination, bleed following sex, have lower abdominal pain, notice discharge from the vagina or penis, or have genital sores or bumps. Be sure to leave time for patients to ask their own questions or air their concerns about their sexual activity.

Interviewing Teenagers Requires Finesse

Assure them that the questions you plan to ask are routine. Keep your questions specific, and use terms familiar to them. Don't assume all teens understand the meaning of "intercourse" or "anal sex." Adolescents who don't understand what you are asking may answer "No" to avoid appearing ignorant. Most young people are willing to discuss their sexual behaviors and concerns with their physician provided they don't have to initiate the conversation and confidentiality is ensured. Nonetheless, teens unwilling to disclose their sexual history to you should be encouraged to confide in an alternate health care provider, whether another clinician or a local health department professional.

Diagnostic Screening

Which STDs are worth screening for? In certain populations, screening for chlamydia is required, but consensus is lacking for BV in pregnant women and for HPV infection.

Chlamydia

Because of the asymptomatic nature of Chlamydia trachomatis infection, its potentially serious ramifications, and its prevalence in the United States, the CDC screening guidelines are very specific. Unmarried, sexually active female patients younger than 20 are automatic candidates for chlamydial testing. Routine screening also is recommended for women aged 20 to 24, particularly those with new or multiple sex partners and who do not use barrier contraceptives regularly. Having more than 1 sex partner remains a uniform risk factor for every STD.

Various reasons have been posited for the delay in popularity of the polymerase chain reaction (PCR) and ligase chain reaction (LCR) tests for chlamydia. For optimal test results, first-voided urine (FVU) specimens are required, which takes testing out of the hands of physicians. These tests also require more extensive follow-up.

Both of these highly accurate techniques allow specimens to be taken from multiple sites (for example, the endocervix, urethra, or urine). The availability of these tests may encourage more men to be screened. Chlamydial screening for this population previously required urethral swabbing—a painful process for patient and clinician. The new methodologies also allow detection of a larger number of silent infections that traditional tests might otherwise miss. Unlike immuno-fluorescent antibody tests and enzyme immunoassays (EIAs), which only uncover about 60% of infections in asymptomatic young women, LCR and PCR tests detect more than 90% of all infections

16

while offering equal specificity. One study comparing the performance of LCR to ETA using FVU obtained from 447 female patients found the sensitivity of LCR to be 96.3% versus 37% for EIA.[4]

The CDC advocates the use of more sensitive screening tests, which can obviate frequent empirical treatment. Yet, older methodologies remain faster, less costly, and less complex. They are also associated with fewer stringent specifications regarding specimen handling and transport.

Besides enhancing outcomes, screening high-risk candidates for *C. trachomatis* infection appears to be a sound strategy for avoiding liability. Claims and settlements totaling millions of dollars have been acquired in instances of preterm births alleged to have been caused by STDs.[5]

Because the risk of contracting chlamydia diminishes with age, routine screening for patients aged 30 and older is usually unnecessary. Exceptions include patients with new or multiple sex partners and those who suspect their partner may have infected them. Similarly, unless you are practicing in an area where a certain infection is prevalent, many experts feel screening nonrisk patients for other STDs is not advisable.

Nonetheless, when a patient is suspected of having a particular STD, testing for other infections is recommended. At minimum, a patient with either gonorrhea, chlamydia, syphilis, or HIV should also be tested for the other 3. Once the decision to screen has been made, using proper diagnostic techniques is critical to appropriate disease management.

Bacterial Vaginosis

Some physicians continue to screen pregnant patients for BV, but this practice has spurred controversy. Authorities question whether the risks associated with this illness are sufficiently high and whether preventive therapy works well enough to warrant universal screening for this population. Current CDC guidelines indicate that it may be worthwhile to screen pregnant women who have had a previous preterm delivery.[6] The recommendation for treatment is with a systemic (as opposed to a vaginal) medication against BV. Others believe more information is required.

Human Papillomavirus Infection

Another active debate involves HPV screening. One camp contends HPV testing should be conducted during routine Pap smears so that more aggressive diagnostic and therapeutic methodologies can be implemented if certain HPV infections are detected. Naysayers argue that searching for the defining silent HPV infection does not help manage a patient and that the precancerous cellular changes themselves are the only important target for treatment. Until inexpensive HPV tests become available, an Institute of Medicine (IOM) 1997 report entitled, "The Hidden Epidemic: Confronting Sexually Transmitted Diseases," IOM's comprehensive study contends that the high incidence of STDs in this country is due largely to inconsistent treatment and that an effective system for STD prevention and control has not yet been established. Another recent study showed that about half of primary care physicians managing a patient with PID were unsure of, or did not follow, CDC guidelines.[2]

In light of its findings, the IOM urges greater guideline dissemination and implementation of CDC protocols by all primary care providers and managed care organizations. Clinicians should resist the temptation, however, to merely look up a drug regimen for a particular STD in the new guidelines. Reading an entire section on a certain infection will help you understand the nuances and weigh the pros and cons of a certain therapeutic option over another.

Since 1993, significant advances have occurred, with key implications for managing STDs. For example, effective single-dose oral therapies are now available for most curable STDs. Infections such as chlamydia can thus be managed in 1 office visit, thereby reducing the time period in which an infected person can transmit the disease to others. Nonetheless, 7-day drug regimens are just as effective and much less costly, though compliance may be an issue with some patients.

Herpes Simplex Virus Infection

Recommendations for treating both primary and recurrent HSV have been revised. Research indicates antiviral drugs such as acyclovir, famciclovir, and valacyclovir have similar efficacy. They decrease duration of symptoms and viral shedding, and they accelerate healing. These agents can also be used to treat recurrences or as suppressive therapy to prevent recurrence.

Pelvic Inflammatory Disease

A significant change in treatment has been the CDC's recognition that not all PID patients require hospitalization for parenteral antibiotic therapy. It was previously believed that such therapy could only be administered to inpatients since they required bed rest and supervised treatment. According to the CDC, patients who still may require hospitalization:

- Are pregnant
- May have a surgical emergency, such as appendicitis, that cannot be excluded
- Fail to respond clinically to oral antimicrobial therapy
- Are unable to follow or tolerate an outpatient oral regimen
- Have severe illness, nausea, vomiting, or high fever
- Have a tubo-ovarian abscess
- Are immunodeficient.[6]

Genital Warts

Patient-applied medications are now available to treat genital warts. These alleviate numerous bothersome symptoms and are simpler to dispense when symptoms flare than traditional therapies. Before prescribing one of these solutions/gels, however be certain your patients can identify and reach all warts; otherwise, therapy will be ineffective.

Bacterial Vaginosis

Although metronidazole has been found to be safe in all stages of pregnancy, most clinicians, on theoretical grounds, would recommend its use only after the first trimester. Systemic metronidazole is probably better to use than vaginal preparations, which have not prevented prematurity. Note that the use of clindamycin vaginal cream during pregnancy is not recommended.[6]

Gonorrhea

Concern is mounting about the future ability of the fluoroquinolones to treat gonorrhea. While the incidence of infections caused by *Neisseria gonorrhoeae* has decreased in this country since 1975, the proportion of gonococcal infections caused by resistant organisms has increased.[7] Various reports indicate that a small percentage of isolates nationwide display lessened susceptibility to fluoroquinolones.[8] Impending changes in antimicrobial susceptibility may lead to the resurgence of this infection and to the emergence of new forms of antibiotic resistance. Fortunately, other medications used to treat gonorrhea show no signs of antimicrobial resistance at this time.

For any patient with an STD, if symptoms persist despite your best treatment efforts, seek assistance from a local health department or an infectious disease specialist. Both resources are available to help you effectively manage your STD population.

STD Prevention

While most Americans are at least somewhat aware of the serious repercussions associated with HIV infection, studies indicate too few people in this country recognize the numerous risks associated with irresponsible sexual behavior. The importance of educating patients on the dangers of STDs cannot be stressed enough. Primary care clinicians are in an optimal position to teach the public how STDs are contracted, what signs and symptoms are associated with these infections, what to do when infection is suspected, and how to practice safer sex. As part of this prevention equation, the CDC's 1998 guidelines highlight the need for clinicians and health care agencies to recognize the sexually transmitted nature of hepatitis B and to endorse this series of immunizations.

References

1. Osujih, M., "The 'Other' Sexually Transmitted Diseases: A Case for Public Health Education."; J. Roy; *Soc Health,* 1997:117:351-354.

2. Gunn, R.A.; Rolfs, R.T.; Greenspan, J.R. et al.; "The Changing Paradigm of Sexually Transmitted Disease Control in the Era of Managed Health Care."; *JAMA,* 1998; 279:680-684.

3. Kamwendo, F.; Forslin, L.; Bodin, L., et al.; "Programmes to Reduce Pelvic Inflammatory Disease—the Swedish Experience."; *Lancet,* 1998;35(suppl III):25-28.

4. LeBar, W.D.; "Keeping Up with New Technology: New Approaches to Diagnosis of Chlamydia Infection."; *Clin Chem,* 1996:42:809-812.

5. McGregor, J.A.; Paul, K.; "Money-Saving Benefits of Screening and Treating for *Chlamydia Trachomatis* in Patients and Partners."; *Sex Transm Dis,* 1998:26:53-54.

6. "Centers for Disease Control and Prevention: 1998 Guidelines for Treatment of Sexually Transmitted Diseases."; *MMWR. Morb Mortal Wkly Rep,* 1998;47(RR-1):i-116.

7. Erbelding, E.; Quinn, T.C.; "The Impact of Antimicrobial Residence on the Treatment of Sexually Transmitted Diseases.";
   Infect Dis Clin North Am, 1997; 11:889-903.

8. Weisfuse, I.B.; "Gonorrhoea Control and Antimicrobial Resistance."; *Lancet,* 1998; 351:928.

Table 2.1. The most common STDs in the United States are here shown according to the approximate number of new cases in Americans each year.

Human papillomavirus infection	750,000
Genital herpes simplex	500,000
Hepatitis B	150,000
Syphilis	120,000
HIV infection	45,000
Chlamydial infection	4 million
Trichomoniasis	3 million
Gonorrhea	1.1 million

STDs and US Teens

Each year, some 3 million teenagers in this country contract a sexually transmitted disease (STD). According to recent studies, 1 in 4 sexually active teens acquires an STD before graduating from high school. Research also shows more adolescents are afflicted with diseases such as human papillomavirus infection, chlamydia, and gonorrhea than any other patient population.[1]

HIV infection appears to be on the increase in this population, too. While the number of AIDS cases among teens remains comparatively small, the incidence of AIDS in people in their 20s is high. This has led authorities to conclude many HIV infections are acquired during adolescence.

A number of factors contribute to this dismal national scenario:

- About 70% of all males and 60% of females have had intercourse by their senior year in high school. About 40% of boys

21

and 30% of girls become sexually promiscuous by the ninth grade.

- Teenagers typically have multiple sex partners, many of whom are more likely to be infected with an STD.

- Young people tend to take risks, such as having unprotected sex.

- Adolescents are at greater risk than other populations for substance abuse and other behaviors that increase the likelihood of STD acquisition.

- Many youths avoid the health care system out of fear their parents will discover they are sexually active.

- Adolescents are biologically more susceptible to infection than adults.

Primary care clinicians are in a favorable position to offer teens preventive education that promotes healthy sexual behavior. Considering the high number of teenagers who are sexually active by age 18, you can reasonably assume your young patients either fall within this group or are seriously considering becoming sexually active. Deal with this reality in a pragmatic, nonjudgmental way, and create opportunities to talk with these patients privately about their sexual relationships. Many states give teenagers the legal right to receive medical treatment for an STD and to consent to HIV testing/counseling without parental knowledge. Avoid the temptation to talk down to teenage-patients. This only spawns anger or distrust and discourages teens from disclosing critical medical information.

1. Krowchuk, D.P.; "Sexually Transmitted Diseases in Adolescents: What's New?"; *South Med J.*, 1998;91:124-131.

The Importance of Partner Notification

According to the CDC, partner referral is one of the best ways to avoid future sexually transmitted disease (STD) transmission/reinfection, particularly when infections are curable or preventable by vaccine. Clinicians should urge all patients with an STD to notify any sex partner(s) of their disease exposure and to encourage them to seek evaluation. This protocol is known as patient referral. If you suspect this process will be ineffective or impossible for a particular client, a local health department will initiate either a contact or provider referral. The former practice allows patients a specific period of time to refer their partners. Referrals that fail to manifest themselves within that time frame are handed over to a health department staff member, who then sets a provider referral in motion.

Many patients prefer that public health officials take charge of partner notifications to ensure confidentiality. Most clinicians welcome this choice since they have neither the time nor the skill required to locate and refer all partners for diagnosis, treatment, and counseling. Partner notifications also can be quite awkward. How do you get the spouse of your male patient (who has just admitted to contracting his infection from a third party) to come in for evaluation without throwing a grenade into the marriage? Health department professionals are highly skilled in soliciting all pertinent information from patients about their social relationships (which can take several meetings) and in discretely obtaining spousal or partner permission to undergo testing. If you suspect your patient is hiding critical information from you, call your local health department for assistance.

When a diagnosis of bacterial vaginosis (BV) or genital warts is made, routine partner rehabilitation is not standard protocol. For instance, a woman's response to therapy for BV and the likelihood of relapse/recurrence are unaffected by treatment of her sex partner(s). Regarding genital warts, the role of reinfection is minimal and, in the absence of a therapeutic cure, treatment to attenuate transmission is impractical.

Consequently, some experts believe partner notification is unnecessary where these 2 infections are concerned. Yet, partners may benefit from a lesson on the implications of having sex with infected partners. They should be cautioned, for instance, that a patient can remain infectious despite wart eradication and reminded about the importance of using condoms for reducing the risk of transmission to uninfected parties and of acquiring another STD.

How many partners from a patient's history should be tracked down? Only those who have had contact with the patient over the past few months—or everyone from the patient's sexual past? It depends on the type of infection being traced. STDs like gonorrhea, which are transmitted from person to person quickly and have very short incubation periods, are lower on the list of health department contact investigations. Syphilis, on the other hand, is much higher on the contact list since it has a much longer incubation period, can cause long-term structural damage, and may lead to congenital syphilis. Nonetheless, use discretion when deciding whom to contact.

Pre-Exposure Immunization and STD Prevention

Vaccines are currently licensed in this country to prevent the spread of infection with hepatitis A virus (HAV) and hepatitis B virus (HBV). Both are safe, effective, and extremely important considering how easily these viruses are channeled from person to person. HBV is about 100 times more infectious than HIV. Over the past decade, sexual transmission has been responsible for up to 60% of the estimated 240,000 new HBV infections reported annually in the United States. HBV infection causes some 6000 deaths in this country every year as a direct result of its chronic complications: cirrhosis and primary hepatocellular carcinoma.

Now that routine infant and adolescent HBV vaccination programs have been set in motion, immunizing high-risk adults has become a top priority. According to the CDC, people who should receive the HBV vaccine include:

- Sexually active homosexual/bisexual men

- Sexually active heterosexual men and women, particularly those in whom another STD has recently been diagnosed, those with multiple sex partners, those who have received treatment in an STD clinic, and prostitutes

- Illegal drug users

- Health care workers

- Recipients of certain blood products

- Household/sexual contacts of people with chronic HBV infection

- Adoptees from countries where HBV is endemic

- Certain international travelers

- Clients/employees of facilities for the developmentally disabled

- Infants, children, and adolescents

- Patients on hemodialysis.[1]

The HBV vaccine is highly immunogenic. Protective levels of antibody are present in about half of all young patients after 1 dose; in about 85%, after 2 doses; and in more than 90%, after 3 doses. (The final dose is required to provide long-term immunity.) A current immunization schedule calls for vaccination at initiation (or, time zero), 1 to 2 months, and 4 to 6 months. Because chronic HBV infection is more likely to develop in patients with HBV-HIV coinfection, and since HIV can impair the effectiveness of the vaccine, HIV patients should be tested for hepatitis B surface antibody 1 to 2 months after receiving the final vaccine.

While HAV infection is not an STD, the CDC still recommends the HAV vaccine for men who have sex with other men and illegal drug users. The inactivated HAV vaccine, administered as a 2-dose series, is both immunogenic and effective. Research indicates almost all patients respond to 1 dose of this vaccine and that the second provides long-term protection.

Clinical trials currently are under way for vaccines against many STDs, including HIV and genital herpes. Several new HSV vaccines, including replication-limited live-virus vaccines, live-virus vectors (where immunogenic HSV genes are inserted into a live viral or bacterial vector), and vaccines containing immunogenic envelope glycoproteins are being developed and evaluated.[2] In addition, the relative simplicity of papillomaviruses bodes well for a successful genital warts vaccine. As clinical trials geared toward prophylactic and therapeutic vaccination for this illness progress, experts estimate a successful vaccine may become available within a few years.[3]

1. "Centers for Disease Control and Prevention: 1998 Guidelines for Treatment of Sexually Transmitted Diseases."; *MMWR Morb Mortal Wkly Rep.*, 1998:47 (RR-): 102.

2. Mindel, A.; "Genital Herpes—How Much of a Pubic-Health Problem?"; *Lancet.*, 1998;351 (suppl. III):16-18.

3. Galloway, D.A.;"Is Vaccination Against Human Papillomavirus a Possibility?"; *Lancet.*, 1998;351 (suppl. III):22-24.

—by Nancy E. Trotto

Chapter 3

STDs: Statistics

The following are the statistics for sexually transmitted diseases in the United States, prepared by the Office of Communications and Public Liaison of the National Institute of Allergy and Infectious Diseases (NIAID).

Overall Statistics

- In the United States, an estimated 15.3 million new cases of sexually transmitted diseases (STDs) occur each year, at least one-quarter of them among teenagers.[1]

- Of the top 11 reportable diseases in the United States in 1996, five are transmitted sexually (chlamydial infection, gonorrhea, AIDS, syphilis and hepatitis B).[2]

- Approximately two-thirds of people who acquire STDs in the United States are younger than 25.[1,3]

- In the United States in 1994, approximately $10 billion was spent on major STDs (other than HIV/AIDS) and their preventable complications. This figure rises to approximately $17 billion if sexually transmitted human immunodeficiency virus (HIV) infections are included.[3]

1998 National Institute of Allergy and Infectious Diseases (NIAID).

- Worldwide, an estimated 333 million new cases of four curable STDs (gonorrhea, chlamydial infection, syphilis and trichomoniasis) occurred in 1997.[4]

HIV/AIDS

- As of December 1998, an estimated 33.4 million people worldwide were living with HIV/AIDS. Cumulative AIDS-related deaths worldwide as of December 1997 numbered approximately 13.9 million.[5]

- In 1997 alone, HIV/AIDS-associated illnesses caused the deaths of approximately 2.5 million people worldwide.[5]

- In the United States, 641,086 cases of AIDS had been reported to the Centers for Disease Control and Prevention (CDC) as of Dec. 31, 1997. Of these people, 390,692 had died by the end of 1997.[6]

- In 1994, the total cost of sexually transmitted HIV infection in the United States was approximately $6.7 billion.[3]

Chlamydial Infection

- Infection with Chlamydia trachomatis is the most common bacterial STD in the United States. Three million new cases are estimated to occur annually in this country.[1]

- As many as 85 percent of women with chlamydial infections are asymptomatic; 40 percent of infected men report no symptoms.[3]

- In 1997, 526,653 chlamydial infections were reported to the CDC, a case rate of 207 per 100,000 population.[7]

- In 1994, the total cost of chlamydial infections in the United States was estimated to be $2.0 billion.[3]

- Worldwide, an estimated 89 million new chlamydial infections occurred in 1997.[4]

- If not adequately treated, 20 to 40 percent of women with genital chlamydial infections develop pelvic inflammatory disease (PID), which in turn causes problems such as infertility, ectopic pregnancy and chronic pelvic pain.[3]

Gonorrhea

- An estimated 650,000 cases of gonorrhea, caused by *Neisseria gonorrhoeae*, occur annually in the United States.[1]

- In 1997, 324,901 cases of gonorrhea in the United States were reported to the CDC, a case rate of 122/100,000.[7]

- Approximately 50 percent of *N. gonorrhoea* infections in women are asymptomatic.[3]

- In 1994, costs associated with gonorrhea in the United States totalled an estimated $1.1 billion.[3]

- Worldwide, an estimated 62 million new cases of gonorrhea occurred in 1997.[4]

- If not adequately treated, 10 to 40 percent of women infected with gonorrhea develop PID.[3]

Pelvic Inflammatory Disease

- At least 1 million cases of PID, an important complication of both gonorrhea and chlamydial infection, occur annually in the United States.[3]

- Of all infertile women, at least 15 percent are infertile because of tubal damage caused by PID.[3]

- Total costs associated with PID in the United States were estimated to be $6 billion in 1996.[8]

- Following PID, scarring will cause approximately 20 percent of women to become infertile, 18 percent to develop chronic pelvic pain, and 9 percent to have ectopic pregnancies.[9]

Genital Herpes

- About one in five people in the United States over age 12 — approximately 45 million individuals — are infected with HSV-2, the virus that causes genital herpes.[10]

- Up to 1 million new HSV-2 infections may be transmitted each year in the United States.[1]

- Costs associated with genital herpes totalled approximately $237 million in 1994.[3]

Hepatitis B

- An estimated 77,000 cases of sexually transmitted hepatitis B infection occur annually in the United States.[1]

- Approximately 750,000 people in the United States are living with sexually acquired hepatitis B infection.[1]

- Costs associated with sexually transmitted hepatitis B in the United States totalled $156 million in 1994.[3]

Human Papillomavirus (HPV) Infection

- An estimated 20 million people in the United states are infected with HPV, and as many as 5.5 million new infections occur each year.[1]

- Cervical infection with oncogenic types of HPV is associated with more than 80 percent of cases of invasive cervical cancer.[11]

- An estimated 13,700 cases of invasive cervical cancer will be diagnosed in the United States in 1998.[12]

- In 1998, an estimated 4,800 American women will die of cervical cancer.[12]

- Worldwide, cervical cancer is the second most common cancer among women. More than 425,000 new cases and 195,000 deaths occurred in 1997.[4]

- In the United States, total costs associated with HPV (excluding HPV-related cervical cancer) were an estimated $3.8 billion in 1994 in the United States.[3]

- Total costs associated with HPV-related cervical cancer totalled approximately $737 million in the United States in 1994.[3]

Syphilis

- An estimated 70,000 sexually transmitted infections with *Treponema pallidum*, the cause of syphilis, occur each year in the United States.[1]

- Globally, an estimated 12 million new cases of sexually acquired syphilis occurred in 1997.[4]

- In 1997, 8,550 cases of primary and secondary syphilis in the United States were reported to the CDC, a case rate of 3.2/100,000.[7]

- Costs associated with syphilis in the United states totalled an estimated $106 million in 1994.[3]

Trichomoniasis

- Globally, an estimated 170 million people acquired *Trichomonas vaginalis*, a sexually transmitted parasite, in 1997.[4]

- Approximately 5 million cases of trichomoniasis occur annually in the United States.[1]

References:

1. American Social Health Association. Sexually Transmitted Diseases in America: How Many Cases and at What Cost? Menlo Park, CA: Kaiser Family Foundation, 1998.

2. Centers for Disease Control and Prevention. Summary of notifiable diseases in the United States, 1996. *MMWR* 1997;45:1-103.

3. Institute of Medicine. Committee on Prevention and Control of Sexually Transmitted Diseases. The Hidden Epidemic: Confronting Sexually Transmitted Diseases. Eng TR and Butler WT, eds. Washington, DC: *National Academy Press*, 1997.

4. World Health Organization. World Health Report 1998. Geneva: *WHO*, 1998.

5. UNAIDS: Report on the Global HIV/AIDS Epidemic, December, 1998.

6. Centers for Disease Control and Prevention. HIV/AIDS Surveillance Report 1997;9(no. 2):1-44.

7. Centers for Disease Control and Prevention. National Center for HIV, STD and TB Prevention. Sexually Transmitted Disease Surveillance, 1997. Atlanta: CDC, 1998.

8. Washington AE and Katz P. Cost of and payment source for pelvic inflammatory disease—trends and projections, 1983 through 2000. *JAMA* 1991;266(18):2565-69.

9. Westrom L, et al. Pelvic inflammatory disease and fertility. A cohort of 1,844 women with laparoscopically verified disease and 657 control women with normal laparoscopic results. *Sex Transm Dis* 1992;19:185-92.

10. Fleming DT, et al. Herpes Simplex Virus type 2 in the United States, 1976 to 1994. *NEJM* 1997;337:1105-11.

11. National Institutes of Health. Consensus Development Statement on Cervical Cancer. Bethesda, Maryland, April 1-3, 1996.

12. American Cancer Society. Cancer Facts and Figures, 1998.

NIAID, a component of the National Institutes of Health, supports research on AIDS, malaria, tuberculosis and other infectious diseases, as well as allergies and immunology.

Chapter 4

The Statistics of STDs among Youth

Of the top ten most frequently reported diseases in the United States in 1995, half—accounting for 87 percent of all cases—were sexually transmitted diseases (STDs). With approximately 12 million new cases occurring annually, rates of curable STDs in the United States are the highest in the developed world.[1]

The public and private costs of STDs are tremendous. A conservative estimate of total costs associated with the most common types is approximately $10 billion. This increases to $17 billion when HIV/AIDS infections are included.[2]

Despite these tremendous health and economic burdens, the scope and impact of the STD epidemic are still under appreciated. And, to a large extent, the diseases are largely hidden from public discourse.[3]

Incidence and Prevalence

- At least 1 person in 4 will contract an STD at some point in his or her life.

- More than 12 million Americans, 3 million of whom are teenagers, are infected with an STD each year.

- As many as 56 million American adults and adolescents may have an incurable viral STD other than HIV.

- Chlamydial infection is the most common bacterial STD. More than 4 million cases occur each year. Just 23 percent of American adults under 65 cite chlamydia when asked to name any STDs.

- About 200,000 to 500,000 new cases of genital herpes occur each year, and 31 million Americans are already infected with the genital herpes virus (herpes simplex virus, or HSV).

- At least 24 million people are infected with human papillomavirus (HPV) or genital warts, and as many as 1 million new infections occur each year. HPV is associated with cervical and other genital and anal cancers.

- Trends in viral STD infections are unknown, but initial visits to doctors for genital warts and herpes have increased steadily over the last 30 years, dropping off slightly in the last five years.

- Between 1987 and 1991, the number of annually reported cases of syphilis—over 100,000—was at its highest levels in 40 years.

- At least 800,000 cases of gonorrhea occur each year.

Health Consequences

- Millions of women, men and children are affected by long-term complications of STDs, including various cancers, infertility, ectopic pregnancy and spontaneous abortion, and other chronic diseases.

- At least 15 percent of all infertile American women are infertile because of tubal damage caused by pelvic inflammatory disease (PID) resulting from an STD.

- Viral STDs result in lifelong incurable infection. Seventeen percent of American adults under 65 think all STDs are curable—but a large majority (80 percent) know that not all STDs are curable.

- STD infections increase susceptibility to HIV. People with an active syphilis, genital herpes, or chancroid infection, or who have chlamydia, gonorrhea, or trichomoniasis are 3 to 5 times more likely to contract HIV than other people. More than half (54 percent) of American adults under 65 do not know that STDs increase susceptibility to HIV.

Impact on Teenagers and Young Adults

- Three million teenagers—about 1 in 4 sexually experienced teenagers—acquire an STD every year. By the end of 1995, there were more than 2,300 teenagers diagnosed with AIDS.

- Young adults are the age groups at greatest risk of acquiring an STD for a number of reasons: they are more likely to have multiple sexual partners; they may be more likely to engage in unprotected intercourse; and their partners may be at higher risk of being infected.

- Compared to older adult women, female teenagers are more susceptible to cervical infections, such as gonorrhea and chlamydial infections, due to their cervical anatomy.

- Chlamydia is more common among teenagers than among adult men and women; in some studies, up to 30 percent of sexually active teenage women and 10 percent of sexually active teenage men tested for STDs were infected with chlamydia.

Critical Components of STD Prevention and Control

Communities need critical prevention and control services to help reduce costly complications of STDs. They should include both these patient-based and population-based approaches:

- *Screening high-risk populations for prevalent STDs.* Because the prevalence of STD infections varies from place to place, private sector providers may benefit from consulting with public health professionals on disease prevalence in their community in order to select cost-effective strategies for providing relevant STD screening services.

- *Treating individuals with diagnosed and presumptive infections.* Recommendations of STD experts on treatment regimens for STDs should be readily available to health care providers.

- *Providing prevention counseling and education.* Both public and private sources are needed to provide STD prevention counseling and education to individual patients in order to reach those affected by STDs. Such services are essential to reach sexual partners, to address future infections, as well as to ensure that medication is taken properly and that patients return for follow-up care. Community education about STD prevention is also important for beginning to change risky behavior before infection occurs,

- *Notifying, treating, and educating partners of persons diagnosed with STDs.* A sexual partner who has been exposed to an STD should be informed of his or her potential infection by the infected person, his or her health care provider, the provider's staff, or public health staff trained in partner notification. In most states, the law protects public health personnel in the notification process but does not protect other persons. Private providers and public health personnel may work together to provide sexual contacts with information on all aspects of needed care. Notification is a key step to prevent reinfection and further spread of STDs.

- *Reporting STD cases to assist in planning, evaluating, resource allocating, and coordinating efforts.* Health departments monitor and analyze reported STDs to identify problems in specific communities, to evaluate the effects of control measures, and to detect changes in trends. Complete and accurate reporting is essential so that the partnership of private providers and public health personnel can appropriately address STD problems. Laws in every state require providers to report some STDs. Most states require reporting of gonorrhea, syphilis, chlamydia, and AIDS. Several require reporting of herpes, HIV infection, or STD complications such as PID. Under-reporting of STDs results in failure to note disease trends and inadequate planning to address STD problems.

These approaches are needed because:

- *Screening and treatment will prevent significant future complications.* When left untreated, STDs can result in severe consequences including infertility, tubal pregnancy, chronic pain, cancer, premature births, low birth weight, congenital infections in newborns, and even death. In addition, HIV transmission is much more likely when other STDs are present, making STD treatment an important intervention for prevention of HIV infection.

In the United States, chlamydia—which infects approximately 4 million people each year—causes the majority of uterine and fallopian tube infections or PID in women. PID is the leading cause of preventable infertility and tubal pregnancy. Tubal pregnancy, in turn, is the leading cause of first-trimester pregnancy-related death in African-American women.

Prospective epidemiological studies have repeatedly demonstrated twofold to fivefold increases of HIV transmission when other STDs are present. In addition, other STDs have been demonstrated to increase HIV susceptibility in women by increasing the cells targeted by HIV CD4 cells in their cervical secretions. Other STDs have also been shown to increase the probability that HIV will be transmitted from an HIV-infected person to another person. A recent study demonstrated that in communities with improved STD treatment, HIV transmission was reduced by 42 percent.

- *Screening and early treatment are cost-effective.* The cost of untreated STDs far exceeds the cost of prevention services. For example, evidence indicates that chlamydia screening and treatment decreases the incidence of costly complications, such as PID. A random trial of chlamydia screening demonstrated a 60 percent reduction in the incidence of PID in the screened group in the 12 months following testing. Treatment of the consequences of chlamydia (e.g., PID, infertility, ectopic pregnancy) is estimated to be 12 times greater than the cost of screening and treatment.

- *These approaches would result in a healthier population.* STDs are strongly linked to long-term health complications. For example, the association between human papillomavirus and cervical cancer is well documented. STDs are one of the most important preventable causes of adverse outcomes of pregnancy, including low birth weight/prematurity, congenital infection, stillbirth, and postpartum infection. The two leading causes of preventable infertility are chlamydia and gonorrhea. Women, adolescents, and people of color are disproportionately affected by STDs and their consequences. STD prevention services could dramatically lower the incidence of STDs, their long-term consequences, and their significant cost. The overall health of Americans would improve with the routine availability of these components of STD prevention.

Resources

For more information about STDs, contact:

American Social Health Association (ASHA)

P.O. Box 13827
Research Triangle Park, NC 27709
Phone: (919) 361-8400
Internet: http://www.ashastd.org

National AIDS/HIV Hotline

(800) 342-AIDS (English)
(800) 344-7432 (Spanish)
(800) 243-7889 TTY Service for the Deaf

National Herpes Hotline

(919) 361-8488

CDC National STD Hotline

(800) 227-8922

ASHA Resource Center

Publications about Herpes and HPV
(800) 230-6039

SIECUS

130 West 42nd Street
Suite 350
New York, NY 10036-7802
Internet: http://www.siecus.org

References

1. The Hidden Epidemic: Confronting Sexually Transmitted Diseases; National Academy Press, Washington, DC, December 1996.

2. Ibid.

3. Ibid.

Chapter 5

The Statistics of STDs among Persons Over Age 50

Early in the human immunodeficiency virus (HIV) epidemic, infection occurred disproportionately among older persons as a result of transmission through receipt of contaminated blood or blood products. Through 1989, receipt of contaminated blood or blood products accounted for only 1% of cases among persons aged 13-49 years; in comparison, this risk factor accounted for 6%, 28%, and 64% of cases among persons aged 50-59 years, 60-69 years, and ≥70 years, respectively[1]. Because of implementation of voluntary donor deferral and routine screening of blood donations in 1985, the number and proportion of acquired immunodeficiency syndrome (AIDS) cases associated with this risk factor decreased among persons aged ≥50 years[2]. However, among persons aged ≥50 years, the number and proportion with AIDS associated with other modes of exposure increased. This report describes the characteristics of persons aged ≥50 years with AIDS reported during 1996 and presents trends in the incidence of AIDS-opportunistic illnesses (AIDS-OIs) diagnosed during 1991-1996 by mode of HIV exposure for persons aged ≥50 years. The findings indicate that, even though the incidence of AIDS-OIs during 1996 was higher among persons aged 13-49 years (89%), the proportion of AIDS-OIs accounted for by those aged ≥50 years (11%) was substantial.

For persons with AIDS reported in 1996, the analysis included only cases reported during January 1 through December 31, 1996. Trends

©1998 U.S. Department of Health and Human Services (DHHS), from *Morbidity and Mortality Weekly Report*, Jan. 23, 1998, Vol.47, No.2, Pg.21(7); reprinted with permission.

in AIDS incidence were based on cumulative AIDS cases among persons aged ≥13 years reported to CDC through June 1997 from the 50 states, the District of Columbia, and the U.S. territories and were analyzed by sex, age, race/ethnicity, mode of exposure, and year of AIDS diagnosis[3]. Estimates were adjusted for delays in reporting and for the anticipated reclassification of cases initially reported without an HIV risk/exposure[3]. To adjust for the 1993 expansion of the AIDS reporting criteria*, estimates of the incidence of AIDS-OIs were calculated from the sum of cases reported with an AIDS-OIs and cases with estimated dates of diagnosis of an AIDS-OI that were reported based only on immunologic criteria[3]. AIDS-OI incidence was estimated quarterly through December 1996 (the most recent annual period for which reliable estimates were available). To calculate annual AIDS incidence rates, mid-year U.S. population estimates were used based on decennial census data[4].

Reported AIDS Cases among Persons Aged >50 Years, 1996

In 1996, of 68,473 persons aged ≥13 years reported with AIDS, 7459 (11%) were aged ≥50 years; this proportion has remained stable since 1991. Of those aged ≥50 years, 48% were aged 50-54 years, 26% were aged 55-59 years, 14% were aged 60-64 years, and 12% were aged ≥65 years. Males accounted for 84% of cases, and blacks accounted for the highest proportion (43%) by race/ethnicity. Although men who have sex with men (MSM) accounted for the highest proportion of cases by exposure category (36%), compared with persons aged 13-49 years, a higher proportion of cases among persons aged ≥50 years were reported without risk information (26%). For both age groups, the highest proportions of cases were in the South (35% and 37%, respectively) and Northeast (32% and 30%, respectively).**

In 1996, persons aged >50 years were more likely than those aged 13-49 years to be reported with an AIDS-OI (e.g., wasting syndrome [7% versus 4%]† and HIV encephalopathy (3% versus 1% †) than to be reported with severe immunosuppression and without an AIDS-OI (53% versus 58%)†. In addition, persons aged ≥50 years were more likely to have died within 1 month of their AIDS diagnosis (13% versus 6%)†, suggesting late diagnosis of HIV infection.

Trends in AIDS-OI Incidence, 1991-1996

From 1991 to 1996, the proportionate increase in incident cases of AIDS-OIs was greater among persons aged ≥50 years (22%; from

5260 cases to 6400 cases)†† than among persons aged 13-49 years (9%; from 46,000 cases to 50,300 cases). From 1991 to 1996, among men aged ≥50 years, the number of incident cases of AIDS-OIs among MSM remained stable (2900 cases each for 1991 and 1996), while incident cases among men whose risk was heterosexual contact increased 94% (from 360 cases to 700 cases) and incident cases among men reporting injecting-drug use (IDU) increased 53% (from 850 cases to 1300 cases). Among male recipients of contaminated blood or blood products, incident cases of AIDS-OIs decreased 48% (from 250 cases to 130 cases). Among women aged >50 years, cases attributed to heterosexual contact and IDU increased 106% (from 340 cases to 700 cases) and 75% (from 160 cases to 280 cases), respectively, while cases among recipients of contaminated blood or blood products decreased 33% (from 120 cases to 80 cases).

In both 1991 and 1996, the rate of AIDS-OIs was higher for persons aged 13-49 years than for persons aged ≥50 years; rates among men in both age groups were higher than among women. The rate ratios of AIDS-OIs for 1996 and 1991 were similar for both age groups of men (1.1, 1.0) and the same for both age groups of women (1.6). (Reported by local, state, and territorial health departments Division of HIV/AIDS Prevention-Surveillance and Epidemiology, National Center for HIV STD, and TB Prevention, CDC.)

Editorial Note: Even though the incidence of AIDS-OIs during 1996 was higher among persons aged 13-49 years, the proportion accounted for by persons aged ≥50 years (11%) was substantial. The findings in this report suggest that persons aged ≥50 years may not be promptly tested for HIV infection following the onset of HIV-related illnesses. Specifically, the finding that a higher proportion of persons aged ≥50 years were reported with an AIDS-OI and died within 1 month of AIDS diagnosis suggests that persons aged ≥50 years had AIDS diagnosed later during the course of HIV infection than persons aged 13-49 years. Although older HIV-infected patients have a shorter observed AIDS-free interval and shorter survival period than younger HIV-infected patients[5], one reason for later diagnosis among persons aged ≥50 years is that physicians may be less likely to consider HIV infection among this group. This may result in missed opportunities for timely use of OI prophylaxis or antiretroviral therapies to prevent progression of disease. For example, AIDS-OIs that occur commonly among persons aged ≥50 years (e.g., HIV encephalopathy and wasting syndrome) mimic other diseases associated with aging (e.g., Alzheimer disease, depression, and malignancies). In addition, in 1996, a survey of primary-care physicians reported they were less likely to discuss symptoms suggestive of HIV infection or to counsel older patients for HIV testing than their younger patients[6]. To increase opportunities for HIV testing of U.S. persons aged ≥50 years, health-care providers should be encouraged to discuss risk factors, obtain sexual and drug histories for patients, and consider HIV infection in the differential diagnosis of clinical illnesses that may represent HIV infection in this age group.

Persons aged ≥50 years also may not be promptly tested for HIV infection because they may not perceive themselves to be at risk for HIV infection. AIDS surveillance data indicate that higher proportions of persons aged ≥50 years with cases of AIDS are reported without an identified risk. In 1994, the prevalence of reported condom use was lower among sexually active persons aged ≥50 years who engaged in high-risk behaviors, and a higher proportion of these persons had never been tested for HIV, compared with younger persons who engaged in the same behaviors[7]. During June 1990 through October 1994, a study in 12 state and local health department clinics indicated that older women with heterosexually acquired AIDS were less likely than younger women to have used a condom before their HIV diagnosis and were less likely to have been tested for HIV before being hospitalized with an AIDS-OI[8].

Because of the frequently long incubation period from HIV infection to AIDS diagnosis, many persons who were diagnosed with AIDS at age ≥50 years were probably infected as younger adults; therefore, prevention efforts also must be directed at adults who engage in high-risk sexual and drug-use behaviors. In addition, because of the impact of recent advances in treatment on AIDS incidence, the AIDS surveillance data in this report may underestimate the current impact of the HIV epidemic both in persons in this age group and younger persons[9]. Therefore, surveillance for HIV infection and AIDS is important for monitoring HIV transmission—particularly among persons aged ≥50 years—and for evaluating the effectiveness of prevention programs. CDC supports HIV surveillance in 31 states and is developing technical guidance to assist all states and territories in conducting HIV and AIDS case surveillance.

*Conditions in HIV-infected persons that were added to the AIDS case definition in 1993 included laboratory measures of severe immunosuppression (i.e., [CD4.sub.+] T-lymphocyte count [is less than] 200 cells/[Mu] L or percentage of total lymphocytes [is less than] 14) and three clinical conditions (pulmonary tuberculosis, recurrent pneumonia, and invasive cervical cancer).

**Northeast-Connecticut, Maine, Massachusetts, New Hampshire, New Jersey, New York, Pennsylvania, Rhode Island, and Vermont; Midwest Illinois, Indiana, Iowa, Kansas, Michigan, Minnesota, Missouri, Nebraska, North Dakota, Ohio, South Dakota, and Wisconsin; South Alabama, Arkansas, Delaware, District of Columbia, Florida, Georgia, Kentucky, Louisiana, Maryland, Mississippi, North Carolina, Oklahoma, South Carolina, Tennessee, Texas, Virginia, and West Virginia; and West Alaska, Arizona, California, Colorado, Hawaii, Idaho, Montana, Nevada, New Mexico, Oregon, Utah, Washington, and Wyoming.

†p [is less than] 0.05 (Chi-square).

††Estimates are adjusted for delays in reporting AIDS cases, the 1993 expansion of the AIDS case definition, and anticipated redistribution of cases initially reported with no identified risk, but not for incomplete reporting of cases. Adult/adolescent and total estimates of [is less than] 200, 200-499, 500-999, and ≥1000 are rounded to the nearest 10, 20, 50, and 100, respectively.

References

1. Ship, J.A., Wolff, A., Selik, R.M., "Epidemiology of acquired immune deficiency syndrome in persons aged 50 years or older." *J Acquir Immune Defic Syndr* 1991;4:84-8.

2. Selik, R.M., Ward, J.W., Buehler, J.W., "Demographic differences in cumulative incidence rates of transfusion-associated acquired immunodeficiency syndrome." *Am J Epidemiol* 1994;140: 105-12.

3. CDC. "HIV/AIDS surveillance report, year-end edition 1996." Atlanta, Georgia: US Department of Health and Human Services, CDC, 1996. (Vol. 7, no. 2).

4. Bureau of the Census. "State population estimates by age, sex, race, and Hispanic origin," 1990-1995. Washington, DC: US Department of Commerce, Economics and Statistics Administration, Bureau of the Census, 1996.

5. Skiest, D.J., Rubinstien, E., Carley, N., Gioiella, L., Lyons, R., "The importance of comorbidity in HIV-infected patients over 55: a retrospective case-control study." *Am J Med* 1996;101:605-11.

6. Skiest, D.J., Keiser, P., "Human immunodeficiency virus infection in patients older than 50 years: a survey of primary care

physicians' beliefs, practices, and knowledge." *Arch Fam Med* 1997;6: 289-94.

7. Stall, R., Catania, J., "AIDS risk behaviors among late middle-aged and elderly Americans: the National AIDS Behavioral Surveys." *Arch Intern Med* 1994;154:57-63.

8. Schable, B., Chu, S.Y., Diaz, T., "Characteristics of women 50 years of age or older with heterosexually acquired AIDS." *Am J Public Health* 1996;86:1616-8.

9. CDC. "Update: trends in AIDS incidence," 1996. *MMWR* 1997;46:861-7.

Part Two

Types of Sexually Transmitted Diseases

Chapter 6

Chancroid

Chancroid ("shan-kroid") is an important bacterial infection caused by *Haemophilus ducreyi*, which is spread by sexual contact. Periodic outbreaks of chancroid have occurred in the United States, the last one being in the late 1980s. These outbreaks are usually seen in minority populations in the inner cities, especially in the southern and eastern portion of the country. Globally, this disease is common in sub-Saharan Africa among men who have frequent contact with prostitutes.

The infection begins with the appearance of painful open sores on the genitals, sometimes accompanied by swollen, tender lymph nodes in the groin. These symptoms occur within a week after exposure. Symptoms in women are often less noticeable and may be limited to painful urination or defecation, painful intercourse, rectal bleeding, or vaginal discharge. Chancroid lesions may be difficult to distinguish from ulcers caused by genital herpes or syphilis. A physician must therefore diagnose the infection by excluding other diseases with similar symptoms. People with chancroid can be treated effectively with one of several antibiotics. Chancroid is one of the genital ulcer diseases that may be associated with an increased risk of transmission of the human immunodeficiency virus (HIV), the cause of AIDS.

Chancroid is endemic in some areas of the United States, and the disease also occurs in discrete outbreaks. Chancroid is a cofactor for HIV transmission, and high rates of HIV infection among patients who

1998 Centers for Disease Control (CDC), excerpted from "1998 Guidelines for Treatment of Sexually Transmitted Disease", *MMWR* 1998, 47(No.RR-1); 1998 National Institute of Allergy and Infectious Disease (NIAID).

have chancroid have been reported in the United States and other countries. An estimated 10% of patients who have chancroid could be coinfected with *T. pallidum* or HSV.

A definitive diagnosis of chancroid requires identification of *H. ducreyi* on special culture media that are not widely available from commercial sources; even using these media, sensitivity is less than or equal to 80%. A probable diagnosis, for both clinical and surveillance purposes, may be made if the following criteria are met:

• the patient has one or more painful genital ulcers

• the patient has no evidence of *T. pallidum* infection by darkfield examination of ulcer exudate or by a serologic test for syphilis performed at least 7 days after onset of ulcers

• the clinical presentation, appearance of genital ulcers, and regional lymphadenopathy, if present, are typical for chancroid and a test for HSV is negative.

The combination of a painful ulcer and tender inguinal adenopathy, which occurs among one third of patients, suggests a diagnosis of chancroid; when accompanied by suppurative inguinal adenopathy, these signs are almost pathognomonic. PCR testing for *H. ducreyi* might become available soon.

Treatment

Successful treatment for chancroid cures the infection, resolves the clinical symptoms, and prevents transmission to others. In extensive cases, scarring can result despite successful therapy.

Other Management Considerations

Patients who are uncircumcised and HIV-infected patients might not respond as well to treatment as those who are circumcised or HIV-negative. Patients should be tested for HIV infection at the time chancroid is diagnosed. Patients should be retested 3 months after the diagnosis of chancroid if the initial test results for syphilis and HIV were negative.

Follow-Up

Patients should be reexamined 3-7 days after initiation of therapy. If treatment is successful, ulcers improve symptomatically within 3 days and objectively within 7 days after therapy. If no clinical improvement is evident, the clinician must consider whether:

- the diagnosis is correct
- the patient is coinfected with another STD
- the patient is infected with HIV
- the treatment was not taken as instructed
- the *H. ducreyi* strain causing the infection is resistant to the prescribed antimicrobial.

The time required for complete healing depends on the size of the ulcer; large ulcers may require greater than 2 weeks. In addition, healing is slower for some uncircumcised men who have ulcers under the foreskin. Clinical resolution of fluctuant lymphadenopathy is slower than that of ulcers and may require drainage, even during otherwise successful therapy. Although needle aspiration of buboes is a simpler procedure, incision and drainage of buboes may be preferred because of less need for subsequent drainage procedures.

Management of Sex Partners

Sex partners of patients who have chancroid should be examined and treated, regardless of whether symptoms of the disease are present, if they had sexual contact with the patient during the 10 days preceding onset of symptoms in the patient.

Special Considerations

Pregnancy

The safety of azithromycin for pregnant and lactating women has not been established. Ciprofloxacin is contraindicated during pregnancy. No adverse effects of chancroid on pregnancy outcome or on the fetus have been reported.

HIV Infection

HIV-infected patients who have chancroid should be monitored closely. Such patients may require longer courses of therapy than those recommended for HIV-negative patients. Healing may be slower among HIV-infected patients, and treatment failures occur with any regimen. Because data are limited concerning the therapeutic efficacy of the recommended ceftriaxone and azithromycin regimens in HIV-infected patients, these regimens should be used for such patients only if follow-up can be ensured. Some experts suggest using the erythromycin 7-day regimen for treating HIV-infected persons.

Chapter 7

Chlamydia

Chapter Contents

Section 7.1

Chlamydial Infection

1998 National Institute of Allergy and Infectious Diseases (NIAID).

Chlamydial ("kla-mid-ee-uhl") infection is the most common bacterial sexually transmitted disease (STD) in the United States today. The U.S. Centers for Disease Control and Prevention estimates that more than 4 million new cases occur each year. The highest rates of chlamydial infection are in 15 to 19-year-old adolescents regardless of demographics or location. Pelvic inflammatory disease (PID), a serious complication of chlamydial infection, has emerged as a major cause of infertility among women of childbearing age. Chlamydial infection is caused by a bacterium, *Chlamydia trachomatis*, and can be transmitted during vaginal, oral, or anal sexual contact with an infected partner. A pregnant woman may pass the infection to her newborn during delivery, with subsequent neonatal eye infection or pneumonia. The annual cost of chlamydial infection is estimated to exceed $2 billion.

Symptoms

Most chlamydial infections are silent, causing no symptoms. However, men and women with *C. trachomatis* may experience abnormal genital discharge or pain during urination. These early symptoms may be mild. If symptoms occur, they usually appear within one to three weeks after exposure. Two of every three infected women and one or two of every four infected men have no symptoms whatsoever. As a result, often the disease may not be diagnosed and treated until complications develop.

Doctors estimate that, in women, one-third of the chlamydial infections result in PID. Often these infections are not diagnosed until PID or other complications develop. In men, rarely, chlamydial infections may lead to pain or swelling in the scrotal area, which is a sign of epididymitis, an inflammation of a part of the male reproductive system located near the testicles. Left untreated, this condition, like PID in women, can cause infertility.

C. trachomatis can cause proctitis (inflamed rectum) and conjunctivitis (inflammation of the lining of the eye). The bacteria also have been found in the throat as a result of oral sexual contact with an infected partner. In tropical climates, a particular strain of *C. trachomatis* causes an STD called lymphogranuloma venereum (LGV), which is characterized by prominent swelling and inflammation of the lymph nodes in the groin. Complications may follow if LGV is not treated; this infection is very rare in the United States.

Diagnosis

Chlamydial infection can be confused with gonorrhea because the symptoms of both diseases are similar; in some populations they occur together. The most reliable way to diagnose chlamydial infection is for a clinician to send a sample of secretions from the patient's genital area to a laboratory that will look for the organism using one of a wide variety of quick and inexpensive laboratory tests. Although attempting to grow the organism in specialized tissue culture in the laboratory is one of the most definitive tests, it is expensive and technically difficult to do, and test results are not available for three or more days.

Scientists have developed several rapid tests for diagnosing chlamydial infection that use sophisticated techniques and a dye to detect bacterial proteins. Although these tests are slightly less accurate, they are less expensive, more rapid, and can be performed during a routine checkup. These tests use a process called DNA amplification to detect the genes of the organisms in genital secretions. Recently, the U.S. Food and Drug Administration approved this process for detection of *C. trachomatis* in urine. This is a major step in diagnosing chlamydial infection because it does not require an invasive sample; it can be used in settings where performing a pelvic examination is not convenient or not feasible, e.g., in college health units and at health fairs. Results from the urine test are available within 24 hours.

Treatment

Doctors usually prescribe antibiotics such as a one-day course of azithromycin or a seven-day course of doxycycline to treat chlamydial infection. Other antibiotics such as erythromycin or ofloxacin also are effective. Pregnant women can be treated with azithromycin or erythromycin. Amoxicillin is also a safe alternative for treating pregnant women. Penicillin, which is often used for treating some other STDs, is not effective against chlamydial infections. New medications are being developed that should greatly simplify treatment and help control the spread of *C. trachomatis* in the population.

A person with chlamydial infection should be sure to take all of the prescribed medication, even after symptoms disappear. If the symptoms do not disappear within one to two weeks after finishing the medicine, the patient should make a follow-up visit to the doctor or clinic. All sex partners of a person with chlamydial infection should be tested and treated to prevent reinfection and further spread of the disease.

Pelvic Inflammatory Disease

Each year up to 1 million women in the United States develop PID, a serious infection of the reproductive organs. As many as half of all cases of PID may be due to chlamydial infection, and many of these occur without symptoms. PID can result in scarring of the fallopian tubes, which can block the tubes and prevent fertilization from taking place. An estimated 100,000 women each year become infertile as a result of PID.

In other cases, scarring may interfere with the passage of the fertilized egg down into the uterus. When this happens, the egg may implant in the fallopian tube. This is called ectopic or tubal pregnancy. This is life threatening for the mother and results in the loss of the fetus. PID is the most common cause of pregnancy-related death among poor teenagers in the inner cites and rural areas of the United States. The annual cost estimates exceed $7 billion.

Effects of Chlamydial Infection in Newborns

A baby who is exposed to *C. trachomatis* in the birth canal during delivery may develop conjunctivitis (eye infection) or pneumonia. Symptoms of conjunctivitis, which include discharge and swollen eyelids, usually develop within the first 10 days of life. Symptoms of pneumonia, including a progressively worsening cough and congestion, most often develop within three to six weeks of birth. Both conditions can be treated successfully with antibiotics. Because of these risks to the newborn, many doctors recommend routine testing of all pregnant women for chlamydial infection.

Prevention

Because chlamydial infection often occurs without symptoms, people who are infected may unknowingly infect their sex partners. Many doctors recommend that all persons who have more than one sex partner, especially women under 25 years of age, be tested for chlamydial infection regularly, even in the absence of symptoms. Using condoms or diaphragms during sexual intercourse may help reduce the transmission of chlamydia.

Research

NIAID researchers are working on two strategies to prevent infection: topical microbicides and a vaccine. Scientists also are looking for better ways to treat people with chlamydial infection. In addition, developing simple, inexpensive tests to diagnose chlamydial infection remains one of the most urgent research priorities.

Scientists also are studying the basic process of how *C. trachomatis* causes disease in the body and why some people suffer more severe complications than others. These studies may lead to insights about how to recognize women at risk for PID and PID-related infertility or other complications of chlamydial infection.

Section 7.2

Age Based Screening for Chlamydia

1998 National Institute of Allergy and Infectious Diseases (NIAID).

Investigators from the National Institute of Allergy and Infectious Diseases (NIAID) and Johns Hopkins University compared three strategies to screen 7,699 women without symptoms who attended two family planning clinics in Baltimore, Md. In addition to the age-based screening found to be most effective, investigators evaluated universal screening and screening with the criteria recommended by the Centers for Disease Control and Prevention (CDC). All women were tested with polymerase chain reaction (PCR). They calculated the cost-effectiveness of chlamydial screening by comparing total costs, including screening program costs, and estimating future medical costs of all sequelae.

"Certainly one of the great values of this study," says Anthony S. Fauci, M.D., director of NIAID, "is the confirmation that screening enables clinicians to identify and treat women with chlamydial infections and no symptoms, thus preventing many occurrences of serious sequelae, such as infertility."

Chlamydial infection is one of the leading sexually transmitted diseases in the United States today. The CDC estimates that more than 4 million new cases occur each year. Pelvic inflammatory disease, a serious complication of chlamydial infection, has emerged as a major cause of infertility among women of childbearing age. Genital chlamydial infection is caused by the bacterium, *Chlamydia trachomatis*, and is transmitted during vaginal or anal sexual contact with an infected partner. A pregnant woman may pass the infection to her newborn during delivery, with subsequent neonatal eye infection or pneumonia. The annual cost of chlamydial infections and their sequelae in the United States exceeds $2.7 billion.

"The majority of women infected with Chlamydia do not have symptoms, and damage to their fallopian tubes resulting in infertility can occur silently over time if the infection remains undiagnosed and not treated," said author Thomas C. Quinn, M.D., of NIAID and Johns Hopkins University, Baltimore, Md. "In our study, 6.6 percent of women attending the Baltimore family planning clinics were found to be infected. Because of the initial lack of symptoms and signs, most of these women would not have been diagnosed or treated if they had not undergone routine screening for Chlamydia using either urine or cervical specimens. New and simple tests make screening easier."

Currently, the CDC recommends testing all women with evidence of an inflamed cervix and all women younger than 20 years of age. They also suggest: (1) testing women 20 to 23 years of age who have not consistently used barrier contraception or have had a new sex partner or more than one sex partner during the past 90 days; and (2) testing women 24 years of age or older who have not consistently used barrier contraception and have had a new sex partner or more than one sex partner during the past 90 days.

The investigators compared each screening strategy's ability to identify women at risk and thus trigger testing and treatment, which in turn would result in fewer or no sequelae and reduced overall medical costs. They defined medical outcomes as prevented cases of pelvic inflammatory disease, chronic pelvic pain, ectopic pregnancy, infertility, male urethritis and epididymitis in adults, and conjunctivitis and pneumonia in infants.

The results were dramatic. Without screening, there would have been 152 cases of pelvic inflammatory disease and other sequelae in women, men and infants with an associated cost of $676,000. Screening according to CDC criteria would have prevented 64 cases of pelvic inflammatory disease and saved $231,000. Screening all women younger than 30 years of age would have prevented 85 cases of pelvic inflammatory disease and saved $305,000. Universal screening would have prevented an additional six cases, but would have cost considerably more than age-based screening—approximately $3,000 more per case of pelvic inflammatory disease prevented.

The authors caution that although the study results suggest that age-based screening provides the greatest cost savings, universal screening is desirable in some situations. In general, screening with any criteria and a highly sensitive diagnostic test should be part of any chlamydial prevention and control program. NIAID has a major commitment to develop new sexually transmitted disease (STD) diagnostic tests that are rapid, inexpensive, easy-to-use and do not require an invasive sample. If such tests were available and acceptable to the patient, screening for "silent" STDs would be even more cost-effective.

Section 7.3

Chlamydia Screening and PID Rates

1996 National Institute of Allergy and Infectious Diseases (NIAID).

Routine screening for a common cervical infection could significantly reduce women's risk for pelvic inflammatory disease (PID), a study supported by the National Institute of Allergy and Infectious Diseases (NIAID) suggests.

Researchers at the University of Washington and Group Health Cooperative of Puget Sound, both in Seattle, found that women who were screened and treated for asymptomatic chlamydial infections were nearly 60 percent less likely than unscreened women to develop PID, an infection of the upper reproductive tract that often leads to infertility, tubal pregnancy and other serious complications. The finding is reported in the May 23 issue of *The New England Journal of Medicine*.

"This finding holds great promise for improving the health of young women," said Department of Health and Human Services Secretary

Donna E. Shalala. "The findings should also remind all of us that regular health screening is the foundation of good health."

PID affects more than 1 million women in the United States each year. Most cases are caused by *Chlamydia trachomatis*, the most common sexually transmitted bacterial pathogen in the United States. According to the Centers for Disease Control and Prevention (CDC), more than 4 million people each year are diagnosed with chlamydia. Experts say the actual number of cases probably is much higher, since chlamydial infections often produce no symptoms and thus frequently go undiagnosed. Research reviewed at a recent NIAID workshop on PID suggests that up to 40 percent of untreated chlamydial infections in women ascend the upper genital tract to cause PID. Scientists have hypothesized that identifying and treating women with asymptomatic chlamydial infections could reduce the burden of PID.

"This is an extremely important finding that potentially could have an enormous impact on a very costly disease," says NIAID Director Anthony S. Fauci, M.D. Dr. Fauci notes that studies have estimated the costs associated with treating PID and its consequences at between $5 billion and $7 billion each year.

In an editorial accompanying the paper, CDC officials praised the result as a "landmark" finding. "Screening for chlamydia should become the standard of care for young, sexually active women," says the CDC's Judith N. Wasserheit, M.D., M.P.H., one of the editorial's authors. The CDC has spearheaded an effort to establish a nationwide chlamydia prevention program.

A prior study of women enrolled in a health maintenance organization (HMO) had shown that certain characteristics, such as being younger than 25 years, unmarried, and having two or more sex partners during the previous year, were associated with a higher than average risk for chlamydia infection. Using these and other criteria, researchers Delia Scholes, Ph.D., Walter E. Stamm, M.D., and their colleagues identified a study population of approximately 2,600 women who were assigned at random to either an intervention or control group.

Throughout the study, women in both groups continued to receive all necessary medical care from their HMO physicians. In addition, women in the intervention group were screened for chlamydial infection and those who tested positive were treated with antibiotics. Women in the control group who presented with symptoms of cervical inflammation were tested for chlamydial infection, then treated.

One year later, follow-up questionnaires and reviews of the participants' medical records revealed that nine cases of PID had occurred among the 1,009 women in the screening group, compared with 33 cases of PID among the 1,598 women who were treated when symptomatic. From these data, the incidence of PID—the rate at which new cases occur during a specific period—was calculated to be 56 percent lower in the screened group as compared with the control group.

"We've provided the most direct evidence to date that early detection and treatment of asymptomatic chlamydial infections can reduce the incidence of PID, at least among certain populations of young women," says Dr. Stamm, the study's principal investigator.

Penelope Hitchcock, D.V.M., chief of NIAID's Sexually Transmitted Diseases Branch, notes that the study represents a significant advance in the Institute's PID research program.

"These results tell us that we can intervene early, during lower genital tract infection, and make a difference by preventing many cases of PID," she says. The finding also underscores the importance of developing better diagnostic tests for STDs. Until recently, she says, difficulties associated with diagnosing asymptomatic chlamydial infection precluded widespread screening. However, since the current study was begun, a non-invasive, urine-based assay developed by Abbott Laboratories working with NIAID investigators allows earlier detection of both asymptomatic and symptomatic cases of chlamydia infection, says Dr. Hitchcock. NIAID researchers currently are trying to develop even faster, less expensive assays for chlamydia and other sexually transmitted pathogens.

Despite the improved prospects for PID prevention, Dr. Hitchcock adds that another critically important issue—finding better ways to diagnose and treat women with asymptomatic PID—remains a formidable research challenge.

"As many as 25 percent of all women of reproductive age have already had an episode of PID, and most of them were undiagnosed and untreated," she says. "Research toward identifying women with subclinical PID could ultimately help prevent many cases of ectopic pregnancy, infertility and other serious consequences of this disease."

Section 7.4

Chlamydia's Quick Cure

1999 July-August, *FDA Consumer Magazine;*
United States Food and Drug Administration (FDA).

Anna Lange (not her real name) had no symptoms when she went to a Wake County, N.C., sexually transmitted diseases clinic earlier this year to pick up her birth control pills. But a routine test revealed that the 20-year-old Lange had chlamydia. "She came in and had no complaints," says Peter Leone, M.D., the clinic's medical director, "and then 'boom'—she was diagnosed with a sexually transmitted disease."

The sexually transmitted disease chlamydia usually comes with no telltale symptoms, so most people don't even know when they are infected. But left untreated, the so-called "silent epidemic" of chlamydia threatens to cause reproductive damage and infertility in many of the 3 million to 4 million Americans who get it each year. "Chlamydia's consequences can be devastating," says Diane Mitchell, M.D., an obstetrician-gynecologist and medical reviewer with the Food and Drug Administration.

Routine chlamydia screening and early, effective treatment are the keys to reducing chlamydia's toll, according to Penny Hitchcock, chief of the National Institutes of Health's sexually transmitted disease branch. Two recent medical advances, she says, constitute "very important breakthroughs" in controlling the rampant disease: a new drug treatment recently approved by FDA to cure chlamydia in a single oral dose, and a urine-based screening test that, unlike other tests, does not require a swab sample of cells from the genital area.

Price of Sex

Caused by the *Chlamydia trachomatis* bacteria and transmitted during vaginal, oral or anal sexual contact with an infected partner, chlamydia is the most reported bacterial infection in the United States and the most common bacterial (and thus curable) sexually transmitted disease by far, ahead of gonorrhea and syphilis.

A person can become infected at any age, but "it's adolescents that we're most worried about," Hitchcock says. "Far and away, the age group most affected are the 15 to 19-year-olds. If you're sexually active and you're in that age group, you're at risk." Studies show that young adults in Lange's age group, 20 to 24, are the second most affected group.

While wearing a condom may help reduce the risk of chlamydia, anyone who is sexually active can get the disease.

Symptoms of chlamydia, when they occur, usually appear within one to three weeks of exposure. In women, signs can include unusual vaginal discharge or bleeding, burning during urination, or lower abdominal pain. Men, like women, may have pain during urination, or they may notice a burning and itching around or discharge from the penis or pain and swelling in the testicles.

More often, though, chlamydia lives up to its reputation for silence. Experts estimate that up to 75 percent of women and 50 percent of men with chlamydia have no symptoms or symptoms so mild that they don't seek medical attention.

Chlamydia is "a very insidious disease," says Hitchcock. "Because it rarely causes symptoms, people don't know they're infected. So they don't get treated, and they infect their partners, who also don't get treated."

Without treatment, the national Centers for Disease Control and Prevention estimates, chlamydia can lead in up to 40 percent of cases to pelvic inflammatory disease, a serious infection of the woman's fallopian tubes that can also damage the ovaries and uterus. Also, women infected with chlamydia may have three to five times the risk of getting infected with HIV if exposed, according to CDC.

It's not known whether chlamydia infection causes fertility problems or other long-term consequences in men. "We are worried—though we don't have a lot of evidence—that chlamydia infection could cause chronic problems in men," Hitchcock says. "But as far as we know, the biggest price is paid by young women."

Babies sometimes pay a price, as well. Babies who are exposed to chlamydia in the birth canal during delivery can be born with pneumonia or an eye infection called conjunctivitis, both of which can be dangerous unless treated early with antibiotics.

Simple Screening and Treatment

Because so many people are at risk for chlamydia and because the disease can ravage a woman's reproductive system without so much as a symptom, experts recommend regular, widespread screening to detect the disease.

Traditional methods of screening require a health professional to collect a swab sample of genital secretions. For women this type of test "minutely prolongs" a pap smear, FDA's Mitchell explains. "At worst, it can feel like a tiny menstrual cramp, but most women don't experience any discomfort." Male samples are obtained by inserting a swab into the end of the penis.

In the past, the sample had to be "cultured" in a laboratory to look for *C. trachomatis*, and it could take three days or more for results to become available. Also, accuracy of results could vary greatly based on the lab staff's level of expertise and experience.

Today, a number of tests are available to supplement or sometimes replace the relatively expensive and slow traditional culture. The three major types of nonculture tests are:

- **Direct fluorescent antibody test.** This oldest alternative to culture uses a scientific method called staining to make chlamydia easier to spot under a microscope. DFA can give quicker results than culture and can be performed on specimens taken from the eye, cervix or penis.

- **Enzyme immunoassays.** This test to detect the presence of the cells of *C. trachomatis* comes in some forms that allow use in small, unsophisticated laboratories that don't have special lab equipment. Because testing can be done where the specimen is collected, results are more rapid than with culture, access to testing is increased, and costs can be lower.

- **Tests to detect the genes of *C. trachomatis* in urine, as well as genital, samples.** Developed and approved in the last few years, these tests can accurately identify even very small numbers of genes in a specimen. These tests can be expensive, but are becoming more popular among public and other labs because of their accuracy and the relative ease of collecting urine samples. "Now we can screen women and men who don't think they are ill without doing an invasive sampling, so people are much more likely to participate in screening programs," Hitchcock says.

No one screening method is best, Leone says. "It's a tradeoff. We're constantly balancing what is the cheapest test with what is the most sensitive, what is easiest to get from the patient versus what will pick up the most infections."

At Leone's clinic, Lange was tested using the enzyme immunoassay method. She doubted the results at first, Leone says. "We explained to her that yes, the test was accurate, and she really needed to be treated even though she had no symptoms."

Lange and her boyfriend both took the antibiotic azithromycin (Zithromax), a prescription drug approved by FDA in 1997 to cure chlamydia in one dose. "It's a breakthrough because we can observe therapy rather than depending on people to adhere to a more complicated regimen," Hitchcock says. Doxycycline (sold under several brand names), the other antibiotic approved and commonly used to treat chlamydia, is generally taken twice a day for seven days.

Underused Tools

Widespread chlamydia screening among women can get results, as was demonstrated in a recent study supported by NIH. Researchers at Seattle's Group Health Cooperative of Puget Sound and the University of Washington found that symptomless women who were screened and treated for chlamydial infection were almost 60 percent less likely than unscreened women to develop pelvic inflammatory disease.

With such effective tools for screening and treatment, why has it proved so difficult to stop the spread of this microorganism? The answer, experts agree, is that not enough at-risk young people are getting tested.

"There are about a million reasons people don't get tested," Mitchell says. "They might feel uncomfortable, or not have insurance, or just not know they should be tested for chlamydia."

Also, doctors often fail to discuss the issue of sexually transmitted diseases with their young patients, according to Gale Burstein, M.D., a chlamydia researcher at Johns Hopkins University. "Physicians have to make a commitment to ask all of their adolescent patients if they are sexually active. But doctors are sometimes uncomfortable pursuing that line of questioning," Burstein says, adding that "a sexually active adolescent woman is more likely to test positive for chlamydia than for tuberculosis, yet TB tests are done much more routinely."

Beyond encouraging more young people to get routinely screened for chlamydia, experts are searching for other avenues to control this sexually transmitted disease. Recently, researchers at Stanford University and the University of California at San Francisco uncovered new information about the chromosomes of *C. trachomatis*, providing promising leads for developing new antibiotics and even a vaccine.

Hitchcock, whose agency supported the study, says she and other STD experts at NIH are "very excited about the new opportunities for vaccine development."

Until the hope of a vaccine is realized, those who choose to be sexually active should use condoms—for what they're worth. "Condom use clearly prevents HIV infection and gonorrhea, as well as pregnancy," Hitchcock says. "Use a condom, but not with blinders on, either. Don't kid yourself that condoms make sex risk-free."

Condoms and Chlamydia

The only sure-fire way to avoid getting chlamydia and other sexually transmitted diseases is by abstaining from sex or being in a mutually monogamous relationship with an uninfected partner. Having multiple partners increases your risk of getting the disease, according to experts.

Anna Lange was especially surprised when she was diagnosed with chlamydia because, besides not having any symptoms, she had been in a monogamous relationship for six months. "We explained to her that the diagnosis didn't mean that either she or her current boyfriend had been unfaithful," says Peter Leone, M.D., medical director at Anna's STD clinic. "We couldn't tell her when or from whom she'd gotten infected. But she did have a history of unprotected sex for a couple of years previously, and she could have become infected at any time during this period."

While even "protected" sex with a condom can't completely prevent transmission of chlamydia or some other sexually transmitted diseases, experts recommend correct and consistent condom use to reduce the chances of getting chlamydia or other STDs.

Should You Get Tested?

The National Centers for Disease Control and Prevention recommends annual chlamydia screening for all sexually active adolescent girls and for other females who may be at high risk for chlamydial infection, such as those who:

- are less than 25 years old
- don't use barrier contraceptives consistently
- have new or multiple sex partners
- have signs of a possible cervical infection
- have previously had an STD.

"Females who are at risk because of their age and sexual activity need to get screened at least once a year," says researcher Gale Burstein, M.D. She and other chlamydia experts have recently questioned whether that is even enough.

Based on a study they conducted in 1998, Burstein and her colleagues at Johns Hopkins University recently recommended a twice-yearly screening of sexually active female adolescents. In tracking more than 3,000 sexually active Baltimore high school girls for three years, they found that more than a quarter of them tested positive for chlamydia at least once in that time frame.

Routine screening is recommended for pregnant women, also, because of the risk that their babies will become infected with chlamydia at birth.

There are no recommendations for routine screening among males, which Burstein says makes it especially likely that their chlamydial infection will be overlooked. "There is a lot of chlamydia in men that we're missing, and they are a major reservoir of infection. We're really only putting a band-aid on the problem because, even if we're screening the women, some are going back to their partners and getting reinfected."

Another Chlamydia Making Headlines

The *Chlamydia trachomatis* bacteria that cause the sexually transmitted disease should not be confused with *Chlamydia pneumoniae*. These other bugs, which can cause colds and pneumonia, have been in the news because investigators are researching their possible link with atherosclerosis, a clogging of the arteries that causes most heart attacks and strokes. Add this type of chlamydia to smoking, a bad diet, and a sedentary lifestyle as possible contributors to heart disease.

—by Tamar Nordenberg

Chapter 8

Cytomegalovirus (CMV)

Chapter Contents

Section 8.1

Cytomegalovirus Facts

1998 National Institute of Allergy and Infectious Diseases (NIAID).

Cytomegalovirus (CMV) is a very common virus that infects approximately one-half of all young adults in the United States. It rarely causes serious consequences except in people with suppressed or impaired immune systems or in infants, whose immune systems are still developing. The virus, a member of the herpesvirus family, is found in saliva, urine, and other bodily fluids. Because it is often found in semen as well as in cervical secretions, the virus can be spread by sexual contact; it also can be easily spread by other forms of physical contact such as kissing. Day-care center staff for children under the age of 3 are at increased risk of CMV infection and should carefully wash their hands after changing diapers. Like other herpesvirus infections, CMV is incurable; people are infected with it for life. Although the virus usually remains in an inactive state, it can reactivate from time to time.

Symptoms

In healthy adults, CMV usually produces no symptoms of infection. Occasionally, however, mild symptoms of swollen lymph glands, fever, and fatigue may occur. These symptoms may be similar to those of infectious mononucleosis.

Diagnosis

The ELISA (enzyme-linked immunosorbent assay) test is commonly used to detect levels of antibodies (disease-fighting proteins of the immune system) in the blood. A number of other blood tests can suggest a diagnosis of CMV infection, but no blood test can reliably diagnose it. Although CMV can be isolated from urine or other body fluids, it may be excreted months or years after an infection; therefore, isolation of the virus from these fluids is not a reliable method of diagnosing recent infection.

Complications

Babies can be infected with CMV in the uterus if their mothers become infected with the virus or develop a recurrence of a previous infection during pregnancy. Although most babies infected with CMV before birth do not develop any symptoms, CMV is the leading cause of congenital infection in the United States. An estimated 6,000 babies each year develop life-threatening complications of congenital CMV infection at birth or suffer serious consequences later in life, including mental retardation, blindness, deafness, or epilepsy. Investigators supported by NIAID are currently studying how the virus interferes with normal fetal development and at which stages the fetus is most susceptible to infection. Congenital CMV is the most common cause of progressive deafness in children.

When CMV is acquired after birth, or if it reactivates, it can be life-threatening for persons with suppressed immune systems, such as those receiving chemotherapy or persons who have received immunosuppressant drugs for organ transplantation. Persons with HIV infection or AIDS may develop severe CMV infections, including CMV retinitis, an eye disease that can lead to blindness.

Treatment

NIAID scientists are testing new antiviral drugs that might be effective against CMV infections. The antiviral drugs foscarnet and ganciclovir have been approved for treating people with AIDS-associated CMV retinitis.

Prevention

There is no intervention to prevent CMV. Use of the male condom may reduce risk although virus in the saliva would be transmitted by kissing or oral intercourse. Some experts believe that primary or first-time exposure during pregnancy is a major cause of CMV infection in newborns. Infants infected before or just after birth are likely to be shedding CMV in saliva and urine, which can infect others. Hand washing and proper handling of diapers may reduce risk. Scientists are working to develop a vaccine and other methods to provide immunity to CMV and offer protection against severe disease.

Section 8.2

Prevention of Cytomegalovirus in Transplant Recipients

© 1995 Lancet Ltd., from *The Lancet*, Nov. 25, 1995, Vol.346, No.8987, Pg.1380(2), by Drew J. Winston; reprinted with permission.

Before 1990, cytomegalovirus (CMV) was the single most common pathogen causing infection in both solid-organ and marrow transplant recipients. Without any available effective antiviral prophylaxis, the overall frequency of CMV infection was about 50%. Many infected patients developed symptomatic CMV disease, manifested by pneumonia, hepatitis, gastrointestinal ulcers, a non-specific febrile illness associated with leucopenia and thrombocytopenia, or less commonly, retinitis. Patients with CMV pneumonia or disseminated infection often died. CMV infection was also found to be associated with an increased risk of other opportunistic infections, allograft injury, and higher transplantation costs.

As a result of successful prophylactic strategies, CMV disease is now being eliminated at most transplant centers. These strategies include use of CMV-seronegative blood products, high-dose acyclovir, CMV hyperimmune or standard intravenous immune globulin, and ganciclovir. Depending on the CMV-serological status of the organ recipient and donor and the degree of immunosuppression after transplant, each of these approaches has certain advantages and limitations.

For CMV-seronegative transplant recipients receiving an organ or bone marrow from a CMV-seronegative donor, exclusive use of CMV-seronegative blood products eliminates most CMV disease.[1] This approach, which has been used mostly in marrow transplants and to a lesser extent in solid-organ transplants, is inexpensive. It is limited only by the need for large volumes of blood products in patients with hemorrhagic complications and the availability of CMV-seronegative blood donors.

For prevention of CMV disease in CMV-seropositive patients or in CMV-seronegative patients with a CMV-seropositive donor, the best results have been achieved by long-term administration of intravenous ganciclovir over 3-4 months after transplantation. The effectiveness of long-term ganciclovir for elimination of almost all CMV disease has been shown in placebo-controlled trials in marrow transplants and by direct comparison with high-dose acyclovir in liver transplant recipients.[2-4] However, long-term ganciclovir prophylaxis is expensive, requires maintenance of intravenous access for a considerable time, and may expose some patients who otherwise may not need long-term prophylaxis to the toxicity of ganciclovir. The most frequent side-effect of ganciclovir is neutropenia, which is far more common in marrow transplants (50%) than in solid-organ transplants (10%). Oral ganciclovir could be an acceptable alternative to intravenous ganciclovir, but the efficacy of this preparation is limited by low bioavailability and it is unproven in transplant patients.

CMV disease has also been prevented in both CMV-seropositive and CMV-seronegative patients by the long-term administration of high-dose acyclovir, CMV hyperimmune or standard intravenous immune globulin, and by short courses of ganciclovir (2-4 weeks) followed by oral acyclovir.[5-8] Acyclovir is considerably less active than ganciclovir in vitro against CMV. Acyclovir's efficacy for CMV prophylaxis continues to be controversial. The reduction of CMV disease achieved by CMV hyperimmune or standard intravenous immunoglobulin is modest compared with prophylactic ganciclovir and these preparations are costly. By contrast with long-term ganciclovir prophylaxis, none of these regimens consistently protects against primary CMV disease when the patient is CMV-seronegative and the donor is CMV-seropositive.

Another new approach for decreasing CMV disease after transplantation is pre-emptive therapy with ganciclovir. Instead of providing prophylaxis in every patient, pre-emptive therapy is designed to limit prophylaxis to patients at greatest risk of CMV disease and thereby to lessen toxicity and cost. High-risk patients include those receiving antilymphocyte antibody therapy for graft rejection and symptom-free individuals who are excreting CMV. In a recent randomized controlled trial, Hibberd and colleagues[9] showed that daily administration of ganciclovir to CMV-seropositive renal transplant recipients during every course of treatment with antilymphocyte antibody reduced the frequency of CMV disease from 33% to 14%. There were no adverse events attributable to ganciclovir. Similarly, at UCLA, we have observed that only one of 45 liver transplant recipients (2.2%) whose [OKT.sub.3] therapy was accompanied by 4-6 weeks of pre-emptive ganciclovir therapy developed CMV disease.[10]

Administration of pre-emptive ganciclovir therapy to symptom-free patients excreting CMV also decreases the subsequent incidence of

CMV disease after bone-marrow and liver transplantation.[11,12] However, this approach is limited by the cost of frequent laboratory tests (an expense that might otherwise be applied to drug costs for prophylaxis of a greater number of patients at risk for CMV disease) and by the development of CMV disease in as many as 60% of transplant patients without previous viral shedding. The use of more sensitive laboratory tests for CMV antigen or DNA leads to an earlier and higher rate of viral detection and so may improve the efficacy of pre-emptive ganciclovir therapy. Nevertheless, when pre-emptive ganciclovir therapy based on detection of CMV antigenaemia was compared with ganciclovir prophylaxis of all bone-marrow transplant patients at engraftment, CMV disease occurred less often among those receiving routine ganciclovir prophylaxis at engraftment.[13] It is also not clear how effective pre-emptive therapy is in CMV-seronegative patients with CMV-seropositive donors.

In view of all these various prophylactic strategies, how should CMV disease be prevented in transplant recipients? Since different types of transplants are associated with different risks for CMV disease and morbidity, one strategy is unlikely to be appropriate for all patients. Prophylaxis will probably need to be tailored. Thus, for those at greatest risk for serious and sometimes fatal CMV disease (lung transplant recipients, CMV-seropositive marrow transplants, and any CMV-seronegative recipient of a CMV-seropositive donor organ), long-term ganciclovir prophylaxis may have the greatest benefit. By contrast, patients with the lowest risk for CMV disease (CMV-seronegative recipients of an organ from a CMV-seronegative donor) may require only CMV-negative blood products. Pre-emptive ganciclovir therapy guided by detection of CMV or use of antilymphocyte antibody therapy may be best suited for settings where the risk of early CMV infection escaping detection is very small and the consequences of CMV disease are moderate and rarely fatal (CMV-seropositive patients receiving a renal, liver, or heart transplant).

1. Bowden RA, Sayers M, Flournoy N, et al. Cytomegalovirus immune globulin and seronegative blood products to prevent cytomegalovirus infection after marrow transplantation. *N Engl J Med* 1986; 314: 1006-10.

2. Winston DJ, Ho WG, Bartoni K, et al. Ganciclovir prophylaxis of cytomegalovirus infection and disease in allogeneic bone marrow transplant recipients. Results of a placebo-controlled, double-blind trial. *Ann Intern Med* 1993; 118: 179-84.

3. Goodrich JM, Bowden RA, Fisher L, Keller C, Schoch G, Meyers JC. Ganciclovir prophylaxis to prevent cytomegalovirus disease after allogeneic marrow transplant. *Ann Intern Med* 1993; 118: 173-78.

4. Winston DJ, Wirin D, Shaked A, Busuttil RW. Randomised comparison of ganciclovir and high-dose acyclovir for long-term cytomegalovirus prophylaxis in liver-transplant recipients. *Lancet* 1995; 346: 69-74.

5. Prentice HG, Gluckman E, Powles R, et al. Impact of long-term acyclovir on cytomegalovirus infection and survival after allogeneic bone marrow transplantation. *Lancet* 1994; 343: 749-53.

6. Snydman DR, Werner BG, Dougherty NN, et al. Cytomegalovirus immune globulin prophylaxis in liver transplantation: a randomized, double-blind, placebo-controlled trial. *Ann Intern Med* 1993; 119: 984-91.

7. Winston DJ, Ho WG, Lin CH, et al. Intravenous immune globulin for prevention of cytomegalovirus infection and interstitial pneumonia after bone marrow transplantation. *Ann Intern Med* 1987; 106: 12-18.

8. Martin M, Manez R, Linden P, et al. A prospective randomized trial comparing sequential ganciclovir-high dose acyclovir to high dose acyclovir for prevention of cytomegalovirus disease in adult liver transplant recipients. *Transplantation* 1994; 58: 225-61.

9. Hibberd PL, Tokoff-Rubin NE, Conti D, et al. Preemptive ganciclovir therapy to prevent cytomegalovirus disease in cytomegalovirus antibody-positive renal transplant recipients: a randomized controlled trial. *Ann Intern Med* 1995; 123: 18-26.

10. Winston DJ, Imagawa DK, Holt CD, et al. Long-term ganciclovir prophylaxis eliminates serious cytomegalovirus disease in liver transplants receiving OKT, therapy for rejection. *Transplantation* (in press).

11. Goodrich JM, Mori M, Gleaves CA, et al. Early treatment with ganciclovir to prevent cylomegalovirus disease after allogeneic bone marrow transplantation. *N Engl J Med* 1991; 325: 1601-07.

12. Singh N, Yu VL, Mieles L, Wagener MM, Miner RC, Gayowski T. High-dose acyclovir compared with short-course preemptive ganciclovir therapy to prevent cytomegalovirus disease in

liver transplant recipients: a randomized trial. *Ann Intern Med* 1994; 120: 375-81.

13. Boeckh M, Gooley T, Stevens-Ayers T, et al. CMV antigenemia-guided ganciclovir early treatment versus ganciclovir at engraftment after allogeneic marrow transplant. In: Programme addendum of 34th Interscience Conference On Antimicrobial Agents and Chemotherapy, Washington, DC. 1994: 7 (abstr 10).

Section 8.3

CMV Infection in Pregnancy

Up to 65% of American women test positive for CMV. Most infected adults are asymptomatic, but congenital CMV infection in newborns can cause serious complications such as deafness and seizures.

Cytomegalovirus (CMV) is a member of the *Herpesviridae* family and shares with other herpes viruses the properties of latency and reactivation. CMV is a common viral pathogen and is not restricted to any particular population group or geographical region, although it is more prevalent in indigent populations. It is the most common cause of congenital infection in the United States. The annual cost for treating complications due to CMV in the US is estimated to approach $2 billion.

Pathophysiology

Infection with CMV may be either primary or secondary. Primary infection is the patient's first encounter with CMV. Secondary infection may occur with a reactivation of the same virus or a new infection with a different strain of CMV.

CMV has been isolated from virtually all body fluids. Infection can therefore occur when susceptible individuals come into direct contact with infected bodily secretions. This may occur through close or intimate physical contact or from receiving infected blood products, vital organs, or bone marrow. In addition, congenital infection may be acquired through transplacental viral transmission, and perinatal infection may be acquired intrapartum or through breastfeeding.

Epidemiology

Overall, approximately 60% to 65% of women in the US are seropositive to CMV by the time they reach their reproductive years, with the highest rate of seroconversion occurring between the ages of 15 and 35. The seropositive rate in lower socioeconomic groups approaches 85%, while in the higher socioeconomic groups it is approximately 55%. This difference appears to be related to poor hygiene, crowded living conditions, and promiscuity. Risk factors include black race, low level of education, age less than 30 years, history of sexually transmitted disease (STD), multiple sexual partners, and close contact with children less than 2 years of age.

Primary CMV infection occurs in 0.7% to 4% of pregnant women, while recurrent infection may occur in up to 13.5%. As with nonpregnant women, seropositivity is higher in pregnant women in the lower socioeconomic groups (70% to 80%) than in women in the higher socioeconomic groups (50% to 60%).

Congenital CMV infection afflicts 1% to 2% of newborns annually in the US. Both primary and recurrent maternal CMV infection may lead to congenital infection of the newborn. However, primary CMV infection in the mother substantially increases risk of viral transmission, with 30% to 40% of fetuses becoming infected, whereas fewer than 1% of fetuses become infected when the mother has recurrent CMV infection. CMV infection also may occur during parturition or with breastfeeding. Approximately half of neonates exposed to infected cervicovaginal secretions or breast milk develop CMV infection.

Infants and toddlers not infected at birth may acquire CMV if placed in a day-care setting. Children in day-care centers have a very high prevalence of CMV shedding, ranging from 23% to 72%. Infected children then become a major source of infection for other family members. The seroconversion rate in families with children in day-care centers approaches 50% of those not previously infected.

Diagnosis

Most CMV-infected patients are minimally symptomatic, although an occasional patient will present with a mononucleosis-like syndrome. Symptoms may include fever, sore throat, myalgias, fatigue, and diarrhea. Patients may exhibit a rash, lymphadenopathy, pharyngitis, and hepatosplenomegaly. Elevated liver enzymes, thrombocytopenia, lymphocystosis, or lymphocytopenia also may be found. A heterophile antibody test will be negative in a CMV-infected patient, and CMV-specific IgG and IgM antibody levels usually are positive. The virus may be detected by culture or antigen testing of body fluids or secretions.

Although seroconversion is a reliable method for diagnosing primary CMV infection, the diagnosis can be problematic. The rise in CMV-specific antibodies may be delayed for up to 4 weeks, and the presence of CMV-specific IgM antibodies can be found in up to 10% of women with recurrent disease. Persistence of CMV-specific IgM antibodies for up to 18 months after a primary infection has been documented as well. Therefore, when seroconversion cannot be documented in a patient, detection of CMV antigen or isolation of the virus is a more reliable method for diagnosing active infection.

Prenatal diagnosis of CMV infection in the fetus also can be problematic. Fetal blood culture and detection of IgM antibodies in fetal blood are not reliable. At present, detection of virus in amniotic fluid by either culture or polymerase chain reaction (PCR) testing remains the most accurate means of diagnosis, with sensitivities ranging from 80% to 100%. Infected fetuses also may have abnormal ultrasound findings. These abnormalities include cerebral ventriculomegaly, periventricular calcifications, hepatomegaly intrauterine growth restriction, ascites or hydrops, and abnormal calcification patterns in the liver or bowel. It should be emphasized, however, that negative studies cannot exclude a CMV infection and that normal prenatal Ultrasound scans do not rule out severe neurologic damage.

Congenital CMV Infection

In utero viral transmission appears to occur with equal frequency throughout pregnancy Intrauterine infection is much higher with primary disease than with recurrent disease. Congenital infection occurs in approximately 40% of pregnant women with primary disease. Approximately 10% of infected fetuses will have clinically apparent disease at birth. Of the remaining infected neonates who are asymptomatic at birth, approximately 5% to 15% will go on to develop sequelae from CMV infection. The prognosis is much better for the offspring of mothers with recurrent disease, with fetuses having only a 1% risk of in utero infection and extremely low risk of developing significant sequelae. Table 8.1 lists common findings in newborns with congenital CMV infection.

Treatment

Fortunately, most CMV infections are asymptomatic or self-limiting. Ganciclovir, foscarnet, and cidofovir are the only antiviral agents currently licensed in the US for treating severe CMV infection. These agents have not been studied in pregnant patients, and information on the use of antiviral agents in pediatric patients is very limited. Currently, the use of ganciclovir in children with symptomatic congenital CMV infection and CNS involvement is being studied in a multicenter trial. CMV-specific monoclonal antibody therapy also is being studied in children with congenital CMV infections.

Prevention

Research on CMV vaccine development is encouraging. Live-attenuated CMV administered to renal transplant patients has been shown to be effective in eliciting an immune response. Safety studies of recombinant vaccines are currently under way. In addition, vaccine administration in pregnant animals has reduced the incidence of congenital infection by CMV.

Until such time as a CMV vaccine is developed, however, susceptible pregnant women must take precautions to prevent transmission of the virus. Since CMV is transmitted through infected body fluids, at-risk pregnant women should practice good hygiene. This includes frequent hand washing, avoiding kissing on the mouth, and not sharing food and utensils. Women who work in situations with potential exposure to children should ascertain their immune status before attempting to conceive. Those who are CMV-IgG negative should consider avoiding such exposure.

Suggested Reading

Adler, S.P.; Current prospects for immunization against cytomegaloviral disease. *Infect Agents Dis.* 1996;5:29-35.

Daniel, Y.; Gull, I.; Peyser, M.R., et al. Congenital cytomegolovirus infection. *Eur J Obstet Gynecol Reprod Biol.* 1995;63:7-16.

Demmler, G.J.; Congenital cytomegalovirus infection and disease. *Adv Pediatr Infect Dis.* 1996;11:135-162.

Hagay, Z.J.; Biran, G.; Ornoy, A., et al. Congenital cytomegalovirus infection: a long-standing problem still seeking a solution. *Am J Obstet Gynecol.* 1996;174:241-245.

Table 8.1. Findings in Newborns with Congenital CMV

Chorioretinitis	Microcephaly
Deafness	Seizures
Hemolytic anemia	Smallness for gestational age
Hepatosplenomegaly	Thrombocytopenia
Intracranial calcifications	

Section 8.4

AIDS-Related CMV

National Institute of Allergy and Infectious Diseases (NIAID), Undated.

What is CMV?

People with HIV may get CMV disease. This chapter explains what CMV is. It also talks about medicines that can be used to help treat the disease and steps you can take to keep yourself healthy.

CMV is short for cytomegalovirus, the germ that causes CMV disease. Many people have this germ in their bodies and may never get sick from it. Because people with HIV have weakened immune systems, they may not be able to fight off CMV and can become seriously ill.

Symptoms of CMV

CMV disease can damage many parts of the body, including the digestive system and lungs. CMV disease most commonly affects the eyes and can cause blindness if it is not treated. A blood test can be used to find out if you have CMV in your body. Other tests may be used to make sure your symptoms are caused by CMV. An eye exam can show CMV even before symptoms appear.

Symptoms of CMV eye disease are:

- Floating spots before the eyes
- Hazy vision, as if looking through a screen
- Blurred or missing areas of vision

Symptoms of CMV digestive disease are:

- Diarrhea
- Loss of appetite
- Fever
- Blood in the stool

- Stomach cramps
- Weight loss
- Painful swallowing
- Pain in center of the chest

Medicines Can Help

Some medicines can help to fight CMV disease. Medicines can be used to:

- *Keep your immune system stronger*. Certain medicines can help the body defend against disease. To keep you healthy, your doctor or clinic nurse may ask you to start taking medicine as soon as you find out you have HIV.

- *Treat the infection*. There are medicines that may keep CMV disease from getting worse. Once you get CMV disease, you may need to continue taking medicine to prevent CMV disease from coming back.

How to Help Yourself

1. *Keep your immune system as strong as you can*. Eat healthy foods. Get enough rest and exercise. Don't use alcohol, cigarettes, and other drugs.

2. *Make sure you keep your clinic appointments*. It's important to get regular checkups to ward off problems BEFORE your eyesight is affected.

3. *Tell your doctor or nurse any symptoms of CMV*. Sudden changes in vision are important warning signs that should be checked out right away.

4. *Follow your care plan.* Take all your medicines as they are prescribed (at the right time and in the right amounts). Be sure you know how to take them. Ask your doctor or clinic nurse if you have any questions. Continue to keep your clinic appointments so that your doctor can check you to make sure that the medicine is working.

5. *Tell your doctor or clinic nurse about any side effects from your medicine.* Medicines used to treat CMV disease can cause fever, diarrhea, nausea, tiredness, or abnormal bruising and bleeding in some people. Your doctor may have to give you another medicine or change the amount that you take to reduce your side effects.

Research: Hope for the Future

Scientists are working to find better drugs to treat and prevent CMV disease. Drugs that may work better and are easier to take than drugs that are now used are being tested in research studies. You may be able to help test one of these new drugs. If you take part in research, you may help yourself—and others with HIV.

Remember:

- CMV is a serious disease that can cause blindness and damage to other organs if not treated.

- Tell your doctor or clinic nurse right away if you have sudden changes in vision or other symptoms of CMV disease.

- Take your medicine as your doctor prescribed.

- Be sure to have regular check-ups.

Chapter 9

Donovanosis (Granuloma Inguinale)

Granuloma inguinale, a rare disease in the United States, is caused by the intracellular gram-negative bacterium *Calymmatobacterium granulomatis*. The disease is endemic in certain tropical and developing areas, including India, Papua New Guinea, central Australia, and southern Africa. The disease presents clinically as painless, progressive, ulcerative lesions without regional lymphadenopathy. The lesions are highly vascular (i.e., a beefy red appearance) and bleed easily on contact. The causative organism cannot be cultured on standard microbiologic media, and diagnosis requires visualization of dark-staining Donovan bodies on tissue crush preparation or biopsy. A secondary bacterial infection might develop in the lesions, or the lesions might be coinfected with another sexually transmitted pathogen.

Treatment

Treatment appears to halt progressive destruction of tissue, although prolonged duration of therapy often is required to enable granulation and re-epithelialization of the ulcers. Relapse can occur 6-18 months later despite effective initial therapy.

Centers for Disease Control and Prevention (CDC), excerpted from 1998 Guidelines for Treatment of Sexually Transmitted Diseases, *MMWR* 1998;47 (No. RR-1).

Recommended Regimens

Trimethoprim-sulfamethoxazole one double-strength tablet orally twice a day for a minimum of 3 weeks, or Doxycycline 100 mg orally twice a day for a minimum of 3 weeks.

Therapy should be continued until all lesions have healed completely.

Alternative Regimens

Ciprofloxacin 750 mg orally twice a day for a minimum of 3 weeks, or Erythromycin base 500 mg orally four times a day for a minimum of 3 weeks.

For any of the above regimens, the addition of an aminoglycoside (gentamicin 1 mg/kg IV every 8 hours) should be considered if lesions do not respond within the first few days of therapy.

Follow-Up

Patients should be followed clinically until signs and symptoms have resolved.

Management of Sex Partners

Sex partners of patients who have granuloma inguinale should be examined and treated if they a) had sexual contact with the patient during the 60 days preceding the onset of symptoms in the patient and b) have clinical signs and symptoms of the disease.

Special Considerations

Pregnancy

Pregnancy is a relative contraindication to the use of sulfonamides. Both pregnant and lactating women should be treated with the erythromycin regimen. The addition of a parenteral aminoglycoside (e.g., gentamicin) should be strongly considered.

HIV Infection

HIV-infected persons who have granuloma inguinale should be treated following the regimens cited previously. The addition of a parenteral aminoglycoside (e.g., gentamicin) should be strongly considered.

Chapter 10

Ectoparasitic Infections

Chapter Contents

Section 10.1

Pubic Lice

Centers for Disease Control and Prevention (CDC), excerpted from
1998 Guidelines for Treatment of Sexually Transmitted Diseases,
MMWR 1998;47(No. RR-1).

Patients who have pediculosis pubis (i.e., pubic lice) usually seek
medical attention because of pruritus. Such patients also usually notice lice or nits on their pubic hair.

Recommended Regimens

Permethrin 1% creme rinse applied to affected areas and washed
off after 10 minutes. Or Lindane 1% shampoo applied for 4 minutes
to the affected area, and then thoroughly washed off. This regimen
is not recommended for pregnant or lactating women or for children
aged less than 2 years. Or Pyrethrins with piperonyl butoxide applied
to the affected area and washed off after 10 minutes.

The lindane regimen is the least expensive therapy. Toxicity, as
indicated by seizure and aplastic anemia, has not been reported when
treatment was limited to the recommended 4-minute period. Permethrin has less potential for toxicity than lindane.

Other Management Considerations

The recommended regimens should not be applied to the eyes.
Pediculosis of the eyelashes should be treated by applying occlusive
ophthalmic ointment to the eyelid margins twice a day for 10 days.

Bedding and clothing should be decontaminated (i.e., either ma-
chine-washed or machine-dried using the heat cycle or dry-cleaned)
or removed from body contact for at least 72 hours. Fumigation of living areas is not necessary.

Follow-Up

Patients should be evaluated after 1 week if symptoms persist. Re-
treatment may be necessary if lice are found or if eggs are observed

at the hair-skin junction. Patients who do not respond to one of the recommended regimens should be re-treated with an alternative regimen.

Management of Sex Partners

Sex partners within the preceding month should be treated.

Special Considerations

Pregnancy

Pregnant and lactating women should be treated with either permethrin or pyrethrins with piperonyl butoxide.

HIV Infection

Patients who have pediculosis pubis and also are infected with HIV should receive the same treatment regimen as those who are HIV-negative.

Section 10.2

Scabies

1998 National Institute of Allergy and Infectious Disease (NIAID).

Scabies is a skin infestation with a tiny mite, *Sarcoptes scabiei*. Scabies has become relatively common throughout the general population. It is highly contagious and is spread primarily through sexual contact, although it also is commonly transmitted by contact with skin, infested sheets, towels, or even furniture.

Symptoms

Scabies causes intense itching, which often becomes worse at night. Small red bumps or lines appear on the body at sites where the female scabies mite has burrowed into the skin to lay her eggs. The areas most commonly affected include the hands (especially between the fingers), wrists, elbows, lower abdomen, and genitals. The skin reaction may not develop until a month or more after infestation. During this time, a person may pass the disease unknowingly to a sex partner or to another person with whom he or she has close contact.

Diagnosis

Scabies may be confused with other skin irritations such as poison ivy or eczema. To make an accurate diagnosis, a doctor takes a scraping of the irritated area and examines it under a microscope, to reveal the presence of the mite.

Treatment

As with pubic lice, lindane is an effective treatment for scabies. Pregnant women should consult a doctor before using this product. Nonprescription remedies such as sulfur ointment also are available. Sulfur is fairly effective but may be objectionable because of its odor and messiness. Itching can persist even after the infestation has been eliminated because of lingering skin irritation. A hydrocortisone cream or ointment or a soothing lotion may provide relief from itching.

Prevention

Family members and sex partners of a person with scabies are advised to undergo treatment. Twenty-four hours after drug therapy, a person with scabies infestation is no longer contagious to others, even though the skin irritation may persist for some time. As with pubic lice, special care must be taken to rid clothing and bedding of any mites.

Chapter 11

Epididymitis

Definition

Inflammation of the epididymis, the long, tightly coiled tube that is located behind each testicle and carries sperm from the testicle to the vas deferens, is called epididymitis. This condition causes fever and pain, developing progressively over several hours in the back portion of the testicles, and the scrotum may be enlarged and red.

Cause

Epididymitis may be caused by a bacterial or chlamydial infection that travels from the urinary tract to the sperm duct. Occasionally an episode of epididymitis is precipitated by extreme straining, which causes urine to back up the reproductive tract to the epididymis.

Among sexually active men aged less than 35 years, epididymitis is most often caused by *C. trachomatis* or *N. gonorrhoeae*. Epididymitis caused by sexually transmitted *E. coli* infection also occurs among homosexual men who are the insertive partners during anal intercourse. Sexually transmitted epididymitis usually is accompanied by urethritis, which often is asymptomatic. Nonsexually transmitted epididymitis associated with urinary tract infections caused by Gram-negative enteric organisms occurs more frequently among men aged greater than 35 years, men who have recently undergone urinary tract instrumentation or surgery, and men who have anatomical abnormalities.

Although most patients can be treated on an outpatient basis, hospitalization should be considered when severe pain suggests other diagnoses (e.g., torsion, testicular infarction, and abscess) or when patients are febrile or might be noncompliant with an antimicrobial regimen.

Diagnostic Considerations

Men who have epididymitis typically have unilateral testicular pain and tenderness; hydrocele and palpable swelling of the epididymis usually are present. Testicular torsion, a surgical emergency, should be considered in all cases but is more frequent among adolescents. Torsion occurs more frequently in patients who do not have evidence of inflammation or infection. Emergency testing for torsion may be indicated when the onset of pain is sudden, pain is severe, or the test results available during the initial examination do not enable a diagnosis of urethritis or urinary tract infection to be made. If the diagnosis is questionable, an expert should be consulted immediately, because testicular viability may be compromised. The evaluation of men for epididymitis should include the following procedures:

- A Gram-stained smear of urethral exudate or intraurethral swab specimen for diagnosis of urethritis (i.e., greater than or equal to 5 polymorphonuclear leukocytes per oil immersion field) and for presumptive diagnosis of gonococcal infection.

- A culture of urethral exudate or intraurethral swab specimen, or nucleic acid amplification test (either on intraurethral swab or first-void urine) for *N. gonorrhoeae* and *C. trachomatis*.

- Examination of first-void urine for leukocytes if the urethral Gram stain is negative. Culture and Gram-stained smear of uncentrifuged urine should be obtained.

- Syphilis serology and HIV counseling and testing.

Treatment

Empiric therapy is indicated before culture results are available. Treatment of epididymitis caused by *C. trachomatis* or *N. gonorrhoeae* will result in a) a microbiologic cure of infection, b) improvement of the signs and symptoms, c) prevention of transmission to others, and d) a decrease in the potential complications (e.g., infertility or chronic pain).

Recommended Regimens

For epididymitis most likely caused by gonococcal or chlamydial infection: Ceftriaxone 250 mg IM in a single dose, plus Doxycycline 100 mg orally twice a day for 10 days.

For epididymitis most likely caused by enteric organisms, or for patients allergic to cephalosporins and/or tetracyclines: Ofloxacin 300 mg orally twice a day for 10 days.

As an adjunct to therapy, bed rest, scrotal elevation, and analgesics are recommended until fever and local inflammation have subsided.

Follow-Up

Failure to improve within 3 days requires reevaluation of both the diagnosis and therapy. Swelling and tenderness that persist after completion of antimicrobial therapy should be evaluated comprehensively. The differential diagnosis includes tumor, abscess, infarction, testicular cancer, and tuberculous or fungal epididymitis.

Management of Sex Partners

Patients who have epididymitis that is known or suspected to be caused by *N. gonorrhoeae* or *C. trachomatis* should be instructed to refer sex partners for evaluation and treatment. Sex partners of these patients should be referred if their contact with the index patient was within the 60 days preceding onset of symptoms in the patient.

Patients should be instructed to avoid sexual intercourse until they and their sex partners are cured. In the absence of a microbiologic test of cure, this means until therapy is completed and patient and partner(s) no longer have symptoms.

Special Considerations

HIV Infection

Patients who have uncomplicated epididymitis and also are infected with HIV should receive the same treatment regimen as those who are HIV-negative. Fungi and mycobacteria, however, are more likely to cause epididymitis in immunosuppressed patients than in immunocompetent patients.

Chapter 12

Gonorrhea

Chapter Contents

Section 12.1

Gonorrhea Facts

1998 National Institute of Allergy and Infectious Disease (NIAID).

In 1995, 392,848 cases of gonorrhea in the United States were reported to the U.S. Centers for Disease Control and Prevention (CDC). The Institute of Medicine, however, estimates that 800,000 cases of gonorrhea occur annually in the United States. The annual cost of gonorrhea and its complications is estimated at close to $1.1 billion.

Gonorrhea is caused by a bacterium, *Neisseria gonorrhoeae*, that grows and multiplies quickly in moist, warm areas of the body including the reproductive tract, the oral cavity, and the rectum. Although in women the cervix usually is the initial site of infection, the disease can spread to and infect the uterus (womb) and fallopian tubes, resulting in pelvic inflammatory disease (PID). This can cause infertility and ectopic (tubal) pregnancy.

The disease is most commonly spread during sexual intercourse—vaginal, oral, and anal. Gonorrhea of the rectum can occur in people who practice anal intercourse and also may occur in women due to spread of the infection from the vaginal area.

Gonorrhea can be passed from an infected woman to her newborn infant during delivery, causing eye infections in the baby. When the infection occurs in the genital tract, mouth, or rectum of a child, it is due most commonly to sexual abuse.

Symptoms

The early symptoms of gonorrhea often are mild, and many women who are infected have no symptoms of the disease. If symptoms of gonorrhea develop, they usually appear within two to 10 days after sexual contact with an infected partner, although a small percentage of patients may be infected for several months without showing symptoms. The initial symptoms in women include a painful or burning sensation when urinating and/or vaginal discharge that is yellow or bloody. More advanced symptoms, which indicate progression to PID, include abdominal pain, bleeding between menstrual periods, vomiting, or fever. Men are more often symptomatic than women. They usually have a discharge from the penis and a burning sensation during urination that may be severe. Symptoms of rectal infection include discharge, anal itching, and sometimes painful bowel movements.

Diagnosis

Three techniques, gram stain, detection of bacterial genes or nucleic acid (DNA), and culture, are generally used to diagnose gonorrhea. Many doctors prefer to use more than one test to increase the chance of an accurate diagnosis. The gram stain is quite accurate for men but is not very sensitive for women. Only one in two women with gonorrhea have a positive gram stain. The test involves placing a smear of the discharge from the penis or the cervix (the opening to the uterus) on a slide and staining the smear with a dye. The slide is examined under a microscope for the presence of the bacteria. A doctor usually can give test results to the patient at the time of an office or clinic visit. More often, urine or cervical swabs are used for a new test that detects the genes of the bacteria. These tests are as accurate as culture and are used widely.

The culture test involves placing a sample of the discharge onto a culture plate and incubating it up to two days to allow the bacteria to multiply. The sensitivity of this test depends on the site from which the sample is taken. Cervical samples detect infection approximately 90 percent of the time. The doctor also can take a throat culture to detect pharyngeal gonorrhea.

Treatment

Because penicillin-resistant cases of gonorrhea are common, other antibiotics are used to treat most patients with gonococcal infections. One of the most effective medicines to treat patients is ceftriaxone, which the doctor can inject in a single dose. Other effective antibiotics that a patient can take by mouth include a single dose of cefixime, ciprofloxacin, or ofloxacin. Pregnant women and patients younger than 18 years old should not take ciprofloxacin or ofloxacin.

Gonorrhea can occur together with chlamydial infection, another common sexually transmitted disease (STD). Therefore, doctors usually prescribe a combination of antibiotics, such as ceftriaxone and doxycycline or azithromycin. Single-dose oral therapy is available. All sexual partners of a person with gonorrhea should be tested and treated if infected whether or not they have symptoms of infection.

Complications

The most common consequence of untreated gonorrhea is PID, a serious infection of the female reproductive organs that occurs in an estimated 1 million American women each year. Gonococcal PID often appears immediately after the menstrual period. PID can scar or damage cells lining the fallopian tubes, resulting in infertility in as many as 10 percent of women affected. If the tube is only partially scarred, proper passage of the fertilized egg into the uterus is prevented. If this happens, the egg may implant in the tube; this is called ectopic or tubal pregnancy and is life-threatening if not detected early. Rarely, untreated gonorrhea can spread to the blood or the joints. An infected pregnant woman may give the infection to her infant as the baby passes through the birth canal during delivery. A doctor can prevent infection of the eye, called ophthalmia neonatorum, by applying silver nitrate or other medications to the baby's eyes immediately after birth. Because of the risks from gonococcal infection to both mother and child, doctors recommend that a pregnant woman have at least one test for gonorrhea.

Gonorrhea also increases the risk of HIV infection (HIV, human immunodeficiency virus, causes AIDS), so prevention and early treatment of gonorrhea is critically important.

Prevention

By using male condoms correctly and consistently during sexual activity, sexually active people can reduce their risk of gonorrhea and its complications.

Research

Scientists supported by the National Institute of Allergy and Infectious Diseases (NIAID) are continuing to learn more about the organism that causes gonorrhea and are working on better methods to prevent, diagnose, and treat it. The dramatic rise of antibiotic-resistant strains of the gonococcus underscores the need for a means of preventing gonorrhea. Scientists have developed a laboratory method to detect these resistant strains, which helps the physician select an appropriate treatment.

An effective vaccine against gonorrhea remains a key research priority for NIAID-supported scientists. Determining the sequence of the bacterial genome is expected to aid scientists in identifying new vaccine candidates.

Section 12.2

Gonorrhea in Females

1999 Clinical Reference Systems Ltd., from *Clinical Reference Systems*, July 1, 1999, Pg.633, by David W. Kaplan; reprinted with permission.

Cause

Gonorrhea is one of the most common sexually transmitted diseases. It is caused by bacteria called *Neisseria gonorrhoeae* and is transmitted through sexual intercourse. Gonorrhea most often starts as an infection of the cervix.

Popular names for gonorrhea are clap, drip, dose, and strain.

Many women infected with gonorrhea have no symptoms. If symptoms occur, they appear 2 to 10 days after exposure to the disease. Symptoms of gonorrhea include:

- thick, creamy, yellow vaginal discharge
- burning during urination
- bleeding or spotting between periods
- heavier than usual menstrual periods
- abdominal pain
- painful intercourse
- fever.

Expected Course

The outcome of a gonorrheal infection depends on:

- the length of time you have been infected
- the extent of the infection; that is, whether the infection has spread to other parts of your body
- the number of previous gonorrheal infections you have had.

If only the cervix is infected, proper treatment should clear up the infection in about 10 days. If not treated, gonorrhea in women can spread through the uterus to the fallopian tubes and ovaries, causing pelvic inflammatory disease (PID). PID can cause infertility, as well as increase the risk of an ectopic (tubal) pregnancy. Further complications of untreated gonorrhea include spread of infection into the bloodstream and to other parts of the body.

Gonorrhea can be transmitted from a mother to her baby during birth.

Treatment

Antibiotics for Gonorrhea

You will need to take the antibiotic prescribed by your physician.

Antibiotics for Chlamydia

Because many women who have gonorrhea also have a chlamydial infection, treatment for gonorrhea also includes treatment for chlamydia. You will need to take the antibiotic prescribed by your physician.

Contacts

Tell everyone with whom you have had sex in the last 3 months about your infection. They must also be treated, even if they have no symptoms. Do not have sex until both you and your partner have finished all the medication.

Follow-up

Return to your physician about 7 days after finishing your medication so that your physician can make sure that the infection is gone.

Prevention

Because gonorrhea is sexually transmitted, there are ways that you can help prevent this infection. Not having sexual intercourse (abstinence) is the best method of prevention. Use of condoms is the next best method. In addition, you are less likely to get a sexually transmitted disease if you have just one sexual partner.

It is possible to be infected with chlamydia or gonorrhea and yet not have any symptoms. If you continue to be sexually active, you should get a test for chlamydia and a gonorrhea culture at your yearly pelvic examination, along with a Pap smear.

Call Your Physician Immediately If:

- You develop severe abdominal pain.
- You vomit and cannot hold the medication down.
- You develop a fever over 100 degrees F (37.8 degrees C).
- You feel you are getting sicker.

Section 12.3

Gonorrhea in Males

©1999 Clinical Reference Systems Ltd., from *Clinical Reference Systems*, July 1, 1999, Pg.NA, by David W. Kaplan; reprinted with permission.

Cause

Gonorrhea is one of the most common sexually transmitted diseases. It is caused by bacteria called Neisseria gonorrhoeae and is transmitted through sexual intercourse. It most often starts as an infection of the urethra. The urethra is the tube that urine passes through in the penis. Popular names for gonorrhea are clap, drip, dose, and strain.

If symptoms occur, they usually appear 2 to 10 days after exposure. Symptoms of gonorrhea include:

- thick, yellow discharge (drip) from the penis
- burning or pain during urination
- urge to urinate often.

Expected Course

The outcome of a gonorrheal infection depends on:

- the length of time you have been infected
- the extent of the infection
- the number of previous infections you have had.

If only the urethra is infected, proper treatment should clear up the infection in 10 days. If untreated, gonorrhea can lead to scarring of the urethra, inability to urinate normally, and inflammation of the testicles. Testicle inflammation can cause sterility.

Treatment

Antibiotics for Gonorrhea

You will need to take the antibiotic prescribed by your physician.

Antibiotics for Chlamydia

Because many men who have gonorrhea also have a chlamydial infection, treatment for gonorrhea also includes treatment for chlamydia. You will need to take the antibiotic prescribed by your physician.

Contacts

Tell everyone with whom you have had sex in the last 3 months about your infection. They must also be treated, even if they have no symptoms. Do not have sex until both you and your partner have finished all the medication.

Follow-up

Return to your physician's office about 7 days after completing your medication so that your physician can make sure that the infection is gone.

Prevention

Because gonorrhea is sexually transmitted, there are ways that you can help prevent this infection. Not having sexual intercourse (abstinence) is the best method of prevention. Use of condoms is the next best method. In addition, you are less likely to get a sexually transmitted disease if you have just one sexual partner.

Call Your Physician during Office Hours If:

- Your symptoms get worse.
- You have other questions or concerns.

Chapter 13

Hepatitis

Chapter Contents

Section 13.1

Viral Hepatitis A

1999 Centers for Disease Control and Prevention (CDC).

General Information

What is hepatitis A?

Hepatitis A is a liver disease caused by hepatitis A virus.

What are the signs and symptoms of hepatitis A?

Persons with hepatitis A virus infection may not have any signs or symptoms of the disease. Older persons are more likely to have symptoms than children. If symptoms are present, they usually occur abruptly and may include fever, tiredness, loss of appetite, nausea, abdominal discomfort, dark urine, and jaundice (yellowing of the skin and eyes). Symptoms usually last less than 2 months; a few persons are ill for as long as 6 months. The average incubation period for hepatitis A is 28 days.

How is hepatitis A diagnosed?

A blood test (IgM anti-HAV) is needed to diagnose hepatitis A. Talk to your doctor or someone from your local health department if you suspect that you have been exposed to hepatitis A or any type of viral hepatitis.

How is hepatitis A virus transmitted?

Hepatitis A virus is spread from person to person by putting something in the mouth that has been contaminated with the stool of a person with hepatitis A. This type of transmission is called "fecal-oral." For this reason, the virus is more easily spread in areas where there are poor sanitary conditions or where good personal hygiene is not observed.

Most infections result from contact with a household member or sex partner who has hepatitis A. Casual contact, as in the usual office, factory, or school setting, does not spread the virus.

What products are available to prevent hepatitis A virus infection?

Two products are used to prevent hepatitis A virus infection: immune globulin and hepatitis A vaccine. Immune globulin is a preparation of antibodies that can be given before exposure for short-term protection against hepatitis A and for persons who have already been exposed to hepatitis A virus. Immune globulin must be given within 2 weeks after exposure to hepatitis A virus for maximum protection.

Hepatitis A vaccine has been licensed in the United States for use in persons 2 years of age and older. The vaccine is recommended (before exposure to hepatitis A virus) for persons who are more likely to get hepatitis A virus infection or are more likely to get seriously ill if they do get hepatitis A.

How are hepatitis A vaccines made?

There is no live virus in hepatitis A vaccines. The virus is inactivated during production of the vaccines, similar to Salk-type inactivated polio vaccine.

Is hepatitis A vaccine safe?

Yes, hepatitis A vaccine has an excellent safety profile. No serious adverse events have been attributed definitively to hepatitis A vaccine. Soreness at the injection site is the most frequently reported side effect.

Any adverse event suspected to be associated with hepatitis A vaccination should be reported to the Vaccine Adverse Events Reporting System (VAERS). VAERS forms can be obtained by calling 1-800-822-7967.

Is immune globulin safe?

Yes. No instance of transmission of HIV (the virus that causes AIDS) or other viruses has been observed with the use of immune globulin administered by the intramuscular route. Immune globulin can be administered during pregnancy and breast-feeding.

Is immune globulin in short supply?

Yes. This shortage is expected to continue necessitating a prioritization of indications for the use of immune globulin.

Can other vaccines be given at the same time that hepatitis A vaccine is given?

Yes. Hepatitis B, diphtheria, poliovirus (oral and inactivated), tetanus, oral typhoid, cholera, Japanese encephalitis, rabies, yellow fever vaccine or immune globulin can be given at the same time that hepatitis A vaccine is given, but at a different injection site.

How long does immunity last after hepatitis A vaccination?

Although data on long-term protection are limited, estimates based on modeling techniques suggest that protection will last for at least 20 years.

When are persons protected after receiving hepatitis A vaccine?

Protection against hepatitis A begins four weeks after the first dose of hepatitis A vaccine. Check with your doctor for when the next dose is due.

Can hepatitis A vaccine be given after exposure to hepatitis A virus?

No, hepatitis A vaccine is not licensed for use after exposure to hepatitis A virus. In this situation, immune globulin should be used.

Should prevaccination testing be done?

Prevaccination testing is done only in specific instances to control cost (e.g., persons who were likely to have had hepatitis A in the past). This includes persons who were born in countries with high levels of hepatitis A virus infection, elderly persons, and persons who have clotting factor disorders and may have received factor concentrates in the past.

Should postvaccination testing be done?

No. We gave our patients the first dose of a 3-dose series of HAVRIX (360 EL.U.) to protect them from hepatitis A.

Can we just give one additional dose of 720 EL.U. to complete the vaccination series?

There are no studies that have looked at this issue. It is recommended that these children complete the 3-dose series with the 360 EL.U. formulation. If this formulation is not available to complete the vaccination series, a single dose of the 720 EL.U. formulation should provide more than adequate protection.

Can a patient receive the first dose of hepatitis A vaccine from one manufacturer and the second (last) dose from another manufacturer?

Yes. Although studies have not been done to look at this issue, there is no reason to believe that this would be a problem.

What should be done if the second dose of hepatitis A vaccine is delayed?

The second dose should be administered as soon as possible. There is no need to repeat the first dose.

Can hepatitis A vaccine be given during pregnancy or lactation?

We don't know for sure, but because vaccine is produced from inactivated hepatitis A virus, the theoretical risk to the developing fetus is expected to be low. The risk associated with vaccination, however, should be weighed against the risk for hepatitis A in women who may be at high risk for exposure to hepatitis A virus.

Can hepatitis A vaccine be given to immunocompromised persons? (e.g., persons on hemodialysis or persons with AIDS)

Yes.

Persons Who Should Receive Hepatitis A Vaccine

Hepatitis A vaccination provides protection before one is exposed to hepatitis A virus. Hepatitis A vaccination is recommended for the following groups who are at increased risk for infection and for any person wishing to obtain immunity.

Persons traveling to or working in countries that have high or intermediate rates of hepatitis A.

All susceptible persons traveling to or working in countries that have high or intermediate rates of hepatitis A should be vaccinated or receive immune globulin before traveling. Persons from developed countries who travel to developing countries are at high risk for hepatitis A. Such persons include tourists, military personnel, missionaries, and others who work or study abroad in countries that have high or intermediate levels of hepatitis A. The risk for hepatitis A exists even for travelers to urban areas, those who stay in luxury hotels, and those who report that they have good hygiene and that they are careful about what they drink and eat.

Children in communities that have high rates of hepatitis A and periodic hepatitis A outbreaks.

Children living in communities that have high rates of hepatitis A (e.g., American Indian, Alaska Native) should be routinely vaccinated beginning at 2 years of age. High rates of hepatitis A are generally found in these populations, both in urban and rural settings. In addition, to effectively prevent epidemics of hepatitis A in these communities, vaccination of previously unvaccinated older children is recommended within 5 years of initiation of routine childhood vaccination programs. Although rates differ among areas, available data indicate that a reasonable cutoff age in many areas is 10-15 years of age because older persons have often already had hepatitis A. Vaccination of children before they enter school should receive highest priority, followed by vaccination of older children who have not been vaccinated.

Men who have sex with men.

Sexually active men (both adolescents and adults) who have sex with men should be vaccinated. Hepatitis A outbreaks among men who have sex with men have been reported frequently. Recent outbreaks have occurred in urban areas in the United States, Canada, and Australia.

Illegal-drug users.

Vaccination is recommended for injecting and noninjecting illegal-drug users if local health authorities have noted current or past outbreaks among such persons. During the past decade, outbreaks have been reported among injecting-drug users in the United States and in Europe.

Persons who have occupational risk for infection.

Persons who work with hepatitis A virus-infected primates or with hepatitis A virus in a research laboratory setting should be vaccinated. No other groups have been shown to be at increased risk for hepatitis

A virus infection because of occupational exposure. Outbreaks of hepatitis A have been reported among persons working with non-human primates that are susceptible to hepatitis A virus infection, including several Old World and New World species.

Primates that were infected were those that had been born in the wild, not those that had been born and raised in captivity.

Persons who have chronic liver disease.

Persons with chronic liver disease who have never had hepatitis A should be vaccinated, as there is a higher rate of fulminant (rapid onset of liver failure, often leading to death) hepatitis A among persons with chronic liver disease. Persons who are either awaiting or have received liver transplants also should be vaccinated.

Persons who have clotting-factor disorders.

Persons who have never had hepatitis A and who are administered clotting-factor concentrates, especially solvent detergent-treated preparations, should be given hepatitis A vaccine. All persons with hemophilia (Factor VIII, Factor IX) who receive replacement therapy should be vaccinated because there appears to be an increased risk of transmission from clotting-factor concentrates that are not heat inactivated.

Groups for Whom Hepatitis A Vaccine Is Not Routinely Recommended

Food Service Workers

Foodborne hepatitis A outbreaks are relatively uncommon in the United States; however, when they occur, intensive public health efforts are required for their control. Although persons who work as food handlers have a critical role in common-source foodborne outbreaks, they are not at increased risk for hepatitis A because of their occupation. Consideration may be given to vaccination of employees who work in areas where community-wide outbreaks are occurring and where state and local health authorities or private employers determine that such vaccination is cost-effective.

Sewerage Workers

In the United States, no work-related outbreaks of hepatitis A have been reported among workers exposed to sewage.

Health-Care Workers

Health-care workers are not at increased risk for hepatitis A. If a patient with hepatitis A is admitted to the hospital, routine infection control precautions will prevent transmission to hospital staff.

Children Under 2 Years of Age

Because of the limited experience with hepatitis A vaccination among children under 2 years of age, the vaccine is not currently licensed for this age-group.

Day-Care Attendees

The frequency of outbreaks of hepatitis A is not high enough in this setting to warrant routine hepatitis A vaccination. In some communities, however, day-care centers play a role in sustaining community-wide outbreaks. In this situation, consideration should be given to adding hepatitis A vaccine to the prevention plan for children and staff in the involved center(s).

Travel and the Prevention of Hepatitis A

Who should receive protection against hepatitis A before travel?

All susceptible persons traveling to or working in countries that have high or intermediate rates of hepatitis A should be vaccinated or receive immune globulin before traveling. Persons from developed countries who travel to developing countries are at high risk for hepatitis A. Such persons include tourists, military personnel, missionaries, and others who work or study abroad in countries that have high or intermediate levels of hepatitis A. The risk for hepatitis A exists even for travelers to urban areas, those who stay in luxury hotels, and those who report that they have good hygiene and that they are careful about what they drink and eat.

How soon before travel should the first dose of hepatitis A vaccine be given?

Protection against hepatitis A virus infection begins four weeks before travel. Check with your doctor about when the next dose is due.

106

What should be done if a person cannot receive hepatitis A vaccine?

Travelers who are allergic to a vaccine component or who elect not to receive vaccine should receive a single dose of immune globulin (0.02 mL/kg), which provides effective protection against hepatitis A for up to 3 months. Travelers whose travel period exceeds 2 months should be administered immune globulin at 0.06 mL/kg; administration must be repeated if the travel period exceeds 5 months. *Note!!* Immune globulin is in very short supply and the supply is often not adequate for use in this setting.

If travel starts sooner than 4 weeks prior to the first vaccine dose, what should be done?

Because protection may not be complete until 4 weeks after vaccination, persons traveling to a high-risk area less than 4 weeks after the initial dose of hepatitis A vaccine should also be given immune globulin (0.02 mL/kg), but at a different injection site. *Note!!* Immune globulin is in very short supply and the supply is often not adequate for use in this setting. Therefore, the first dose of hepatitis A vaccine should be administered as soon as travel to a high-risk area is planned.

What should be done for travelers who are less than 2 years of age to protect them from hepatitis A virus infection?

Immune globulin is recommended for travelers less than 2 years of age because the vaccine is currently not licensed for use in this age group. *Note!!* Immune globulin is in very short supply and the supply is often not adequate for use in this setting.

107

Section 13.2

Viral Hepatitis B

1999 Centers for Disease Control and Prevention (CDC).

General Information

Who is at risk?

Hepatitis B can affect anyone. Each year in the United States, more than 200,000 people of all ages get hepatitis B and close to 5,000 die of sickness caused by HBV. If you have had other forms of hepatitis, you can still get hepatitis B. Get vaccinated! Hepatitis B is preventable.

How great is your risk for hepatitis B?

One out of 20 people in the United States will get hepatitis B some time during their lives. Your risk is higher if you:

- have sex with someone infected with HBV

- have sex with more than one partner

- are a man and have sex with a man

- live in the same house with someone who has lifelong HBV infection

- have a job that involves contact with human blood

- shoot drugs

- are a patient or work in a home for the developmentally disabled

- have hemophilia

- travel to areas where hepatitis B is common

Your risk is also higher if your parents were born in Southeast Asia, Africa, the Amazon Basin in South America, the Pacific Islands, and the Middle East.

If you are at risk for HBV infection, ask your health care provider about hepatitis B vaccine.

How do you get hepatitis B?

You get hepatitis B by direct contact with the blood or body fluids of an infected person; for example, you can become infected by having sex or sharing needles with an infected person. A baby can get hepatitis B from an infected mother during childbirth. Hepatitis B is not spread through food or water or by casual contact.

Who is a carrier of hepatitis B virus?

Sometimes, people who are infected with HBV never recover fully from the infection; they carry the virus and can infect others for the rest of their lives. In the United States, about one million people carry HBV.

How do you know if you have hepatitis B?

You may have hepatitis B (and be spreading the disease) and not know it; sometimes a person with HBV infection has no symptoms at all. If you have symptoms:

- your eyes or skin may turn yellow
- you may lose your appetite
- you may have nausea, vomiting, fever, stomach or joint pain
- you may feel extremely tired and not be able to work for weeks or months.

Is there a cure for hepatitis B?

There is no cure for hepatitis B; this is why prevention is so important. Hepatitis B vaccine is the best protection against HBV.

Three doses are needed for complete protection. If vaccine was never given, children 11-12 years of age should get hepatitis B vaccine.

If you are pregnant, should you worry about hepatitis B?

If you have HBV in your blood you can give hepatitis B to your baby. Babies who get HBV at birth may have the virus for the rest of their lives, can spread the disease, and can get cirrhosis of the liver or liver cancer. All pregnant women should be tested for HBV early in their pregnancy. If the blood test is positive, the baby should receive vaccine along with another shot, hepatitis B immune globulin (called H-BIG), at birth. The vaccine series should be completed during the first 6 months of life.

Who should get vaccinated?

- All babies, at birth.

- All children 11-12 years of age who have not been vaccinated.

- Persons of any age whose behavior puts them at high risk for HBV infection.

- Persons whose jobs expose them to human blood.

Section 13.3

Viral Hepatitis C

1999 Centers for Disease Control and Prevention (CDC).

Diagnosis and Testing

What is hepatitis C?

Hepatitis C is a liver disease caused by the hepatitis C virus (HCV), which is found in the blood of persons who have this disease. HCV is spread by contact with the blood of an infected person.

What blood tests are available to check for hepatitis C?

There are several blood tests that can be done to determine if you have been infected with HCV. Your doctor may order just one or a combination of these tests. The following are the types of tests your doctor may order and the purpose for each:

- *Anti-HCV (antibody to HCV)*

  EIA (enzyme immunoassay). This test is usually done first. If positive, it should be confirmed.

  RIBA (recombinant immunoblot assay). Supplemental test used to confirm a positive EIA test.

Anti-HCV does not tell whether the infection is new (acute), chronic (long-term) or is no longer present.

110

- *Qualitative tests to detect presence or absence of virus (HCV RNA)*
    Generic polymerase chain reaction (PCR)
    Amplicor HCV
- *Quantitative tests to detect amount (titer) of virus (HCV RNA)*
    Amplicor HCV Monitor
    Quantiplex HCV RNA (bDNA)

PCR and other tests to directly detect virus are not licensed tests and are only available on a research-basis. A single positive PCR test indicates infection with HCV. A single negative test does not prove that a person is not infected. Virus may be present in the blood and just not found by PCR. Also, a person infected in the past who has recovered may have a negative test. When hepatitis C is suspected and PCR is negative, PCR should be repeated.

Can you have a "false positive" anti-HCV test result?

Yes. A false positive test means the test looks as if it is positive, but it is really negative. This happens more often in persons who have a low risk for the disease for which they are being tested. For example, false positive anti-HCV tests happen more often in persons such as blood donors who are at low risk for hepatitis C. Therefore, it is important to confirm a positive anti-HCV test with a supplemental test as most false positive anti-HCV tests are reported as negative on supplemental testing.

Can you have a "false negative" anti-HCV test result?

Yes. Persons with early infection may not as yet have developed antibody levels high enough that the test can measure. In addition, some persons may lack the (immune) response necessary for the test to work well. In these persons, research-based tests such as PCR may be considered.

How long after exposure to HCV does it take to test positive for anti-HCV?

Anti-HCV can be found in 7 out of 10 persons when symptoms begin and in about 9 out of 10 persons within 3 months after symptoms begin. However, it is important to note that many persons who have hepatitis C have no symptoms.

How long after exposure to HCV does it take to test positive with PCR?

It is possible to find HCV within 1 to 2 weeks after being infected with the virus.

Who should get tested for hepatitis C?

- persons who ever injected illegal drugs, including those who injected once or a few times many years ago

- persons who were treated for clotting problems with a blood product made before 1987 when more advanced methods for manufacturing the products were developed

- persons who were notified that they received blood from a donor who later tested positive for hepatitis C

- persons who received a blood transfusion or solid organ transplant before July 1992 when better testing of blood donors became available

- long-term hemodialysis patients

- persons who have signs or symptoms of liver disease (e.g., abnormal liver enzyme tests) healthcare workers after exposures (e.g., needle sticks or splashes to the eye) to HCV-positive blood on the job

- children born to HCV-positive women

What is the next step if you have a confirmed positive anti-HCV test?

Measure the level of ALT (alanine aminotransferase, a liver enzyme) in the blood. An elevated ALT indicates inflammation of the liver and you should be checked further for chronic (long-term) liver disease and possible treatment. The evaluation should be done by a healthcare professional familiar with chronic hepatitis C.

Can you have a normal liver enzyme (e.g., ALT) level and still have chronic hepatitis C?

Yes. It is common for persons with chronic hepatitis C to have a liver enzyme level that goes up and down, with periodic returns to normal or near normal. Some persons have a liver enzyme level that is normal for over a year but they still have chronic liver disease. If the liver enzyme level is normal, persons should have their enzyme level re-checked several times over a 6 to 12 month period. If the liver enzyme level remains normal, your doctor may check it less frequently, such as once a year.

How is HCV spread from one person to another?

How could a person have gotten hepatitis C?

HCV is spread primarily by direct contact with human blood. For example, you may have gotten infected with HCV if:

- you ever injected street drugs, as the needles and/or other drug "works" used to prepare or inject the drug(s) may have had someone else's blood that contained HCV on them.

- you received blood, blood products, or solid organs from a donor whose blood contained HCV.

- you were ever on long-term kidney dialysis as you may have unknowingly shared supplies/equipment that had someone else's blood on them.

- you were ever a healthcare worker and had frequent contact with blood on the job, especially accidental needlesticks.

- your mother had hepatitis C at the time she gave birth to you. During the birth her blood may have gotten into your body.

- you ever had sex with a person infected with HCV.

- you lived with someone who was infected with HCV and shared items such as razors or toothbrushes that might have had his/her blood on them.

Is there any evidence that HCV has been spread during medical or dental procedures done in the United States?

Medical and dental procedures done in most settings in the United States do not pose a risk for the spread of HCV. There have, however, been some reports that HCV has been spread between patients in hemodialysis units where supplies or equipment may have been shared between patients.

Can HCV be spread by sexual activity?

Yes, but this does not occur very often.

Can HCV be spread by oral sex?

There is no evidence that HCV has been spread by oral sex.

Can HCV be spread within a household?

Yes, but this does not occur very often. If HCV is spread within a household, it is most likely due to direct exposure to the blood of an infected household member.

Since more advanced tests have been developed for use in blood banks, what is the chance now that a person can get HCV infection from transfused blood or blood products?

1 chance out of 100,000, per each transfused unit.

Pregnancy and Breast Feeding

Should pregnant women be routinely tested for anti-HCV?

No. Pregnant women have no greater risk of being infected with HCV then non-pregnant women. If pregnant women have risk factors for hepatitis C, they should be tested for anti-HCV.

What is the risk that HCV infected women will spread HCV to their newborn infants?

About 5 out of every 100 infants born to HCV infected women become infected. This occurs at the time of birth, and there is no treatment that can prevent this from happening. Most infants infected with HCV at the time of birth have no symptoms and do well during childhood. More studies are needed to find out if these children will have problems from the infection as they grow older. There are no licensed treatments or guidelines for the treatment of infants or children infected with HCV. Children with elevated ALT (liver enzyme) levels should be referred for evaluation to a specialist familiar with the management of children with HCV-related disease.

Should a woman with hepatitis C be advised against breast-feeding?

No. There is no evidence that breast-feeding spreads HCV. HCV-positive mothers should consider abstaining from breast-feeding if their nipples are cracked or bleeding.

When should babies born to mothers with hepatitis C be tested to see if they were infected at birth?

Children should not be tested for anti-HCV before 12 months of age as anti-HCV from the mother may last until this age. If testing is desired prior to 12 months of age, PCR could be performed at or after an infant's first well-child visit at age 1-2 months.

Counseling

How can persons infected with HCV prevent spreading HCV to others?

Do not donate blood, body organs, other tissue, or semen. Do not share personal items that might have your blood on them, such as toothbrushes, dental appliances, nail-grooming equipment or razors. Cover your cuts and skin sores to keep from spreading HCV.

How can a person protect themselves from getting hepatitis C and other diseases spread by contact with human blood?

Don't ever shoot drugs. If you shoot drugs, stop and get into a treatment program. If you can't stop, never reuse or share syringes, water, or drug works, and get vaccinated against hepatitis A and hepatitis B. Do not share toothbrushes, razors, or other personal care articles. They might have blood on them. If you are a healthcare worker, always follow routine barrier precautions and safely handle needles and other sharps. Get vaccinated against hepatitis B. Consider the health risks if you are thinking about getting a tattoo or body piercing: You can get infected if:

- the tools that are used have someone else's blood on them.

- the artist or piercer doesn't follow good health practices, such as washing hands and using disposable gloves.

HCV can be spread by sex, but this does not occur very often. If you are having sex, but not with one steady partner:

- You and your partners can get other diseases spread by having sex (e.g., AIDS, hepatitis B, gonorrhea or chlamydia).

- You should use latex condoms correctly and every time.

- You should get vaccinated against hepatitis B.

Should patients with hepatitis C change their sexual practices if they have only one long-term steady sex partner?

No. There is a very low chance of spreading HCV to that partner through sexual activity. If you want to lower the small chance of spreading HCV to your sex partner, you may decide to use barrier precautions such as latex condoms. Ask your doctor about having your sex partner tested.

What can persons with HCV infection do to protect their liver?

- Stop using alcohol.

- See your doctor regularly.

- Don't start any new medicines or use over-the-counter, herbal, and other medicines without a physician's knowledge.

- Get vaccinated against hepatitis A if liver damage is present.

What other information should patients with hepatitis C be aware of?

HCV is not spread by sneezing, hugging, coughing, food or water, sharing eating utensils or drinking glasses, or casual contact. Persons should not be excluded from work, school, play, child-care or other settings on the basis of their HCV infection status. Involvement with a support group may help patients cope with hepatitis C.

Should persons with chronic hepatitis C be vaccinated against hepatitis B?

If persons are in risk groups for whom hepatitis B vaccine is recommended, they should be vaccinated.

Long-term Consequences of HCV Infection

What are the chances of persons with HCV infection developing long term infection, chronic liver disease, cirrhosis, liver cancer, or dying as a result of hepatitis C?

Of every 100 persons infected with HCV about:

- 85 persons may develop long-term infection,

- 70 persons may develop chronic liver disease,

- 15 persons may develop cirrhosis over a period of 20 to 30 years,

- 5 persons may die from the consequences of long term infection (liver cancer or cirrhosis).

Do medical conditions outside the liver occur in persons with chronic hepatitis C?

A small percentage of persons with chronic hepatitis C develop medical conditions outside the liver (this is called extrahepatic). These conditions are thought to occur due to the body's natural immune system fighting against itself. Such conditions include: glomerulonephritis, essential mixed cryoglobulinemia, and porphyria cutanea tarda.

Management and Treatment of Chronic Hepatitis C

When might a specialist (gastroenterologist or hepatologist) be consulted in the management of HCV-infected persons?

A referral to or consultation with a specialist for further evaluation and possible treatment may be considered if a person is anti-HCV positive and has elevated liver enzyme levels. Any physician who manages a person with hepatitis C should be knowledgeable and current on all aspects of the care of a person with hepatitis C.

What is the treatment for chronic hepatitis C?

Antiviral drugs such as interferon used alone or in combination with ribavirin, are approved for the treatment of persons with chronic hepatitis C. Interferon works in 10 to 20 persons out of 100 treated. Interferon combined with ribavirin works (on the viral strain that is mostly found in the U.S.) in about 30-40 persons out of 100. Ribavirin, when used alone, does not work.

What are the side effects of interferon therapy?

Most persons have flu-like symptoms (fever, chills, headache, muscle and joint aches, fast heart rate) early in treatment, but these lessen with continued treatment. Later side effects may include tiredness, hair loss, low blood count, trouble with thinking, moodiness, and depression. Severe side effects are rare (seen in less than 2 out of 100 persons). These include thyroid disease, depression with suicidal thoughts, seizures, acute heart or kidney failure, eye and lung problems, hearing loss, and blood infection.

Although rare, deaths have occurred due to liver failure or blood infection, mostly in persons with cirrhosis. An important side effect of interferon is worsening of liver disease with treatment, which can be severe and even fatal. Interferon dosage must be reduced in up to 40 out of 100 persons because of severity of side effects, and treatment must be stopped in up to 15 out of 100 persons. Pregnant women should not be treated with interferon.

What are the side effects of combination (ribavirin + interferon) treatment?

In addition to the side effects due to interferon described above, ribavirin can cause serious anemia (low red blood cell count) and can be a serious problem for persons with conditions that cause anemia, such as kidney failure. In these persons, combination therapy should be avoided or attempts should be made to correct the anemia. Anemia caused by ribavirin can be life-threatening for persons with certain types of heart or blood vessel disease. Ribavirin causes birth defects and pregnancy should be avoided during treatment. Patients and their healthcare providers should carefully review the product manufacturer information prior to treatment.

Can anything be done to reduce symptoms or side effects due to antiviral treatment?

You should report what you are feeling to your doctor. Some side effects may be reduced by giving interferon at night or lowering the dosage of the drug. In addition, flu-like symptoms can be reduced by taking acetaminophen before treatment.

Can children receive interferon therapy for chronic hepatitis C?

Antiviral drugs are not licensed for persons under 18 years of age. Children with hepatitis C should be referred to a children's specialist in liver diseases. You may want to ask your doctor about clinical trials that may be on-going for children.

Genotype

What does the term genotype mean?

Genotype refers to the genetic make-up of an organism or a virus. There are at least 6 distinct HCV genotypes identified. Genotype 1 is the most common genotype seen in the United States.

Is it necessary to do genotyping when managing a person with chronic hepatitis C?

Yes, as there are 6 known genotypes and more than 50 subtypes of HCV, and genotype information is helpful in defining the epidemiology of hepatitis C. Knowing the genotype or serotype (genotype-specific antibodies) of HCV is helpful in making recommendations and counseling regarding therapy. Patients with genotypes 2 and 3 are almost three times more likely than patients with genotype 1 to respond to therapy with alpha interferon or the combination of alpha interferon and ribavirin. Furthermore, when using combination therapy, the recommended duration of treatment depends on the genotype. For patients with genotypes 2 and 3, a 24-week course of combination treatment is adequate, whereas for patients with genotype 1, a 48-week course is recommended. For these reasons, testing for HCV genotype is often clinically helpful. Once the genotype is identified, it need not be tested again; genotypes do not change during the course of infection.

Why do most persons remain infected?

Persons infected with HCV mount an antibody response to parts of the virus, but changes in the virus during infection result in changes that are not recognized by preexisting antibodies. This appears to be how the virus establishes and maintains long-lasting infection.

Can persons become infected with different genotypes?

Yes. Because of the ineffective immune response described above, prior infection does not protect against reinfection with the same or different genotypes of the virus. For the same reason, there is no effective pre- or postexposure prophylaxis (i.e., immune globulin) available.

Hepatitis C and Healthcare Workers

What is the risk for HCV infection from a needle-stick exposure to HCV contaminated blood?

After needle stick or sharps exposure to HCV positive blood, about 2 (1.8%) healthcare workers out of 100 will get infected with HCV (range 0%-10%).

What are the recommendations for follow-up of healthcare workers after exposure to HCV positive blood?

1. Anti-viral agents (e.g., interferon) or immune globulin should not be used for postexposure prophylaxis.

2. For the person exposed to an HCV-positive source, baseline and follow-up testing including:

   - baseline testing for anti-HCV and ALT activity; and

   - follow-up testing for anti-HCV (e.g., at 4-6 months) and ALT activity. (If earlier diagnosis of HCV infection is desired, testing for HCV RNA may be performed at 4-6 weeks.)

3. Confirmation by supplemental anti-HCV testing of all anti-HCV results reported as positive by enzyme immunoassay.

Should HCV-infected healthcare workers be restricted in their work?

No, there are no recommendations to restrict a healthcare worker who is infected with HCV. The risk of transmission from an infected healthcare worker to a patient appears to be very low. As recommended for all healthcare workers, those who are HCV positive should follow strict aseptic technique and standard precautions, including appropriate use of hand washing, protective barriers, and care in the use and disposal of needles and other sharp instruments.

Section 13.4

Viral Hepatitis D

1999 Centers for Disease Control and Prevention (CDC).

HDV is a defective single-stranded RNA virus that requires the helper function of HBV to replicate. HDV requires HBV for synthesis of envelope protein composed of HBsAg, which is used to encapsulate the HDV genome.

Delta Hepatitis: Clinical Features

HDV infection can be acquired either as a coinfection with HBV or as a superinfection of persons with chronic HBV infection. Persons with HBV-HDV coinfection may have more severe acute disease and a higher risk of fulminant hepatitis (2%-20%) compared with those infected with HBV alone; however, chronic HBV infection appears to occur less frequently in persons with HBV-HDV coinfection.

Chronic HBV carriers who acquire HDV superinfection usually develop chronic HDV infection. In long-term studies of chronic HBV carriers with HDV superinfection, 70%-80% have developed evidence of chronic liver diseases with cirrhosis compared with 15%-30% of patients with chronic HBV infection alone.

Modes of Transmission

The modes of HDV transmission are similar to those for HBV, with percutaneous exposures the most efficient. Sexual transmission of HDV is less efficient than for HBV. Perinatal HDV transmission is rare.

HBV-HDV Coinfection: Typical Serologic Course

The serologic course of HDV infection varies depending on whether the virus is acquired as a coinfection with HBV or as a superinfection of a person with chronic HBV infection. In most persons with HBV-HDV coinfection, both IgM antibody to HDV (anti-HDV) and IgG anti-HDV are detectable during the course of infection. However, in

121

about 15% of patients the only evidence of HDV infection may be the detection of either IgM anti-HDV alone during the early acute period of illness or IgG anti-HDV alone during convalescence. Anti-HDV generally declines to subdetectable levels after the infection resolves and there is no serologic marker that persists to indicate that the patient was ever infected with HDV. Hepatitis Delta antigen (HDAg) can be detected in serum in only about 25% of patients with HBV-HDV coinfection. When HDAg is detectable it generally disappears as HBsAg disappears and most patients do not develop chronic infection. Tests for IgG anti-HDV are commercially available in the United States. Tests for IgM anti-HDV, HDAg and HDV RNA by PCR are only available in research laboratories.

HBV-HDV Superinfection: Typical Serologic Course

In patients with chronic HBV infection who are superinfected with HDV several characteristic serologic features generally occur, including: 1) the titer of HBsAg declines at the time HDAg appears in the serum, 2) HDAg and HDV RNA remain detectable in the serum because chronic HDV infection generally occurs in most patients with HDV superinfection, unlike the case with coinfection, 3) high titers of both IgM and IgG anti-HDV are detectable, which persist indefinitely.

Geographic Distribution of HDV Infection

In general, the global pattern of HDV infection corresponds to the prevalence of chronic HBV infection; however, several distinct features of the distribution of HDV infection have been identified. In countries with a low prevalence of chronic HBV infection, HDV prevalence is generally low among both asymptomatic HBV carriers (<10%) and among patients with chronic HBV-related liver disease (<25%). HDV infection in these countries occurs most commonly among injecting drug users and persons with hemophilia. In countries with moderate and high levels of chronic HBV prevalence, the prevalence of HDV infection is highly variable. In southern Italy and in parts of Russia and Romania, the prevalence of HDV infection is very high among both asymptomatic HBV carriers (>20%) and among patients with HBV-related chronic liver disease HBV (>60%). Other countries, including northern Italy, Spain, Turkey, and Egypt, have a moderate prevalence of HDV infection among asymptomatic HBV carriers (10%-19%) and among patients with chronic HBV-related liver disease (30%-50%). However, in most of Southeast Asia and China, where the prevalence of chronic HBV infection is very high, HDV infection is uncommon. In some South American countries in the Amazon River Basin, periodic epidemics of HDV infection have occurred among chronic HBV carriers in relatively isolated regions. Disease related to HDV infection in these outbreaks has been very severe, with rapid progression to fulminant hepatitis and case-fatality rates of 10%-20%. The cause of the atypical course of HDV infection in these populations is unknown.

Delta Hepatitis: Prevention

Because HDV is dependent on HBV for replication, HBV-HDV coinfection can be prevented with either pre- or postexposure prophylaxis for HBV. However, no products exist to prevent HDV superinfection of persons with chronic HBV infection. Thus, prevention of HDV superinfection depends primarily on education to reduce risk behaviors.

Section 13.5

Viral Hepatitis E

1999 Centers for Disease Control and Prevention (CDC).

Hepatitis E virus (HEV), the major etiologic agent of enterically transmitted non-A, non-B hepatitis worldwide, is a spherical, nonenveloped, single stranded RNA virus that is approximately 32 to 34 nm in diameter. Based on similar physicochemical and biologic properties, HEV has been provisionally classified in the Caliciviridae family; however, the organization of the HEV genome is substantially different from that of other caliciviruses and HEV may eventually be classified in a separate family.

Clinical Features

The incubation period following exposure to HEV ranges from 15 to 60 days (mean, 40 days). Typical clinical signs and symptoms of acute hepatitis E are similar to those of other types of viral hepatitis and include abdominal pain anorexia, dark urine, fever, hepatomegaly, jaundice, malaise, nausea, and vomiting. Other less common symptoms include arthralgia, diarrhea, pruritus, and urticarial rash. The period of infectivity following acute infection has not been determined but virus excretion in stools has been demonstrated up to 14 days after illness onset. In most hepatitis E outbreaks, the highest rates of clinically evident disease have been in young to middle-age adults; lower disease rates in younger age groups may be the result of anicteric and/or subclinical HEV infection. No evidence of chronic infection has been detected in long-term follow-up of patients with hepatitis E.

Typical Serologic Course

The typical serologic course following HEV infection has been characterized using experimental models of infection in nonhuman primates and human volunteer studies. In two human volunteer studies, liver enzyme elevations occurred 4-5 weeks after oral ingestion and persisted for 20-90 days. Virus excretion in stools occurred approximately 4 weeks after oral ingestion and persisted for about 2 weeks. Both IgM and IgG antibody to HEV (anti-HEV) are elicited following HEV infection. The titer of IgM anti-HEV declines rapidly during early convalescence; IgG anti-HEV persists and appears to provide at least short-term protection against disease. No serologic tests to diagnose HEV infection are commercially available in the United States. However, several diagnostic tests are available in research laboratories, including enzyme immunoassays and Western blot assays to detect IgM and IgG anti-HEV in serum, polymerase chain reaction tests to detect HEV RNA in serum and stool, and immunofluorescent antibody blocking assays to detect antibody to HEV antigen in serum and liver.

Epidemiologic Features

HEV is transmitted primarily by the fecal-oral route and fecally contaminated drinking water is the most commonly documented vehicle of transmission. Although hepatitis E is most commonly recognized to occur in large outbreaks, HEV infection accounts for >50% of acute sporadic hepatitis in both children and adults in some high endemic areas. Risk factors for infection among persons with sporadic cases of hepatitis E have not been defined. Unlike hepatitis A virus, which is also transmitted by the fecal-oral route, person-to-person transmission of HEV appears to be uncommon. However, nosocomial transmission, presumably by person-to-person contact, has been reported to occur. Virtually all cases of acute hepatitis E in the United States have been reported among travelers returning from high HEV-endemic areas.

Geographic Distribution of Hepatitis E

Outbreaks of hepatitis E have occurred over a wide geographic area, primarily in developing countries with inadequate environmental sanitation. The reservoir of HEV in these areas is unknown. The occurrence of sporadic HEV infections in humans may maintain transmission during interepidemic periods, but a nonhuman reservoir for HEV is also possible. In the United States and other nonendemic areas, where outbreaks of hepatitis E have not been documented to occur, a low prevalence of anti-HEV (<2%) has been found in healthy populations. The source of infection for these persons is unknown.

Prevention and Control Measures for Travelers to HEV-Endemic Regions

Prevention of hepatitis E relies primarily on the provision of clean water supplies. Prudent hygienic practices that may prevent hepatitis E and other enterically transmitted diseases among travelers to developing countries include avoiding drinking water (and beverages with ice) of unknown purity, uncooked shellfish, and uncooked fruits or vegetables that are not peeled or prepared by the traveler. No products are available to prevent hepatitis E. IG prepared from plasma collected in non-HEV-endemic areas is not effective in preventing clinical disease during hepatitis E outbreaks and the efficacy of IG prepared from plasma collected in HEV-endemic areas is unclear. In studies conducted to date with prototype vaccines in animals, vaccine-induced antibody attenuated HEV infection, but did not prevent virus excretion in stools. If a vaccine is developed, the epidemiology of hepatitis E needs to be further defined in order to determine whether vaccination strategies could be effectively used to prevent this disease.

Chapter 14

Herpes

Chapter Contents

Section 14.1

Herpes Simplex Facts

2000 National Institute on Dental Research (NIDR);
National Institutes of Health (NIH).

Eight out of every 10 American adults are infected with the herpes simplex virus, or HSV. The virus is either dormant within a variety of tissues or is activated and highly contagious. As a contagious virus, HSV is either the direct cause or a cofactor associated with a number of different diseases and disorders. Its best-known manifestation: the common cold sore. The cold sore, or herpetic lesion, typically shows redness, swelling, pain and heat over an eight-to-10 day period. After that, its clinical signs and symptoms appear resolved, leaving no apparent scar. But the virus leaves with a promise to return.

The virus, infecting the lips, oral mucosa or tongue, can be transmitted to the hand or eyes-and it can be transmitted to another person, expanding the sphere of influence of this highly contagious microbe.

HSV also can be associated with other diseases or disorders that compromise the immune system such as protein-calorie malnutrition and AIDS. The virus provides oral health professionals an excellent opportunity to reassess their appreciation of infection and immunity. We can learn from HSV.

For thousands of years, redness and swelling, with pain and heat, have been recognized as the four cardinal signs of inflammation. Aulus Cornelius Celsus in the first century described the typical reaction of flesh to microbes. Since then, astute health care professionals have appreciated that inflammation is the host's response to traumatic injuries as well as to microbe infections. Inflammation is our protective response to dilute, destroy or compartmentalize both the infectious agent (infectious microbes such as viral, bacterial, fungal or parasitic invasion) and the injured tissue.

Redness, swelling, pain, heat and loss of function are clinical characteristics of HSV. Microscopically, the virus involves:

- dilation or injury to capillaries, arterioles and venules;

- exudation of fluids including plasma proteins;

- leukocytic migration into the inflamed area with the release of cytokines.

The "simple" cold sore has many lessons to teach. Humanity's recognition of cold sores is so long-standing that it has led to complacent acceptance. Descriptions of the infection have been documented in early Greek manuscripts, particularly in the writings of Hippocrates (460-377 B.C.). Scholars of Greek civilization define the word herpes to mean "creep or crawl," describing the spreading nature of the visual skin lesion. The early, imprecise visual descriptions of the sore ended in the 20th century when, in 1919, Lowenstein described the infectious nature of the causative virus (herpes simplex) and demonstrated that the virus retrieved from the lesions of the sore produced a similar lesion on the cornea of a rabbit.

Herpes viruses are ubiquitous and have been isolated from baboons, chimpanzees, monkeys, cows, horses, birds and fish. Most animal species have yielded at least one herpes virus upon examination. Nearly 100 herpes viruses, from all sources, have been characterized, at least partially.

In humans, six members of the virus family Herpesviridae have been isolated:

- HSV type 1 (cold sores) and type 2 (genital lesions);

- varicella-zoster, or VZV (chickenpox, shingles);

- human cytomegalovirus, or HCMV;

- Epstein-Barr virus, or EBV (mononucleosis);

- human herpes virus 6, or HHV-6 (roseola);

- herpes B virus, an old-world monkey virus that results from the bite of a monkey, is highly pathogenic in humans but rarely passes from one person to another.

A new herpes virus identified in 1996, human herpes virus 8, or HHV-8, is associated with Kaposi's sarcoma, or KS. KS produces purplish lesions throughout the body as a result of uncontrolled growth of blood vessels. Proof of HHV-8's role in KS will require many additional long-term studies.

Like many viruses, the herpes viruses take up permanent residence in the body once they are introduced. After an initial infection, the virus goes into hiding, escaping the host's immune system by remaining latent in a specific group of cells, causing no apparent harm to the host. The exact cell in which they remain latent varies from one virus type to the next. In cells harboring the latent virus, the viral genomes take the form of closed molecules and only a small subset of virus genes are expressed. Production of infectious progeny virus is invariably accompanied by the irreversible destruction of the infected cell. All of the human herpes viruses have been detected in the saliva sometime during infection.

The HSV types 1 and 2 are the best known. Type 1 is usually responsible for the sores on or near the face (cold sores, fever blisters or oral herpes). Most adults in the United States carry this virus and some suffer periodic bouts of cold sores.

Type 2 usually is involved in producing genital sores (genital herpes). About 16 percent of Americans between 15 and 74 years of age (30 million people) carry this virus. The two virus types are very similar, and either type can infect the mouth and genitals. Some people are infected with both types.

Most people infected with HSV never develop any symptoms. Reports from a number of studies indicate that about half of the people with HSV-2 antibodies do not know that they're infected, yet they are still capable of transmitting the infection.

Primary infection with HSV can produce great variability in clinical symptoms-from being totally asymptomatic to suffering with combinations of sore throat, ulcerative and vesicular lesions, gingivostomatitis, edema of the mucosal membranes, localized lymphadenopathy, anorexia and malaise.

The incubation period for HSV ranges from two to 12 days. In children, the infection characteristically involves a swelling of the gingival and buccal mucosa, making it difficult or impossible to swallow liquids. The clinical illness, accompanied by fever and pain from the lesion, generally lasts two to three weeks. After infection, the virus goes into hiding, entering nerve endings and traveling to ganglia (clusters of nerve cells).

How often the viral infection recurs varies from patient to patient. Factors that trigger recurrence in humans are poorly defined but include fever, stress and exposure to ultraviolet light. Infection recurs when the virus is activated in the ganglia and travels down the nerve to the surface of the skin where it replicates.

Recurrence takes place in phases:

- *prodrome:* warning symptoms that last less than six hours and include tingling and itching at the site of outbreak;

- *inflammation:* swelling and redness at the site before outbreak, indicating that both virus and antibodies have arrived;

- *blisters:* appearance within 24 to 48 hours after prodrome of one or several small fluid-filled vesicles or tiny red bumps or tenderness most commonly at the vermilion border of the lip;

- *ulcers:* occurring within 72 hours after prodrome, often accompanied by pain; the blisters leak fluid, leaving wet-looking sores;

- *crusts:* sores dry within 96 hours, forming a scab that indicates healing; virus diminishes, with healing over two to three days;

- *healing:* complete within eight to 10 days; new skin forms; virus replication is complete, and the virus retreats back up to the host ganglia where it remains, protected from the host's immunological attack.

The virus in the inflamed site can be transmitted to a new site on the host's body or to another person through contact with any part of the body where the virus finds a way to penetrate the skin. For most people, a herpes outbreak is confined to recognizable variations of the classical symptoms. While outbreaks can be physically and emotionally uncomfortable, and sometimes painful, the infection is usually self-limiting and results in complete healing of the infected site. The virus in the inflamed site, however, is infectious and can be transmitted to a new site on the host's body (autoinoculation) or to another person through contact with any part of the body where the virus finds a way to penetrate the skin.

Transmission in most cases requires direct skin-to-skin contact between the infected site and a receptive site. Risk of transmission is highest when the virus is active. But first outbreaks or primary lesions are the most infectious because they include more virus particles on the skin, and the lesions persist for a longer period.

HSV also can be transmitted when the infected person is asymptomatic. About 1 percent of the time, most people asymptomatically shed traces of the virus, sometimes from lesions that are too small to be noticed.

Autoinoculation and transmission by skin contact can have serious complications. Dental professionals are at particular risk of developing a complication known as herpetic whitlow. Caused by HSV-1 or -2, whitlow develops on the hand and is found often among health professionals who treat herpes-infected patients. It is the same disease as oral or genital herpes with the same symptoms, but it is very visible and often very painful. The constant use of protective gloves and other universal precautions, including sterilization and disinfection techniques, can prevent herpetic transmission in the dental office.

Ocular herpes, an infection of the eye, is most often caused by autoinoculation. Fortunately, ocular herpes resolves itself without treatment about half the time and does not recur. Still, the infection can lead to serious damage and even blindness.

Ocular herpes can take the form of conjunctivitis or "pink eye," an inflammation of the mucous membrane under the eyelid and over the whole sclera of the eyeball. Conjunctivitis is irritating but causes no permanent damage.

Herpetic infection of the cornea is called keratitis, which causes superficial branching ulcerations called "dendrites." This condition is often self-limiting and may or may not cause permanent damage.

Herpetic iritis, an infection of the iris and other parts of the inner eye, becomes chronic and can lead to opacification of the cornea and blindness. Early treatment is key to averting the more serious consequences of all forms of ocular HSV.

Eight of 10 people with first-time HSV infections-and a few with recurrences-also contract viral meningitis. The virus inflames the meninges surrounding the brain, but not the brain itself. Symptoms include severe headaches, aversion to light and nausea, which go away on their own, leaving no permanent damage.

Among the rarest of complications is herpes encephalitis, affecting fewer than one in 65,000 Americans each year. In adults, this encephalitis is usually caused by HSV-1, and in newborns by HSV-2. The brain infection causes swelling and inflammation—and unless quickly controlled can result in permanent brain damage and death.

Herpes viruses, as permanent residents of the body, affect several other diseases. Recent research shows that HSV may cause acute, idiopathic facial paralysis (Bell's palsy), though more studies are needed to confirm this observation.

A number of studies dating back to the late 1970s suggest that women with a history of genital herpes are at greater risk of contracting cervical cancer. Here, too, further study is needed. As noted earlier, herpes may have a link to Kaposi's sarcoma. It is also being investigated for a possible causal relationship with the human immunodeficiency virus, which causes AIDS. These examples underscore the interest research scientists have in determining whether the often-dismissed "cold sore" virus has a more devious and influential role in the pathologies of the human body.

Diagnosis of an HSV infection is often done by the naked eye. But there are several more definitive diagnostic methods, some of which can distinguish between HSV-1 and HSV-2. The gold standard for diagnosing a virus is always isolation and culture. But this takes several days, and a negative culture does not necessarily mean absence of virus.

Other methods include:

- immunofluorescence, or IF, where cells are scraped from the lesion, placed on a slide and stained with fluorescent-tagged HSV antibodies, which bind specifically to any HSV present in the cells;

- immunoperoxidase, or IP, which also binds with cells but can amplify the virus content for easier identification;

- the enzyme-linked immunosorbent assay, or ELISA, which is more sensitive than either IF or IP; the infected specimen is combined with commercial HSV antibodies, an enzyme and their chemicals and followed for a color change that occurs only in the presence of HSV.

Still other serological assays measure antibodies that show prior infection with either HSV-1 or HSV-2, although the distinction between types is difficult.

Research on drug therapies for HSV has focused mainly on treating genital herpes to prevent sexual transmission and the effects on newborns. Since its introduction in 1985, oral acyclovir has been the preferred treatment for genital herpes. It also has been found effective in treating oral herpes. The U.S. Food and Drug Administration is reviewing an application that would extend oral acyclovir's use in treating oral herpes.

People who suffer from frequent bouts of HSV can take acyclovir daily for up to one year. Unfortunately, though, it is not a cure for the virus that remains in the body. The drug interferes with virus expression; it doesn't kill it.

Foscarnet also disrupts HSV replication but must be given intravenously because it is not readily absorbable in the stomach. Idoxuridine and vidarabine have been effective in treating ocular herpes but are ineffective in treating other forms of HSV.

Vidarabine is useful in treating herpes encephalitis, herpes zoster and neonatal herpes. Many other compounds have been reported as having anti-HSV impact in the laboratory, but further studies are needed to determine their effectiveness in humans.

Oral herpes is usually treated by the time-tried methods of keeping the blisters clean and dry, being careful not to touch the sores and spread the virus to new sites, and avoiding contacts with people in ways that could transmit the virus.

Researchers at the National Institute of Dental Research confirmed that sunscreen on the lips can prevent sun-induced recurrences of herpes. Most other preventive measures have not been examined under controlled studies.

In late September 1996, the first topical antiviral cream for treating cold sores received FDA approval. Marketed as Denavir, the cream contains penciclovir, which, like acyclovir, is active against HSV replication. Denavir is reported to reduce the duration of HSV pain and speed lesion healing.

The central goal in researching the herpes virus is the development of a vaccine because prevention is the best defense. A vaccine would be effective only in people who have not contracted HSV. It would offer protection and start to break an infectious cycle that involves so much of the population.

Small clinical studies show that a new vaccine consisting of viral glycoproteins found on the virus' exterior is capable of safely stimulating an immune response in both infected and uninfected study participants. Larger studies are needed to demonstrate the vaccine's effectiveness in preventing infection. Other potential vaccines would use a live-virus preparation in which the HSV virulence factors have been removed.

Section 14.2

Genital Herpes Facts

1998 National Institute of Allergy and Infectious Disease (NIAID).

Genital herpes is a contagious viral infection that affects an estimated one out of four (or 45 million) Americans. Doctors estimate that as many as 500,000 new cases may occur each year. The infection is caused by the herpes simplex virus (HSV). There are two types of HSV, and both can cause genital herpes. HSV type 1 most commonly causes sores on the lips (known as fever blisters or cold sores), but it can cause genital infections as well. HSV type 2 most often causes genital sores, but it also can infect the mouth.

Both HSV 1 and 2 can produce sores in and around the vaginal area, on the penis, around the anal opening, and on the buttocks or thighs. Occasionally, sores also appear on other parts of the body where broken skin has come into contact with HSV. The virus remains in certain nerve cells of the body for life, causing periodic symptoms in some people.

Genital herpes infection usually is acquired by sexual contact with someone who unknowingly is having an asymptomatic outbreak of herpes sores in the genital area. People with oral herpes can transmit the infection to the genital area of a partner during oral-genital sex. Herpes infections also can be transmitted by a person who is infected with HSV who has noticeable symptoms. The virus is spread only rarely, if at all, by contact with objects such as a toilet seat or hot tub.

Symptoms

Eighty percent of people with genital herpes are unaware of their disease because they never develop any symptoms or do not recognize them. When symptoms do occur, they vary widely from person to person. Symptoms of a first episode of genital herpes usually appear within two to 10 days of infection, and first episodes last an average of two to three weeks. Early symptoms can include an itching or burning sensation; pain in the legs, buttocks, or genital area; vaginal discharge; or a feeling of pressure in the abdominal region.

Within a few days, sores (also called lesions) appear at the site of infection. Lesions also can occur inside the vagina and on the cervix in women, or in the urinary passage of women and men. Small red bumps appear first, develop into blisters, and then become painful open sores. Over a period of days, the sores become crusted and then heal without scarring. Other symptoms that may accompany the first or primary episode of genital herpes can include fever, headache, muscle aches, painful or difficult urination, vaginal discharge, and swollen glands in the groin area.

Recurrences

In genital herpes, after invading the skin or mucous membranes, the virus travels to the sensory nerves at the end of the spinal cord. Even after the skin lesions have disappeared, the virus remains inside the nerve cells in an inactive, latent state. In most people, the virus will reactivate monthly. It travels along the nerves to the skin, where it multiplies on the surface at or near the site of the original herpes sores, causing new sores to erupt. It also can reactivate without causing any visible sores. At these times, small amounts of the virus may be shed at or near sites of the original infection, in genital secretions, or from barely noticeable lesions. This shedding occurs without any pain or discomfort, it may last only a day, but it is possible to infect a sex partner during this time.

The symptoms of recurrent episodes usually are milder than those of the first episode and typically last about a week. A recurrent outbreak may be signaled by a tingling sensation or itching in the genital area, or pain in the buttocks or down the leg. These are called prodromal symptoms, and, for some people, they can be the most painful and annoying part of a recurrent episode. Sometimes only the prodrome is present and no visible sores develop. At other times, blisters appear that may be very small and barely noticeable, or they may break into open sores that crust over and then disappear.

The frequency and severity of the recurrent episodes vary greatly. While some people recognze only one or two recurrences in a lifetime, others may experience several outbreaks a year. The number and pattern of recurrences often change over time for an individual. Scientists do not know what causes the virus to reactivate. Although some people with herpes report that their recurrences are brought on by other illness, stress, or menstruation, recurrences often are not predictable. In some cases, exposure to sunlight is associated with recurrences.

Diagnosis

The sores of genital herpes in its active stage may be visible to the naked eye. Several laboratory tests may be needed, however, to distinguish herpes sores from other infections. The most accurate method of diagnosis is by viral culture, in which a new sore is swabbed or scraped and the sample is added to a laboratory culture containing healthy cells. When examined under a microscope after one to two days, the cells show changes that indicate growth of the herpes virus.

A newer, more rapid, but somewhat less accurate way of diagnosing herpes involves detection of viral protein components in lesion swabs. These tests should be done when the sores first appear to ensure the most reliable results. Other laboratory tests also are available to physicians. It is important to recognize that the virus is hard to find and that although clinicians commonly fail to detect the virus in an active sore, this does not mean that a person does not have genital herpes.

A blood test cannot determine whether a person has an active genital herpes infection. A blood test, however, can detect antibodies to the virus, which indicate that the person has been infected with HSV at some time and has produced antibodies to it. (Antibodies are proteins made by a person's immune system to fight infections.) Unlike antibodies to some other viruses, however, antibodies to HSV only partially protect an individual against another infection with a different strain or a different type of herpes virus, and they do not prevent a reactivation of the latent virus. The standard blood tests only reliably indicate whether a patient has had a herpes infection, but it cannot tell if it is oral or genital.

New blood tests have been developed that can distinguish whether a person has had prior type 1 or type 2 infection, or both. These tests, however, are available mainly in research hospitals and are not currently available in the doctor's office.

Treatment

During an active herpes episode, whether primary or recurrent, it is important to follow a few simple steps to speed healing and to avoid spreading the infection to other sites of the body or to other people:

- Keep the infected area clean and dry to prevent secondary infections from developing.

- Try to avoid touching the sores; wash hands after contact with the sores.

- Avoid sexual contact from the time symptoms are first recognized until the sores are completely healed, i.e., the scab has fallen off and new skin has formed over the site of the lesion.

Researchers have shown that the oral form of acyclovir (Zovirax® is a superior and safe treatment that helps patients with first or recurrent episodes of genital herpes. The oral form of the drug is taken five times a day and markedly shortens the course of the first episode, and limits the severity of recurrences, particularly if taken within 24 hours of onset of symptoms. People who have very frequent recurrent episodes of the disease can take oral acyclovir twice daily to suppress the virus' activity and prevent most recurrences. Acyclovir is not a cure for herpes-the virus remains in the body for life; but while taken regularly, the medicine interferes with the virus' ability to reproduce itself. This type of therapy also may reduce the risk of transmission to sexual partners.

The U.S. Food and Drug Administration recently approved two new drugs, famciclovir and valacyclovir, to treat recurrent episodes of genital herpes. Famciclovir also has been approved for use in suppressing viral activity and preventing recurrences. These two drugs are taken less frequently than acyclovir, i.e., three times a day for an episode and once a day to help stop further recurrences.

Complications

Usually, genital herpes infections do not cause permanent disability or long-term damage in healthy adults. In people who have suppressed immune systems, however, HSV episodes can be long-lasting and unusually severe. A pregnant woman who develops a first episode of genital herpes can pass the virus to her fetus and may be at higher risk for premature delivery. Half of the babies infected with herpes either die or suffer neurologic damage. A baby born with herpes can develop encephalitis (inflammation of the brain), severe rashes, and eye problems. Acyclovir can greatly improve the outcome for babies with neonatal herpes, particularly if they are treated immediately. With early detection and treatment, most of these serious complications can be lessened.

The newborn's chances of infection depend on whether the mother is having a recurrent or a first outbreak. If the mother is having her first outbreak (especially with HSV 1) near or at the time of a vaginal birth, the baby's risk of infection is approximately one in three. If the outbreak is a recurrence, the baby's risk is very low (less than one in 30). Because of the danger of infection to the baby, however, the physician will perform a cesarean section if herpes lesions are detected in or near the birth canal during labor. Some physicians also perform a viral culture at the time of delivery to detect viral shedding in women known to have had genital herpes outbreaks in the past.

But because it takes days to weeks to get results, and because culture of virus is very difficult, this approach has limited usefulness.

It is important to remember that most women with genital herpes do not have signs of active infection with the virus at delivery.

HSV and AIDS

Genital herpes, like other genital ulcer diseases, increases the risk of acquiring HIV, the virus that causes AIDS, by providing an accessible point of entry for HIV. Also, prior to effective therapy for AIDS, persons with HIV had severe herpes outbreaks, and this may help transmit both herpes and HIV infections to others.

Prevention

People with early signs of a herpes outbreak or with visible sores should not have sexual intercourse until the sores have healed completely. Between outbreaks, using condoms during sexual intercourse may offer partial protection. Use of chronic suppressive acyclovir therapy offers promise for reducing transmission.

Research

Scientists supported by NIAID are concentrating their efforts in several areas of investigation, including determining what causes the virus to reactivate, finding better treatments to prevent transmission and recurrence of HSV, and developing and testing a safe and effective vaccine and safe, effective topical microbicides.

Other scientists have developed an experimental test that can be used to screen blood samples for evidence of herpes infection and can accurately distinguish type 1 from type 2 infections. Rapid diagnostic tests have been developed that can detect active virus in a pregnant woman at the time of delivery. These tests may be able to identify exposed infants who should be observed carefully or receive immediate care.

Emotional Support

Recurrences of genital herpes can be distressing, inconvenient, and sometimes painful. Concern about transmitting the disease to others and disruption of sexual relations during active outbreaks of the sores can affect personal relationships. Patients can cope with and manage the disease effectively, however, with proper counseling, improved treatments, and preventive measures. Counseling and help for those who have genital herpes is often available from local or state health departments.

Section 14.3

Genital Herpes among Pregnant Women

Centers for Disease Control and Prevention (CDC), excerpted from 1998 Guidelines for Treatment of Sexually Transmitted Diseases.

The safety of systemic acyclovir and valacyclovir therapy in pregnant women has not been established. Glaxo-Wellcome, Inc., in cooperation with CDC, maintains a registry to assess the use and effects of acyclovir and valacyclovir during pregnancy.

Current registry findings do not indicate an increased risk for major birth defects after acyclovir treatment (i.e., in comparison with the general population). These findings provide some assurance in counseling women who have had prenatal exposure to acyclovir. The accumulated case histories represent an insufficient sample for reaching reliable and definitive conclusions regarding the risks associated with acyclovir treatment during pregnancy. Prenatal exposure to valacyclovir and famciclovir is too limited to provide useful information on pregnancy outcomes.

The first clinical episode of genital herpes during pregnancy may be treated with oral acyclovir. In the presence of life-threatening maternal HSV infection (e.g., disseminated infection, encephalitis, pneumonitis, or hepatitis), acyclovir administered IV is indicated. Investigations of acyclovir use among pregnant women suggest that acyclovir treatment near term might reduce the rate of abdominal deliveries among women who have frequently recurring or newly acquired genital herpes by decreasing the incidence of active lesions. However, routine administration of acyclovir to pregnant women who have a history of recurrent genital herpes is not recommended at this time.

Perinatal Infection

Most mothers of infants who acquire neonatal herpes lack histories of clinically evident genital herpes. The risk for transmission to the neonate from an infected mother is high among women who acquire genital herpes near the time of delivery (30%-50%) and is low among women who have a history of recurrent herpes at term and women who acquire genital HSV during the first half of pregnancy (3%). Therefore, prevention of neonatal herpes should emphasize prevention of acquisition of genital HSV infection during late pregnancy. Susceptible women whose partners have oral or genital HSV infection, or those whose sex partners' infection status is unknown, should be counseled to avoid unprotected genital and oral sexual contact during late pregnancy. The results of viral cultures during pregnancy do not predict viral shedding at the time of delivery, and such cultures are not indicated routinely.

At the onset of labor, all women should be examined and carefully questioned regarding whether they have symptoms of genital herpes. Infants of women who do not have symptoms or signs of genital herpes infection or its prodrome may be delivered vaginally. Abdominal delivery does not completely eliminate the risk for HSV infection in the neonate.

Infants exposed to HSV during birth, as proven by virus isolation or presumed by observation of lesions, should be followed carefully. Some authorities recommend that such infants undergo surveillance cultures of mucosal surfaces to detect HSV infection before development of clinical signs. Available data do not support the routine use of acyclovir for asymptomatic infants exposed during birth through an infected birth canal, because the risk for infection in most infants is low. However, infants born to women who acquired genital herpes near term are at high risk for neonatal herpes, and some experts recommend acyclovir therapy for these infants. Such pregnancies and newborns should be managed in consultation with an expert. All infants who have evidence of neonatal herpes should be promptly evaluated and treated with systemic acyclovir.

Section 14.4

Genital Herpes and the Newborn

© 1997 U.S. News and World Report Inc., from *U.S. News and World Report,*
Nov. 10, 1997, Vol.123, No.18, Pg.78(4), by Betsy Carpenter;
reprinted with permission.

Fifteen years ago, genital herpes had the sexually permissive in a panic. One in 10 adults was thought to be stricken with this ancient, incurable venereal disease and its accompanying blisters and sores. Suddenly, "free" sex seemed very costly; here was a consequence of a one-night stand that the pill couldn't avert and penicillin couldn't remedy. Then herpes seemed to vanish, eclipsed in the public's mind by the swift, deadly rise of AIDS.

But the virus didn't go away: It surged to create an epidemic. According to a study published in the *New England Journal of Medicine,* since the late 1970s, the proportion of Americans infected with the herpes simplex type 2 virus (HSV-2) has increased by almost one third. Today, 45 million people over the age of 12 carry it—about 1 in 5. Women generally are more susceptible to sexually transmitted diseases (STDs), so the numbers climb even higher for women. One in five white women is infected, versus one in seven white men. One in two black women has the virus, compared with one in three black men.

To Anna Wald, medical director of the Virology Research Clinic at the University of Washington in Seattle, "Herpes has become a major public health problem." In addition to causing sufferers periodic pain and discomfort, genital herpes is potentially devastating to newborns exposed during delivery. Herpes has also been shown to confound the lives of people with suppressed immune systems, such as burn victims and transplant patients. Recent studies show that people with herpes are more susceptible to a variety of STDs, including HIV—the virus that causes AIDS.

Dangerous Myths

Several misconceptions about herpes are fueling the epidemic, according to public-health experts. Most Americans think the virus is uncommon, for instance, afflicting 1 percent or less of the population, says Peggy Clarke, former president of the American Social Health Association in Research Triangle Park in North Carolina. "People just don't know how likely they are to pick it up [from a prospective partner] unless they take precautions."

Many people also hold the mistaken belief that the herpes virus that infects the mouth is benign (herpes simplex type 1 or HSV-1) and that the one that infects the genitals is malevolent (HSV-2). There are differences between the two: HSV-1, which is far more prevalent, infecting about 7 in 10 people, often is acquired in childhood and usually infects the mouth; HSV-2 is typically acquired sexually and usually infects the genitals. But the two are clinically indistinguishable and can inhabit each other's territory. Oral-genital sex is an increasing source of infections, with perhaps 15 percent of genital sores really a manifestation of an HSV-1 infection. "People need to think of [lip] cold sores as infectious to newborns and sexual partners, too," says virologist Rhoda Ashley of the University of Washington in Seattle.

In addition, studies have shown that 2 out of 3 people with the virus don't know they are infected and potentially contagious. How can they miss clusters of itching, painful blisters? For many, a first outbreak is hard to ignore—like a bad case of the flu plus lesions. But others, especially individuals who already harbor HSV-1, often experience only a mild primary infection with HSV-2—with symptoms more like paper cuts or pimples than blisters. According to Ashley, the symptoms can be so variable that "even skilled practitioners can miss [herpes]." Some people also may be refusing to face facts. According to one study, 40 percent to 75 percent of the people with genital herpes who claim to have never experienced symptoms are able to identify them after a doctor delivers the news that they are infected.

No "Safe" Time

Many believe that people who carry herpes are infectious only during acute episodes, when blisters erupt. Yet infected people can shed virus particles from the genital area—and enough of them to infect a sexual partner—even when they are lesion free. Recent research with a new, sensitive test reveals that even when women with HSV-2 have no visible symptoms, they are shedding the virus "subclinically" about 1 in every 6 days. This "subclinical" shedding is generally greatest in the first six months after a person contracts the virus. The shedding rate declines slightly over the next six months and appears to fluctuate thereafter. Most people today with a first-time infection appear to have contracted it from sexual partners who were not aware of any symptoms. (Similarly, people with recurring cold sores in the mouth can transmit the virus between outbreaks.) "It's a tough message to have to tell people, but there's no 'safe' time [for people with the virus] to have [unprotected] sex," says one counselor at the National Herpes Hotline (919-361-8488).

The herpes virus can be devastating to newborns, as Barbara Wilkop of Birmingham, Mich., knows too well. Her 10-year-old son, Jimmy, has an IQ of 35 as a result of contracting herpes from his mother at birth. Jimmy can hear, but he can't understand words. He can ride a bicycle, but he can't always figure out what to do at the end of a dead-end street. He has to be reminded to zip up his pants whenever he goes to the bathroom, and he has so little impulse control that at one family gathering he bit a cousin on the shoulder. "Sometimes I get so sad," says Wilkop. "Jimmy will never get a chance to drive a car, get married, buy a house, or see his first child born."

About 1 in 3,000 infants nationally contracts the herpes virus during delivery, says David Kimberlin of the University of Alabama at Birmingham. Women who have had herpes for several years before having children rarely infect their infants during delivery, thanks to protective antibodies passed from mother to child in the womb. Only about 2 in 100 such infants pick up the virus during birth, and, in most instances, it infects only the skin, eyes, or mouth.

Infants at High Risk

But one third to one half of infants delivered to women who contract the virus for the first time late in their pregnancies contract herpes. In these cases, herpes often attacks the brain, causing death or severe neurological impairment, ranging from blindness and deafness to mental retardation. Because the consequences of infection can be so severe, obstetricians usually recommend delivery by Caesarean section if they spot even the hint of a lesion at the time of delivery. "The general rule is: 'No lesion, vaginal delivery; lesion, C-section,'" according to Larry Gilstrap, chairman of the committee on Obstetrics at the American College of Obstetricians and Gynecologists. As a result, genital herpes is one of the leading causes of C-sections nationally. Although precise figures are not available, Gilstrap estimates that herpes may be fourth or fifth on the list.

Doctors are debating whether pregnant women should be screened for herpes at their first prenatal visit to the doctor, as most are for syphilis, German measles, and a host of other diseases. Zane Brown of the University of Washington in Seattle contends that adding a blood test for herpes to the list makes good sense. "I can go from one end of a decade to the other and not see [a case of] syphilis or gonorrhea, but 35 percent of my patients have genital herpes," he says of his largely middle-class practice. It's especially important to identify high-risk couples, in which the man is infected and the woman isn't. Typically, he tells such couples to use condoms and prescribes for the men an antiviral drug, such as acyclovir or famciclovir, to suppress outbreaks and subclinical shedding, or he counsels couples to abstain from intercourse for the duration of the pregnancy. Physicians who oppose prenatal screening for herpes argue that test results aren't that useful clinically. Even women who test positive in early pregnancy won't necessarily be shedding the virus during delivery, Gilstrap says. And a woman who tests negative at the start of her pregnancy could have picked up the virus by the end.

The opposition of many doctors to prenatal testing seems to stem from a reluctance to deal with the messy emotions that crop up after the diagnosis of an incurable disease—which herpes remains. One prominent obstetrician says that with herpes, "Ignorance is bliss. What am I supposed to say to a wife who tests positive and asks, 'Where did I get this from? I've only had relations with my husband'?"

There are dramatic reasons why all health care providers should deal with the topic. Besides inflicting health problems on infants, adults can find themselves in a fierce struggle with the virus. People with compromised immune systems are the most vulnerable. In burn victims, a herpes skin infection can spread bodywide. "Though rare, it's a well-recognized complication that can kill you," says University of Washington's David Koelle. Bone-marrow-transplant patients and people with lupus can succumb to herpes infections too, although hefty doses of antiviral drugs usually will keep the virus in check. Most AIDS patients—particularly in the disease's early stages—have sufficiently intact immune systems that lesions stay localized. But outbreaks can become the size of silver dollars or larger and be slow to heal.

Public-health experts are deeply concerned about studies finding that getting herpes sores puts sufferers at a much greater risk of contracting HIV—up to nine times as great—by providing portals for HIV to enter the body. "Especially in inner-city populations [which have a high incidence of herpes], it's plausible that herpes is fueling the spread of HIV," says Sharilyn Stanley at the National Institute of Allergy and Infectious Diseases (NIAID) in Bethesda, Md.

Despite the many health threats posed by herpes, few weapons are available to fight the disease. The diagnostic tests commercially available today are unreliable. People with active lesions can have them swabbed and cultured, but such "viral culture" tests are accurate only when lesions are newly formed and teeming with virus particles. Because many people don't get in to see their doctors until their blisters are partly healed, about half the herpes-infected people who take the test are falsely assured that they don't have the virus.

Testing the Blood

Doctors can give patients with no current symptoms a blood test for antibodies to HSV. But the tests currently on the market can't diagnose a case of genital herpes because they don't distinguish between HSV-1 and HSV-2. An accurate, reliable blood test that can tell HSV-1 from HSV-2 is being reviewed by the Food and Drug Administration.

Several studies of couples in which one person is infected and the other isn't have shown that transmission is not inevitable, even after years of sexual contact—although often it takes only a few months for the uninfected partner to catch the virus. Herpes is a "very serious infection," according to Penelope Hitchcock, chief of the division of Microbiology and Infectious Diseases at NIAID, but "[it] is not the most infectious disease in the world."

Still, there is no reliable way to prevent transmission of the virus. Condoms provide only partial protection because the virus can be shed from parts of the body not covered by condoms. "Condoms work pretty well for HIV [which is found in body fluids], and not so very well with HSV," says Andre Nahmias of Emory University School of Medicine in Atlanta. Until recently, researchers hoped that nonoxynol-9, a spermicide often used with condoms and diaphragms, would prove to be an effective chemical barrier, wiping out virus particles as handily as it does sperm cells. But recent studies have shown that nonoxynol-9 is so irritating to the mucosal membranes of the female genital tract that it may increase a woman's susceptibility to infections by damaging these protective membranes. "This is the frustration of clinicians," says Nahmias. "What do you tell people to do?"

To reduce the risk of contracting herpes, Hitchcock of NIAID recommends a few sensible precautions. If a person is not in a monogamous relationship with an uninfected person, he or she should always use condoms. If one partner carries the virus, the couple should never have sex when the partner has lesions, and they should use condoms at other times. If a partner has recurring lip sores, unprotected oral sex should be avoided. Women should abstain when they have vaginal yeast or bacterial infections, which can wipe out healthy microbes.

NIAID has begun funding a host of research projects aimed at developing new tools for stemming the epidemic. A promising area of inquiry is whether daily doses of acyclovir can help carriers of genital herpes protect their partners and infants from infection. A preliminary study published by Laurie Scott, of the University of Texas Southwestern Medical Center in Dallas, and her colleagues suggests that women may be able to protect their babies from infection by taking acyclovir during the last month of pregnancy. Similarly, a study by Anna Wald and colleagues showed that acyclovir therapy reduced viral shedding between outbreaks in women by 94 percent. Wald says, "The transmission study hasn't been done yet, but these results do suggest that the drug may interrupt transmission [between sexual partners]."

Many herpes experts say that only a safe, effective vaccine will be able to decrease the number of people infected each year. But while many potential vaccines are being developed, all are at least a decade away.

Chapter 15

Human Immunodeficiency Virus (HIV)

Chapter Contents

Section 15.1

HIV Infection and AIDS

1999 National Institute of Allergy and Infectious Disease (NIAID).

AIDS—acquired immune deficiency syndrome—was first reported in the United States in 1981 and has since become a major worldwide epidemic. AIDS is caused by the human immunodeficiency virus (HIV). By killing or impairing cells of the immune system, HIV progressively destroys the body's ability to fight infections and certain cancers. Individuals diagnosed with AIDS are susceptible to life-threatening diseases called opportunistic infections, which are caused by microbes that usually do not cause illness in healthy people.

More than 600,000 cases of AIDS have been reported in the United States since 1981, and as many as 900,000 Americans may be infected with HIV. The epidemic is growing most rapidly among minority populations and is a leading killer of African-American males. According to the U.S. Centers for Disease Control and Prevention (CDC), the prevalence of AIDS is six times higher in African-Americans and three times higher among Hispanics than among whites.

Transmission

HIV is spread most commonly by sexual contact with an infected partner. The virus can enter the body through the lining of the vagina, vulva, penis, rectum or mouth during sex.

HIV also is spread through contact with infected blood. Prior to the screening of blood for evidence of HIV infection and before the introduction in 1985 of heat-treating techniques to destroy HIV in blood products, HIV was transmitted through transfusions of contaminated blood or blood components. Today, because of blood screening and heat treatment, the risk of acquiring HIV from such transfusions is extremely small.

HIV frequently is spread among injection drug users by the sharing of needles or syringes contaminated with minute quantities of blood of someone infected with the virus. However, transmission from patient to health-care worker or vice-versa via accidental sticks with contaminated needles or other medical instruments is rare.

Women can transmit HIV to their fetuses during pregnancy or birth. Approximately one-quarter to one-third of all untreated pregnant women infected with HIV will pass the infection to their babies. HIV also can be spread to babies through the breast milk of mothers infected with the virus. If the drug AZT is taken during pregnancy, the chance of transmitting HIV to the baby is reduced significantly. If AZT treatment of mothers is combined with cesarean sectioning to deliver infants, infection rates can be reduced to 1 percent.

Although researchers have detected HIV in the saliva of infected individuals, no evidence exists that the virus is spread by contact with saliva. Laboratory studies reveal that saliva has natural compounds that inhibit the infectiousness of HIV. Studies of people infected with HIV have found no evidence that the virus is spread to others through saliva such as by kissing. No one knows, however, the risk of infection from so-called "deep" kissing, involving the exchange of large amounts of saliva, or by oral intercourse. Scientists also have found no evidence that HIV is spread through sweat, tears, urine or feces.

Studies of families of HIV-infected people have shown clearly that HIV is not spread through casual contact such as the sharing of food utensils, towels and bedding, swimming pools, telephones or toilet seats. HIV is not spread by biting insects such as mosquitoes or bedbugs.

HIV can infect anyone who practices risky behaviors such as:

- sharing drug needles or syringes;

- having sexual contact without using a latex male condom with an infected person or with someone whose HIV status is unknown.

Having another sexually transmitted disease such as syphilis, herpes, chlamydial infection, gonorrhea or bacterial vaginosis appears to make someone more susceptible to acquiring HIV infection during sex with an infected partner.

Early Symptoms

Many people do not develop any symptoms when they first become infected with HIV. Some people, however, have a flu-like illness within a month or two after exposure to the virus. They may have fever, headache, malaise and enlarged lymph nodes (organs of the immune system easily felt in the neck and groin). These symptoms usually disappear within a week to a month and are often mistaken for those of another viral infection. People are very infectious during this period, and HIV is present in large quantities in genital secretions.

More persistent or severe symptoms may not surface for a decade or more after HIV first enters the body in adults, or within two years in children born with HIV infection. This period of "asymptomatic" infection is highly variable. Some people may begin to have symptoms in as soon as a few months, whereas others may be symptom-free for more than 10 years. During the asymptomatic period, however, HIV is actively multiplying, infecting and killing cells of the immune system. HIV's effect is seen most obviously in a decline in the blood levels of CD4+ T cells (also called T4 cells)—the immune system's key infection fighters. The virus initially disables or destroys these cells without causing symptoms.

As the immune system deteriorates, a variety of complications begin to surface. One of the first such symptoms experienced by many people infected with HIV is large lymph nodes or "swollen glands" that may be enlarged for more than three months. Other symptoms often experienced months to years before the onset of AIDS include a lack of energy, weight loss, frequent fevers and sweats, persistent or frequent yeast infections (oral or vaginal), persistent skin rashes or flaky skin, pelvic inflammatory disease that does not respond to treatment, or short-term memory loss.

Some people develop frequent and severe herpes infections that cause mouth, genital or anal sores, or a painful nerve disease known as shingles. Children may have delayed development or failure to thrive.

AIDS

The term AIDS applies to the most advanced stages of HIV infection. Official criteria for the definition of AIDS are developed by the CDC in Atlanta, Georgia, which is responsible for tracking the spread of AIDS in the United States.

In 1993, CDC revised its definition of AIDS to include all HIV-infected people who have fewer than 200 CD4+ T cells. (Healthy adults usually have CD4+ T-cell counts of 1,000 or more.) In addition, the definition includes 26 clinical conditions that affect people with advanced HIV disease. Most AIDS-defining conditions are opportunistic infections, which rarely cause harm in healthy individuals. In people with AIDS, however, these infections are often severe and sometimes fatal because the immune system is so ravaged by HIV that the body cannot fight off certain bacteria, viruses and other microbes.

Opportunistic infections common in people with AIDS cause such symptoms as coughing, shortness of breath, seizures, mental symptoms such as confusion and forgetfulness, severe and persistent diarrhea, fever, vision loss, severe headaches, weight loss, extreme fatigue, nausea, vomiting, lack of coordination, coma, abdominal cramps, or difficult or painful swallowing. Although children with AIDS are susceptible to the same opportunistic infections as adults with the disease, they also experience severe forms of the bacterial infections to which children are especially prone, such as conjunctivitis (pink eye), ear infections and tonsillitis.

People with AIDS are particularly prone to developing various cancers, especially those caused by viruses such as Kaposi's sarcoma and cervical cancer, or cancers of the immune system known as lymphomas. These cancers are usually more aggressive and difficult to treat in people with AIDS. Hallmarks of Kaposi's sarcoma in light-skinned people are round brown, reddish or purple spots that develop in the skin or in the mouth. In dark-skinned people, the spots are more pigmented.

During the course of HIV infection, most people experience a gradual decline in the number of CD4+ T cells, although some individuals may have abrupt and dramatic drops in their CD4+ T-cell counts. A person with CD4+ T cells above 200 may experience some of the early symptoms of HIV disease. Others may have no symptoms even though their CD4+ T-cell count is below 200. Many people are so debilitated by the symptoms of AIDS that they are unable to hold steady employment or do household chores. Other people with AIDS may experience phases of intense life-threatening illness followed by phases of normal functioning.

A small number of people (less than 50) initially infected with HIV 10 or more years ago have not developed symptoms of AIDS. Scientists are trying to determine what factors may account for their lack of progression to AIDS, such as particular characteristics of their immune systems, or whether they were infected with a less aggressive strain of the virus or if their genetic make-up may protect them from the effects of HIV. Scientists hope that understanding the body's natural method of control may lead to ideas for protective HIV vaccines and use of vaccines to prevent disease progression.

Diagnosis

Because early HIV infection often causes no symptoms, it is primarily detected by testing a person's blood for the presence of antibodies (disease-fighting proteins) to HIV. HIV antibodies generally do not reach detectable levels until one to three months following infection and may take as long as six months to be generated in quantities large enough to show up in standard blood tests. HIV testing may also be performed on saliva and urine samples, in addition to blood samples. People exposed to HIV should be tested for HIV infection as soon as they are likely to develop antibodies to the virus. Such early testing will enable them to receive appropriate treatment at a time when they are most able to combat HIV and prevent the emergence of certain opportunistic infections. Early testing also alerts HIV-infected people to avoid high-risk behaviors that could spread HIV to others.

HIV testing is done in most doctors' offices or health clinics and should be accompanied by counseling. Individuals can be tested anonymously at many sites if they have particular concerns about confidentiality. In addition, blood samples for anonymous HIV testing may now be collected at home. Home-based test kits are available by telephone order or over the counter at pharmacies.

Two different types of antibody tests, ELISA and Western Blot, are used to diagnose HIV infection. If a person is highly likely to be infected with HIV and yet both tests are negative, a doctor may test for the presence of HIV itself in the blood. The person also may be told to repeat antibody testing at a later date, when antibodies to HIV are more likely to have developed.

Babies born to mothers infected with HIV may or may not be infected with the virus, but all carry their mothers' antibodies to HIV for several months. If these babies lack symptoms, a definitive diagnosis of HIV infection using standard antibody tests cannot be made until after 15 months of age. By then, babies are unlikely to still carry their mothers' antibodies and will have produced their own, if they are infected. New technologies to detect HIV itself are being used to more accurately determine HIV infection in infants between ages 3 months and 15 months. A number of blood tests are being evaluated to determine if they can diagnose HIV infection in babies younger than 3 months.

Treatment

When AIDS first surfaced in the United States, no drugs were available to combat the underlying immune deficiency and few treatments existed for the opportunistic diseases that resulted. Over the past 10 years, however, therapies have been developed to fight both HIV infection and its associated infections and cancers.

Human Immunodeficiency Virus (HIV)

The Food and Drug Administration has approved a number of drugs for the treatment of HIV infection. The first group of drugs used to treat HIV infection, called nucleoside analog reverse transcriptase inhibitors (NRTIs), interrupt an early stage of virus replication. Included in this class of drugs are zidovudine (also known as AZT), zalcitabine (ddC), didanosine (ddI), stavudine (D4T), lamivudine (3TC) and abacavir succinate. These drugs may slow the spread of HIV in the body and delay the onset of opportunistic infections. Importantly, they do not prevent transmission of HIV to other individuals. Non-nucleoside reverse transcriptase inhibitors (NNRTIs) such as delavirdine, nevirapine and efavirenz are also available for use in combination with other antiretroviral drugs.

A third class of anti-HIV drugs, called protease inhibitors, interrupts virus replication at a later step in its life cycle. They include ritonavir, saquinivir, indinavir and nelfinavir. Because HIV can become resistant to each class of drugs, combination treatment using both is necessary to effectively suppress the virus.

Currently available antiretroviral drugs do not cure people of HIV infection or AIDS, however, and they all have side effects that can be severe. AZT may cause a depletion of red or white blood cells, especially when taken in the later stages of the disease. If the loss of blood cells is severe, treatment with AZT must be stopped. DdI can cause an inflammation of the pancreas and painful nerve damage.

The most common side effects associated with protease inhibitors include nausea, diarrhea and other gastrointestinal symptoms. In addition, protease inhibitors can interact with other drugs resulting in serious side effects. Investigators also recently have reported cases of abnormal redistribution of body fat among some individuals receiving protease inhibitors.

A number of drugs are available to help treat opportunistic infections to which people with HIV are especially prone. These drugs include foscarnet and ganciclovir, used to treat cytomegalovirus eye infections, fluconazole to treat yeast and other fungal infections, and TMP/SMX or pentamidine to treat *Pneumocystis carinii* pneumonia (PCP).

In addition to antiretroviral therapy, adults with HIV whose CD4+ T-cell counts drop below 200 are given treatment to prevent the occurrence of PCP, which is one of the most common and deadly opportunistic infections associated with HIV. Children are given PCP preventive therapy when their CD4+ T-cell counts drop to levels considered below normal for their age group.

Regardless of their CD4+ T-cell counts, HIV-infected children and adults who have survived an episode of PCP are given drugs for the rest of their lives to prevent a recurrence of the pneumonia.

155

HIV-infected individuals who develop Kaposi's sarcoma or other cancers are treated with radiation, chemotherapy or injections of alpha interferon, a genetically engineered naturally occurring protein.

Prevention

Since no vaccine for HIV is available, the only way to prevent infection by the virus is to avoid behaviors that put a person at risk of infection, such as sharing needles and having unprotected sex.

Because many people infected with HIV have no symptoms, there is no way of knowing with certainty whether a sexual partner is infected unless he or she has been repeatedly tested for the virus or has not engaged in any risky behavior. CDC recommends that people either abstain from sex or protect themselves by using male latex condoms whenever having oral, anal or vaginal sex. Only male condoms made of latex should be used, and water-based lubricants should be used with latex condoms.

Although some laboratory evidence shows that spermicides can kill HIV organisms, in clinical trials, researchers have not found that these products can prevent HIV.

The risk of HIV transmission from a pregnant woman to her fetus is significantly reduced if she takes AZT during pregnancy, labor and delivery, and her baby takes it for the first six weeks of life.

Research

NIAID-supported investigators are conducting an abundance of research on HIV infection, including the development and testing of HIV vaccines and new therapies for the disease and some of its associated conditions. More than a dozen HIV vaccines are being tested in people, and many drugs for HIV infection or AIDS-associated opportunistic infections are either in development or being tested. Researchers also are investigating exactly how HIV damages the immune system. This research is suggesting new and more effective targets for drugs and vaccines. NIAID-supported investigators also continue to document how the disease progresses in different people.

Section 15.2

Women and HIV

1997 National Institute of Allergy and Infectious Disease (NIAID).

The number of women with HIV and AIDS in the United States is steadily rising. From 1985 to 1996, the proportion of reported U.S. AIDS cases occurring among women increased from 7 percent to 20 percent. HIV infection is now the third leading cause of death among women ages 25 to 44 and the leading cause of death among black women in this age group.

In addition to conditions such as *Pneumocystis carinii* pneumonia that afflict HIV-infected people of both genders, women suffer gender-specific manifestations of HIV disease, such as recurrent vaginal yeast infections and pelvic inflammatory disease.

Women with HIV frequently have great difficulty accessing health care, and carry a large burden of caring for children and other family members who may also be HIV-infected. They often lack social support and face other challenges that may interfere with their ability to adhere to treatment regimens.

To confront the growing problem of HIV and AIDS in women, the National Institute of Allergy and Infectious Diseases (NIAID) has made woman-focused research an important component of the Institute's AIDS research program.

NIAID supports studies in the United States and abroad of the natural history and manifestations of HIV infection in both non-pregnant and pregnant women, as well as the factors that influence the transmission of HIV to women. Investigators are studying the unique features of HIV/AIDS in women and developing new treatment regimens for women with these conditions.

Scientists also are developing and testing new methods to prevent women from becoming infected with HIV. These include creams or gels that women would apply before intercourse to protect themselves from HIV as well as other sexually transmitted organisms. A recent study supported by NIAID found that one vaginal contraceptive film, N-9, did not offer women any protection against HIV, gonorrhea or chlamydia.

Other studies will be conducted as part of NIAID's overall HIV/STD prevention program.

In addition, researchers are studying the mechanisms of mother-to-child HIV transmission and are devising interventions to reduce such transmission. Notably, NIAID-funded investigators have shown that a specific regimen of zidovudine (AZT), given to an HIV-infected woman during pregnancy and to her baby after birth, can reduce mother-to-infant HIV transmission by two-thirds.

Researchers now are assessing other antiretroviral regimens that may prove even more effective, as well as simpler and less costly regimens that may have broader applications.

Scope of the Problem

An analysis from the National Cancer Institute estimates that between 107,000 and 150,000 women in the United States are living with HIV infection (many of whom have not developed AIDS).

As of Dec. 30, 1996, the Centers for Disease Control and Prevention (CDC) had received reports of 85,500 cases of AIDS among female adults and adolescents in the United States, 48,186 of whom have died. Minority women in the United States are disproportionately affected by AIDS: in 1996, 56 percent of reported female U.S. AIDS cases were among black women, and 20 percent among Hispanic women. These women tend to be poor, young and residents of disenfranchised communities in inner-city neighborhoods.

Approximately 42 percent of the 21 million adults living with HIV/AIDS worldwide are women, according to the World Health Organization (WHO).

Transmission of HIV to Women

In the United States, most HIV-infected women are exposed to the virus during sex with an HIV-infected man or while using HIV-contaminated syringes for the injection of drugs such as heroin, cocaine and amphetamines.

Of U.S. AIDS cases among women reported in 1996, 40 percent were attributed to heterosexual contact and 34 percent to injection drug use; most of the other cases reported in 1996 were attributed to "no known exposure." In recent years, the majority of such unclassified cases upon further investigation have been reclassified as cases attributable to heterosexual exposure. Worldwide, the WHO estimates that about 75 percent of adult HIV infections are due to heterosexual transmission of the virus through sexual intercourse.

During unprotected heterosexual intercourse with an HIV-infected partner, women in general appear to be more easily infected with the virus than do men. Studies in the United States and abroad have demonstrated that other sexually transmitted diseases (STDs), particularly infections that cause ulcerations of the mucosal surfaces (e.g., syphilis and chancroid), greatly increase a woman's risk of becoming infected with HIV. Anal sex also increases a woman's risk of becoming HIV-infected.

NIAID-sponsored cohort studies in the United States have found a number of other factors to be associated with an increased risk of heterosexual HIV transmission including alcohol use, history of childhood sexual abuse, current domestic abuse and use of crack/cocaine.

The consistent use of condoms greatly reduces the risk of becoming infected with HIV. In studies of discordant heterosexual couples (one individual HIV-positive, the other HIV-negative) who report regular condom use, HIV transmission rates have been extremely low.

Signs and Symptoms of HIV

Many manifestations of HIV disease are similar in men and women. Both men and women with HIV may have nonspecific symptoms even early in disease, including low-grade fevers, night sweats, fatigue and weight loss. In the United States, the most common AIDS-associated condition in both women and men is a lung infection called *Pneumocystis carinii* pneumonia (PCP). Anti-HIV therapies, as well as treatments for the infections associated with HIV (so-called opportunistic infections), appear to be similarly effective in men and women.

Other conditions occur in different frequencies in men and women. HIV-infected men, for instance, are eight times more likely than HIV-infected women to develop a skin cancer known as Kaposi's sarcoma. In some studies, women have had higher rates of esophageal candidiasis (yeast infections of the windpipe) and herpes simplex infections than men.

Data from a study conducted by NIAID's Terry Beirn Community Programs for Clinical Research on AIDS (CPCRA) found that HIV-infected women were more likely than HIV-infected men to develop bacterial pneumonia. This finding may be explained by factors such as a delay in care-seeking among HIV-infected women as compared to men, and/or less access to anti-HIV therapies or preventive therapies for PCP.

Woman-Specific Symptoms of HIV Infection

Women also experience HIV-associated gynecologic problems, many of which also occur in uninfected women but with less frequency or severity.

Vaginal yeast infections, common and easily treated in most women, often are particularly persistent and difficult to treat in HIV-infected women. Data from the NIAID-supported Women's Interagency Health Study (WIHS) suggest that these infections are considerably more frequent in HIV-infected women.

A drug called fluconazole is commonly used to treat yeast infections. A CPCRA study demonstrated that weekly doses of fluconazole can also safely prevent vaginal and esophageal candidiasis, without resulting in resistance to the drug.

Other vaginal infections may occur more frequently and with greater severity in HIV-infected women, including bacterial vaginosis and common STDs such as gonorrhea, chlamydia and trichomoniasis.

Severe herpes simplex virus ulcerations, sometimes unresponsive to therapy with the standard drug, acyclovir, can severely compromise a woman's quality of life.

Idiopathic genital ulcers—those with no evidence of an infectious organism or cancerous cells in the lesion—are a unique manifestation of HIV disease. These ulcers, for which there is no proven treatment, are sometimes confused with those caused by herpes simplex virus.

NIAID is currently assessing, in a study known as AIDS Clinical Trials Group (ACTG) 842, the prevalence of idiopathic genital ulcer disease in HIV-infected women and the effect of thalidomide treatment. Thalidomide has previously proven effective in the treatment of oral aphthous ulcers in HIV-infected people.

Human papillomavirus (HPV) infections, which cause genital warts and can lead to cervical cancer, occur with increased frequency in HIV-infected women. A precancerous condition associated with HPV called cervical intraepithelial neoplasia (CIN) also is more common and more severe in HIV-infected women, and more apt to recur after treatment.

Three studies within NIAID's ACTG address CIN in HIV-infected women. A study known as ACTG 200 is assessing topical vaginal 5-fluorouracil maintenance therapy to prevent the recurrence of moderate-to-severe cervical dysplasia. ACTG 293 is evaluating oral isotretinoin for prevention of progression of low-grade (mild) dysplasia to high-grade dysplasia or invasive cancer of the cervix in HIV-positive women. ACTG 866 is assessing the effect of the protease inhibitor indinavir on the progression of cervical dysplasia and HPV infections in HIV-infected women, and on the amount of HIV in vaginal secretions.

Pelvic inflammatory disease (PID) appears to be more common and more aggressive in HIV-infected women than in uninfected women. PID may become a chronic and relapsing condition as a woman's immune system deteriorates.

Menstrual irregularities frequently are reported by HIV-infected women and are being actively studied by NIAID-supported scientists. Although menstrual irregularities were equally common in HIV-infected women and at-risk HIV-negative women in a recent WIHS survey, women with CD4+ T cell counts below 50 per cubic millimeter (mm3) of blood were more likely to report amenorrhea (no menses within the last three months) than uninfected women, or HIV-infected women with higher CD4+ T cell counts.

Because megace, an FDA-approved drug often prescribed for HIV-associated wasting, can cause significant, irregular vaginal bleeding in HIV-infected women, NIAID is planning a trial to assess an alternate drug, nandrolone, in women with HIV-associated weight loss.

Gynecologic Screening

The Public Health Service currently recommends that HIV-positive women have a complete gynecologic evaluation, including a Pap smear, as part of their initial HIV evaluation, or upon entry to prenatal care, and another Pap smear six months later. If both smears are negative, annual screening is recommended thereafter in asymptomatic women. However, more frequent screening—every six months—is recommended for women with symptomatic HIV infection, prior abnormal Pap smears, or signs of human papillomavirus infection.

Early Diagnosis Important

Some women in the United States have poor access to health care. In addition, women may not perceive themselves to be at risk for HIV infection. Because of these reasons and other psychosocial factors, symptoms that could serve as warning signals of HIV infection—such as recurrent yeast infections—may go unheeded. PID, CIN and the other symptoms discussed above should signal caregivers to offer women HIV testing accompanied by counseling.

Early diagnosis of HIV infection allows women to take full advantage of antiretroviral therapies and preventive drugs for opportunistic infections, both of which can forestall the development of AIDS-related symptoms and prolong life in HIV-infected men and women. Early diagnosis also allows women to make informed reproductive choices. Health care workers should be alert to early signs of HIV infection in women, and all women should consider HIV testing if they have engaged in high-risk activities.

Survival among HIV-Infected Women

Women whose HIV infections are detected early and who receive appropriate treatment survive as long as infected men. However, because women may be less likely than men to receive an early diagnosis and treatment, survival times for women as compared to men have been shorter in several studies.

In a CPCRA study of more than 4,500 people with HIV, HIV-infected women were one-third more likely than HIV-infected men to die within the study period. The CPCRA investigators could not definitively identify the reasons for excess mortality among women in this study, but they speculated that poorer access to or use of health care resources among HIV-infected women as compared to men, domestic violence, homelessness and lack of social supports for women may have been important factors.

Perinatal Transmission of HIV

In the United States, approximately 25 percent of pregnant HIV-infected women not receiving AZT therapy have passed on the virus to their babies.

Most perinatal transmission, an estimated 50 to 80 percent of infections, probably occurs late in pregnancy or during birth. Although the precise mechanisms are unknown, scientists think HIV may be transmitted when maternal blood enters the fetal circulation, or by mucosal exposure to virus during labor and delivery. The role of the placenta in maternal-fetal transmission is unclear and the focus of considerable research.

The risk of perinatal transmission is significantly increased if the mother has advanced HIV disease, large amounts of HIV in her bloodstream, or few of the immune system cells—CD4+ T cells—that are the main targets of HIV.

Other factors that may increase the risk of perinatal transmission are maternal drug use, severe inflammation of fetal membranes, or a prolonged period between membrane rupture and delivery. A recent study sponsored in part by NIAID found that HIV-infected women who gave birth more than four hours after the rupture of the fetal membranes were nearly twice as likely to transmit HIV to their infants, as compared to women who delivered within four hours of membrane rupture. In the same study, HIV-infected women who used heroin or crack/cocaine during pregnancy were also twice as likely to transmit HIV to their offspring as HIV-infected women who did not use drugs.

HIV also may be transmitted from a nursing mother to her infant. A recent analysis suggested that breast-feeding introduces an additional risk of HIV transmission of approximately 14 percent. However, the WHO still recommends breast-feeding of infants in developing countries because the benefits are believed to far outweigh the potential risk of HIV transmission.

A Role for AZT

A study conducted by NIAID's Pediatric AIDS Clinical Trials Group demonstrated that AZT, given to HIV-infected pregnant women who had very little or no prior antiretroviral therapy and CD4+ T cell counts above 200/mm3, reduced the risk of maternal-infant transmission by two-thirds.

In the study, known as ACTG 076, AZT therapy was initiated in the second or third trimester and continued during labor, and infants were treated for six weeks following birth. AZT produced no serious side effects in mothers or infants; long-term follow-up of the infants and mothers is ongoing.

Researchers have subsequently shown that this AZT regimen has reduced perinatal transmission in other populations in which AZT has been used. However, the AZT regimen used in ACTG 076 is not always available because of cost and logistical demands. Therefore, NIAID also is pursuing a global strategy that includes the examination of simpler and less costly regimens for preventing mother-to-infant transmission of HIV.

Because a significant amount of perinatal HIV transmission occurs around the time of birth, and the risk of maternal-fetal transmission depends, in part, on the amount of HIV in the mother's blood, it may be possible to reduce transmission using drug therapy only around the time of birth. NIAID-supported researchers are studying the effect of this approach and also whether immunoglobulin preparations containing large quantities of antibodies to HIV can prevent perinatal HIV transmission when given to the mother and/or the neonate. This strategy—known as passive immunization—has been used successfully in reducing perinatal transmission of hepatitis B virus.

Section 15.3

HIV, AIDS, and Pregnancy

© 1999 Clinical Reference Systems Ltd., from *Clinical Reference Systems*, July 1, 1999, Pg.650, by Phyllis G. Cooper; reprinted with permission.

What is AIDS and what is its effect during pregnancy?

Acquired immunodeficiency syndrome, or AIDS, is caused by a virus that attacks your immune system. The AIDS virus is called the human immunodeficiency virus, or HIV. When your immune system can't fight disease, you may become sick with many infections that the body would normally fight off. Such infections are called opportunistic infections.

If you are pregnant and you are infected with HIV, your baby may be infected by the virus before or during birth. The baby can also get the virus from the breast milk of an infected mother. If the baby does get the virus, he or she may become very sick and die.

Between 20% and 40% of the babies born to HIV-infected mothers become infected with the virus. Half or more of these infections occur during labor and delivery. You should ask to be tested for HIV at your first prenatal visit.

How does HIV infection occur?

HIV infection is passed through unprotected sexual activity with an infected partner, transfusion with infected blood, shared needles, or contact with infected body fluids (for example, blood or breast milk). HIV can be passed to an unborn baby through the placenta, by exposure to blood and body fluids during labor and at delivery, or through breast-feeding.

What are the symptoms?

You can be infected with HIV and not have any symptoms. Or you may have one or more of the following signs and symptoms:

- unexplained weight loss

- tiredness and just not feeling well
- fever that lasts from a few days to longer than a month, with no other disease present and no other obvious cause
- diarrhea, especially if it lasts longer than a month and no other disease is present
- unexplained, prolonged swelling of the lymph nodes
- a certain kind of sores or changes in the skin that last more than 4 weeks, including persistent or recurring herpes infections
- oral, esophageal, lung, or vaginal yeast infections
- abnormal Pap tests.

Infants infected with HIV may not have symptoms until they are 9 months old. However, half of all children infected by their mothers will develop symptoms before they are 1 year old. Most infected children will have symptoms before they are 3 years old. Some of the symptoms infants may have include:

- poor growth and weight gain
- enlarged spleen and liver
- chronic pneumonia (lung infections)
- enlarged lymph nodes
- chronic or recurrent diarrhea
- low blood counts
- birth weight less than 5 pounds
- recurrent ear infections
- rash
- failure to develop normally
- small brain.

How is HIV infection diagnosed?

The screening test for HIV is a blood test called the ELISA test. When this test is positive, another more specific blood test, usually the Western blot test, is done to confirm the diagnosis. If both tests are positive, you are infected with HIV. Tests can usually detect HIV infection within several weeks of your exposure to the virus. Sometimes, however, you may not test positive for several months.

A baby is given the ELISA and Western blot tests after birth. However, because some of the mother's antibodies to HIV are passed on to the baby, the test results are not always completely accurate. If a newborn's tests are negative, you cannot be sure that the child is not infected with HIV until many months later.

How is it treated?

If you test positively for HIV, you may have more tests such as:

- tests for other sexually transmitted diseases, including hepatitis B and syphilis
- test for tuberculosis
- blood tests for previous cytomegalovirus (CMV) and toxoplasmosis infections
- ultrasound scans to check for normal growth of the baby in your womb
- nonstress tests during the latter part of the pregnancy to monitor the baby's heartbeat for signs of stress
- tests of your immune system.

If you are pregnant and have tested positively for the HIV virus, your doctor will probably prescribe the drug zidovudine (also called ZDV or AZT). Other drugs may be prescribed as well. Taking these drugs during pregnancy and labor significantly reduces the risk that you will give the infection to your baby. You may be treated with medication for an opportunistic infection such as pneumonia or herpes.

During labor and delivery you do not need to be isolated. All hospital personnel now use special precautions when they handle blood or other body fluids to prevent the spread of AIDS. Make sure that you tell all your health care providers that you are HIV positive.

You should not breast-feed your baby. Give formula to your baby instead to prevent passage of the virus to the baby.

What can be done to help prevent HIV infection during pregnancy?

Ask for counseling and testing if you are pregnant or plan to become pregnant and are in any of the following high-risk groups:

- women with signs of HIV infection

- intravenous (IV) drug abusers and other drug abusers, such as cocaine addicts

- sexual partners of men who are infected with HIV

- prostitutes

- women with more than one sexual partner or whose sexual partner is sexually active outside the relationship (especially women who live in areas where there is a high occurrence of HIV infection)

- sexual partners of men who are drug abusers, bisexual (they have sex with men and women), hemophiliacs, or were born in countries where transmission of HIV to heterosexuals is high

- women who received transfusions of blood between 1978 and 1985 that were not screened for HIV

- women from countries where there is a high occurrence of AIDS in heterosexuals, such as Haiti, the Dominican Republic, central Africa, and Brazil

- women who received semen from a sperm bank for artificial insemination.

Know Your Partner

Ask about your partner's sexual history and if he or she has ever used IV drugs. Do not share toothbrushes, razors, and other implements that may be contaminated with body fluids.

If you have a high risk of being infected with HIV, you should be tested for HIV before you try to get pregnant.

If you know that you are infected with HIV, you should seriously consider the grief and high cost of having a baby born infected with HIV. Try to avoid becoming pregnant. Follow safe sex practices (including the use of latex condoms) to prevent transmission of the infection to others.

If you are already pregnant and infected with HIV and your baby does not become infected with HIV during your pregnancy or delivery, the child may stay free of the infection if you do not breast-feed.

Section 15.4

HIV in Older Adults

What is AIDS?

AIDS is a life-threatening illness caused by infection with the human immunodeficiency virus (HIV). The HIV organism destroys part of the immune system, which is the body's natural defense against infection and disease.

It takes 6 weeks to several months for the body to form antibodies, which are proteins produced in response to the virus. These antibodies can be detected in the blood. When the antibodies are found in your blood you are said to be HIV-positive. When you begin to lose the ability to fight off serious infection, you are said to have AIDS.

How does it occur?

HIV is spread by direct intimate contact with infected blood, semen, or vaginal secretions. This includes sex with an infected person, sharing needles with an infected person, or receiving HIV-infected blood or organ transplants. The virus is also found in smaller amounts in tears, saliva, brain/spinal fluid, breast milk, urine, and feces, although contact with these bodily fluids is not likely to transmit the virus.

HIV is NOT spread by casual contact such as by shaking hands, touching an infected person, touching something that the person has handled, using public toilets or telephones, or using swimming pools.

How does HIV infection affect older adults?

Society generally may not consider older adults to be at risk for AIDS. However, of reported cases of HIV infection, 10% are in people over age 55, and this rate is increasing. Approximately 1 in 25 cases of AIDS in the U.S. now occurs in persons 65 years of age and older.

Among those over age 55 diagnosed with AIDS, the main cause (65%) has been male-to-male homosexual contact. Blood transfusions contaminated with the HIV virus has been the second most frequent cause. These blood transfusions generally occurred before 1985, when reliable testing for the virus was developed. The blood supply now is very safe.

What are the symptoms of AIDS?

The symptoms of AIDS are the symptoms of the diseases that attack the body because of a weakened immune system. Symptoms may include:

- fever, sweats, chills
- fatigue
- loss of appetite, weight loss
- nausea, vomiting
- sore throat
- diarrhea
- body rash.

These symptoms mimic many other illnesses such as cancer, tuberculosis, influenza, mononucleosis, or stomach flu. A physical exam is necessary to rule out other illnesses.

How do you test for HIV infection?

The ELISA test and the Western blot tests are blood tests used to detect HIV antibodies. A negative test does not guarantee that a person is not infected. If the person has only recently been infected, the antibodies may not yet have been formed. It may take up to 6 months for someone to develop antibodies after exposure to the virus. A positive test indicates that the person has been exposed to the virus and has developed antibodies.

Testing can be done at the local Department of Health clinic or at your private physician's office. It is very important that counseling is done before and after the testing to explain results.

Who is at high risk for HIV infection?

- men who have sex with men
- sexual partners of people who are infected
- people who received blood transfusions before 1985
- babies born to mothers who are infected
- people who use IV drugs and share needles
- sexual partners of IV drug users who share needles

- hemophiliacs

- prostitutes and their sex partners

- people who have had oral, anal, or vaginal sex without a condom with multiple partners.

Older persons who have multiple sexual partners, including heterosexuals, may not use condoms because they consider them birth control devices rather than a means of preventing HIV infection. After the death of a long-term partner, older gay men may turn to younger men as sexual partners, increasing their risks of contracting disease.

HIV-infected elderly often suffer due to social and emotional isolation and lack of a support network. They may also have to face informing family members.

How can I avoid exposure to HIV?

You are safest if you are in a stable relationship with one partner and both of you are uninfected.

- Use latex condoms with a water-based lubricant and spermicide containing nonoxynol-9 if you engage in male homosexual practices or if you or your partner have more than one sexual partner.

- Do not use IV drugs or share needles with anyone.

- If you expect to have surgery, you may want to talk to your doctor about banking your own blood for transfusions.

At this time, there is no cure or immunization that will prevent HIV infection. Anyone engaging in at-risk behaviors should contact a physician to arrange for a complete physical examination and blood tests.

All information for HIV testing is strictly confidential. Health care providers may not give test results to anyone other than the patient.

The best way to protect yourself is to obtain as much knowledge as you can about HIV infection and follow guidelines for protection.

Section 15.5

Uncharted Territory: AIDS in the Older Patient

© 1998 Medical Economics Publishing, from *Patient Care*, Nov. 30, 1998, Vol.32, Issue 19, Pg.84(1), by Lori D. Talarico; reprinted with permission.

HIV infection, including AIDS, is generally regarded as a young person's disease, particularly affecting those in young adulthood and early middle age. But the epidemiology is changing. According to the Centers for Disease Control and Prevention (CDC), the number of AIDS cases is rising fastest among heterosexuals older than 50, and this group now accounts for 10% of all patients with AIDS.[1]

The sharp increase is related primarily to IV drug use and sexual transmission (heterosexual and homosexual) not to receiving blood or blood products, which has been deemed safe since the late 1980s. Before that time, hemophiliacs and others who had received transfusions or blood products made up a larger percentage of the older HIV-positive population. The increase in sexually transmitted AIDS cases is expected to continue because at-risk people older than 50 are one sixth as likely as younger adults to use condoms during sex and one fifth as likely to be tested for HIV.[2]

A recent report by the CDC also indicates that the prevalence of AIDS-related opportunistic infections (OIs) in those aged 50 and older is substantial.[3] Another factor that has increased the number of older adults living with AIDS is the advent of better medications. Many who are HIV positive, or who have had full-blown AIDS for years and were not expected to survive long, are living into old age.

For those growing older with AIDS as a chronic disease, as well as for those contracting it in later years, much still needs to be learned. As the many similarities between AIDS pathology and the normal aging process unfold, studies may provide insight into the role of immune activation and replicative senescence in both aging and AIDS. If scientists can find the biological link in what turns on the aging process, they may be one step closer to slowing down some of the degenerative processes of AIDS. More research may also help to identify how the natural history of HIV disease differs in older patients and who is most or least likely to benefit from new treatment regimens.

In the meantime, there are issues—some clinical, some psychosocial—that the physician and the older patient with AIDS must deal with now. The ramifications affect the patient and the physician, the partner or spouse, the immediate family, and sometimes even the community at large.

Problems in Diagnosis

Perhaps the biggest barrier to diagnosing HIV disease in the elderly is that many physicians still don't suspect, never mind test for, HIV in older patients, resulting in delayed diagnosis and treatment and sometimes premature death. Physicians should not make the mistake of assuming that older adults—single, married, or widowed—are not sexually active or that they are heterosexual, monogamous, or using recommended measures to prevent infection with HIV. They should always consider the possibility of infection in the older population, recommend safer sex precautions, and test at-risk elders for HIV. Remember, too, that IV drug abuse does occur in older adults.

Early possible signs of immunosuppression that are frequently overlooked or mistakenly attributed to aging include thrush and skin problems—especially seborrheic dermatitis, herpes zoster, and recurrent herpes simplex virus type 2 (HSV-2)—in a person who doesn't have a history of it. HSV-2 is most commonly associated with skin lesions in the anogenital area. Recurrent episodes may be accompanied by less typical findings such as redness of the skin, cutaneous discomfort or burning, or dysuria. When HIV disease isn't recognized and treated, the most typical OIs are *Pneumocystis carinii* pneumonia (PCP) and recurrent bacterial pneumonia, cytomegalovirus, and Mycobacterium tuberculosis or *Mycobacterium avium* complex (also known as MAC). In a recent study, higher mortality in older patients with AIDS was associated with increased severity of illness at presentation, underrecognition of HIV infection by physicians, and delay in initiating therapy for.[4]

Even though the initial manifestations of HIV disease are the same in all age groups, older patients are often farther along in the disease process when first seen. Although the patient may have waited too long to see a doctor out of fear, ignorance, or denial, physicians are still unlikely to think first of AIDS even when older patients present with more serious AIDS-related conditions like PCP. Elderly persons with undiagnosed HIV disease often have nonspecific signs and symptoms, such as weight loss, fatigue, and diminished physical and mental capabilities. These can be caused by diseases other than HIV infection—malignancy or depression, for instance— or considered an inevitable part of growing.[2] PCP can look like a bacterial pneumonia, bronchitis, or congestive heart failure. Or, because heart failure has already been diagnosed, no underlying cause, like HIV, is ever looked for.

Mild cognitive dysfunction may be assumed to be a result of Alzheimer's disease and not a manifestation of early HIV encephalopathy. AIDS-related dementia progresses more rapidly (over months) than Alzheimer's disease and is more often associated with motor symptoms, gait disorders, peripheral neuropathies, myelopathies, and general physical complaints (mild headache, weight loss, fatigue). Other relatively common neurologic processes overlooked in older HIV patients include opportunistic CNS infections—especially cryptococcal meningitis and toxoplasmosis—and primary brain lymphoma. Eventually, but only after much wasted time, effort, and money, AIDS may be finally diagnosed through a process of elimination. By then the patient often has more serious complications and is close to death, or has already died.

In terms of disease progression, HIV is a virulent pathogen in people of all ages. But, as with almost all viral or bacterial diseases, clinical deterioration is more rapid among older HIV-infected patients than younger ones. And, like other infections in the elderly, HIV is more difficult to diagnose, more severe, and more difficult to treat; has a more rapid progression; and more frequently leads to death.[5] The rate of progression of the illness is dependent on the rate of loss of the CD4 cell population.[6] Older HIV-infected patients lose these cells at a faster rate than do younger patients; therefore the span of time from diagnosis to death is often much shorter.[5]

Problems in Treatment

It's not yet clear which treatment options for older people with AIDS produce the best outcomes. No studies have specifically considered the safety or effectiveness of antiretroviral agents in this population. For now, older patients should be placed on the same retroviral therapy regimens as younger patients.[7] What is known is that older patients have more comorbid illness and are more vulnerable to drug toxicities and interactions than younger patients. This can be problematic in the age of protease inhibitors, when single drug regimens are no longer recommended, drug interactions are common, and dose reduction is often associated with the development of viral resistance.[8]

Since decreased hepatic function is often a natural consequence of aging—one that makes patients more susceptible to toxic hepatic effects—treating multiple diseases with multiple medications, especially while also giving protease inhibitors, can be extremely difficult. Careful monitoring of drug levels is necessary for those taking many of the drugs typically prescribed for older patients, including anticoagulants, antiarrhythmics, anticonvulsants, GI stimulants, benzodiazepines, and tricyclic antidepressants.

There are other indications that treatment and care can be difficult for older people with AIDS. Many patients are less able to comply with antiretroviral therapy. The reasons may include concomitant diseases of aging, poverty, memory failure, and health beliefs that favor the use of nontraditional medications. Increased compliance is seen, however, when there is no history of IV drug use, the older patient is not severely depressed, and the clinical team makes adherence education a care priority.[9]

Long-term protease inhibitor therapy has been associated with hyperlipidemia (particularly hypertriglyceridemia), hyperglycemia, and insulin resistance—a problem that has particular significance in the elderly, for whom control of lipid and glucose levels is often a significant concern. Treatment-induced diabetes mellitus has also been reported, although most patients have a mild hyperglycemia not requiring treatment.

According to *The Geneva Report* from this year's 12th World AIDS Conference, patients who are candidates for protease inhibitors should be warned of these potential side effects and appropriate risk assessment should be made for both diabetes and cardiovascular disease. There are no existing guidelines for monitoring, but some authorities have suggested obtaining baseline glucose, cholesterol, and triglyceride levels with repeat determinations at 3- to 4-month intervals during the first year of treatment. Suggested interventions include dietary modification and lipid-lowering drugs, but the preliminary data on response to these interventions have not been impressive. Measuring glucose tolerance routinely in an attempt to diagnose diabetes is not recommended.[10]

Several distinct and possibly related clinical syndromes have been observed in those taking protease inhibitors, including peripheral lipodystrophy (loss of subcutaneous fat tissue in the face and extremities), with and without increased abdominal girth, and dorsocervical fat pad enlargement, or buffalo hump.[10] Although these physical changes appear to be only cosmetic, the cause remains obscure.

Psychosocial and Emotional Issues

In persons of every age group, living with AIDS complicates various aspects of social support and care. Most of these patients must rely on supportive and personal care services provided at home or in other residential settings. For the majority of those in need, such services remain in short supply, unless the person is resourceful and prosperous enough to locate and purchase care privately. To add to the burden for older patients, Medicare does not cover the necessary medications used for AIDS treatment; so patients are dependent on whatever subsidized support or charity they might be able to find. And, according to many specialists, some health care facilities, especially nursing homes, deny services to those bearing the stigma of AIDS on the grounds that they are not equipped to deal with the disease—even when having appropriate health care coverage is not the issue.

Older adults may also find that the services offered to persons with HIV disease are aimed at younger populations and that providers of these services are not knowledgeable about the specific needs of older patients. And, many services available through the aging network may not have staff knowledgeable in the emotional and psychosocial issues affecting persons with HIV.

Many older AIDS patients live alone or rely for care upon persons who also are old and vulnerable to illness and dependency, such as partners who may themselves have HIV disease. In the older population in general, almost all patients primarily depend on an informal network of relatives and friends to provide help with eating, bathing, shopping, and so on. The burden on informal caregivers can be considerable, and the quality of care for the sick person may be poor and/or inconsistent.

Although having HIV/AIDS is probably always humiliating and unnerving, it seems especially so for older adults. They may perceive the disease as punishment for some action taken many years ago that they are ashamed to divulge or explain. Entire families have to deal with finding out that a parent, partner, or spouse is or was an IV drug user, a bisexual or homosexual, or unfaithful or promiscuous. Psychological counseling for everyone involved is highly recommended. And, referring the patient to an AIDS support group can really help to destigmatize the problem.

Some older gay men who are surviving longer because of antiretroviral therapy are suffering from survivor's guilt because they have outlived so many friends and partners with the same disease. As AIDS becomes a chronic condition, younger gay men may be spared these feelings. Many infected older gay men assumed they wouldn't live to old age and have spent pensions and savings and lost a foothold in the workplace. Treatments have continued to improve, so they now face unexpected potentially productive years unprepared—financially, psychologically, and spiritually. Instead of preparing to die they need to prepare to continue living.

HIV/AIDS Awareness

Even though the majority of AIDS cases in older Americans are a result of the sexual transmission of HIV, sexual behavior in general, not to mention risky sexual behavior, has been virtually ignored in studies of HIV/AIDS within this age group. The bulk of the research examines dementia or other OIs as they manifest themselves in the aging population.

Many older people are repeatedly putting themselves at significant risk of becoming infected with HIV. In the one behavioral study that has been done, the prevalence of having at least 1 risk factor for HIV infection was about 10% among Americans aged 50 or older. Very small proportions of Americans older than 50 with a known behavioral risk for HIV infection used condoms during sexual intercourse or had ever undergone HIV testing.[2]

CDC data show that the percentages of persons older than 50 with AIDS whose transmission risk category is unidentified are increasing. Of those 50 to 54 years old, 10% have no identifiable risk factor at the time of AIDS diagnosis. This figure increases to 12% in those 55 to 59 years old and to 17% in those 65 and older. These numbers indicate that many older adults with HIV are unaware of when or how they were infected or are reluctant to provide this information because of stigma or some other reason.

A sexual history and a drug history should always be a part of the routine background discussion with all patients, especially since heterosexual contact has become the most likely mode of transmission of HIV in this population. It is sexual behavior that determines sexual risk for HIV, not sexual identity, so it is essential to let patients know that you're open to anything that they need to tell you. Physicians should ask specific questions about the gender and number of partners, use of condoms, history of sexually transmitted diseases (STDs), and history of blood transfusions or intravenous drug use. Ask open-ended questions:

- Are you sexually active?

- Are you sexually active with men, women, or both?

- Is your sexual activity limited to your marital relationship or not?

- Are you or have you ever been involved in using IV drugs?

- Have you ever had a sexually transmitted disease?

- Have you ever been sexually active with anyone you know to be or who has been an IV drug user?

- Have you ever had a blood transfusion or received any other blood products?

Counseling is vitally needed for older patients about HIV risk in general and condom use in particular. It is as important to dispel the myths about HIV/AIDS as it is to educate on safer sex. Explain that AIDS is not transmitted by the following:

- Nonsexual contact with infected people

- Clothes, drinking fountains, phones, or toilet seats

- Foods prepared by an infected person

- Mosquito bites, bedbugs, lice, flies, or other insects

- Contact with sweat, saliva, or tears

- Becoming a blood donor.

Increasing the effectiveness of prevention programs for older women who are at risk of HIV infection will also need to involve greater consideration of the distinct characteristics of this age group. For example, older women with heterosexually acquired AIDS were less likely than younger women to have used condoms before they learned of their infection.[2] Negotiating condom use with partners or discussing HIV risk behaviors with health care providers may be especially difficult for women who grew up in a time when sexual matters were not openly discussed. In a study of the characteristics of women aged 50 or older with heterosexually acquired AIDS, these women reported less noninjection drug use (including crack) and fewer sex partners, and they were less likely to have a history of an STD.[13] Thus, if older women go less often to drug or STD clinics that routinely offer HIV counseling and testing, they may be less likely to perceive risk and may have fewer opportunities for access to HIV information.

References

1. El-Sadr, W.; Gettler, J. Unrecognized human immunodeficiency virus infection in the elderly. *Arch Intern Med.* 1995:155:184-186.

2. Stall, R.; Catania, J. AIDS risk behaviors among late middle-aged and elderly Americans: the national AIDS behavioral surveys. *Arch Intern Med.* 1994:154: 57-53.

3. Centers for Disease Control and Prevention. AIDS among persons aged greater than or equal to 50 years—United States, 1991-1996. *MMWR Morb Mortal Wkly Rep.* 1998:47(2): 21-27.

4. Keitz, S.A.; Bastian, L.A.; Bennett, C.L., et al. AIDS-related *Pneumocystis carinii* pneumonia in older patients. *J Gen Intern Med.* 1996:11:591-595.

5. Adler, W.H.; Regal, J.E. Acquired immunodeficiency syndrome in the elderly. *Drugs Aging.* 1994;4:41 0-416.

6. Chen, H.X.; Ryan, P.A.; Ferguson, R.P., et al. Characteristics of acquired immunodeficiency syndrome in older adults: *J Am Geriatr Soc.* 1998:46:153-156.

7. Carpenter, C.C.J.; Fischl, M.A.; Hammer, S.M., et al. Antiretroviral therapy for HIV infection in 1996: recommendations of an international panel. *JAMA.* 1996:276: 146-154.

8. Singh, N.; Squler, C.; Sleek, C., et al. Determinants of compliance with antiretroviral therapy in patients with human immunodeficiency virus: prospective assessment with implications for enhancing compliance. *AIDS Care.* 1996:8:261-269.

9. Volberding, P.A.; Deeks, S.G., Antiretroviral therapy for HIV infection., *JAMA.* 1998; 279:1343-1344.

10. Highlights from Geneva: Conference News at a Glance. Available at http://www.hopkins-aids.edu/geneva/hilites_bart.html#lypod. Accessed, August 19,1998.

11. Centers for Disease Control and Prevention. *HIV/AIDS Surveillance Report*, year end edition. 1995.

12. Feldman, M.D., Sex, AIDS, and the elderly. *Arch Intern Med.* 1994:154:19- 20.

13.   Schable, B.; Chu, S.Y.; Diaz, T., Characteristics of women SD years of age or older with heterosexually-acquired AIDS. *Am J Public Health*. 1996:86:1616-1618.

Resources on HIV/AIDS

The following organizations and Web sites contain information specifically related to HIV/AIDS and aging.

AIDS Education Global Information System
http://www.aegis.com

American Association of Retired Persons (AARP)
http://www.aarp.org

Center for AIDS Prevention Studies
http://chanane.ucsf.edu/capsweb

CDC National AIDS Clearinghouse (CDC NAC)
(Reference Department)
(800) 458-5231
http://www.cdcnpin.org

Fenway Community Health Center (Boston)
http://www.fchc.org

Gay and Lesbian Medical Association
(415) 255-4547
http://www.glma.org

Gay and Lesbian National Hotline
(888) 843-4564

Gayellow Pages—Youth, Family & Senior Resources
http://gayellowpages.com/webfam.htm

HIV/AIDS Treatment Information Service (ATIS)
(800) 448-0440
http://www.hivatis.org

Lesbian and Gay Aging Issues Network of the American Society on Aging (ASA)
http://www.asaging.org/lgain.html

National Association of HIV Over 50
http://www.hivoverfifty.org

National Institute on Aging
http://www.nih.gov/nia

Senior Action in a Gay Environment (SAGE)
(212) 741-2247
http://www.sageusa.org

Sexuality Information and Education Council of the United States
(SIECUS)
(212) 819-9770
http://www.siecus.org/library

Section 15.6

AIDS in Infants and Children

2000 National Institute of Allergy and Infectious Diseases (NIAID).

The National Institute of Allergy and Infectious Diseases (NIAID)
has a lead role in research devoted to children infected with the human immunodeficiency virus (HIV), the virus that causes the acquired
immunodeficiency syndrome (AIDS).

NIAID-supported researchers are developing and refining treatments to prolong the survival and improve the quality of life of HIV-infected infants and children. Many promising therapies are being
tested in the Pediatric AIDS Clinical Trials Group (ACTG), a nationwide clinical trials network jointly sponsored by NIAID and the National Institute of Child Health and Human Development (NICHD).
Scientists also are improving tests for diagnosing HIV infection in
infants soon after birth so that therapy can begin as soon as possible.

Epidemiologic studies are examining risk factors for transmission
as well as the course of HIV disease in pregnant women and their
babies in an era of antiretroviral therapy. Researchers have helped
illuminate the mechanisms of HIV transmission as well as the distinct features of pediatric HIV infection and how the course of disease and the usefulness of therapies can differ in children and adults.

Researchers also are studying ways to prevent transmission of HIV
from mother to infant. Notably, Pediatric ACTG investigators have

demonstrated that a specific regimen of zidovudine (AZT) treatment, given to an HIV-infected woman during pregnancy and to her baby after birth, can reduce maternal transmission of HIV by two-thirds.[1] Many consider this finding to be one of the most significant research advances to date in the fight against HIV and AIDS.

A Global Problem

According to UNAIDS (The Joint United Nations Programme on HIV/AIDS) and the World Health Organization (WHO),[2,3] at the end of 1998, an estimated 1.2 million children worldwide under age 15 were living with HIV/AIDS. Approximately 3.2 million children under 15 had died from the virus or associated causes. The number of children who had lived with HIV from the start of the epidemic through 1997 was estimated to be 3.8 million. As HIV infection rates rise in the general population, new infections are increasingly concentrating in younger age groups.

Statistics for the year 1998 alone show that:

- 590,000 children under age 15 were newly infected with HIV.

- One-tenth of all new HIV infections were in children under age 15.

- Approximately 7,000 young people aged 10 to 24 became infected with HIV every day-that is, five each minute.

- Nine out of 10 new infections in children under 15 were in sub-Saharan Africa.

- An estimated 510,000 children under 15 died of AIDS-related causes, up from 460,000 in 1997.

More than 95 percent of all HIV-infected people now live in developing countries, which have also suffered 95 percent of all deaths from AIDS. In countries with the longest-lived AIDS epidemics, some doctors report that children ill from HIV occupy three-quarters of pediatric hospital beds, and childrens' life expectancy has been shortened dramatically. In Botswana, for example, because of AIDS, the life expectancy of children born early in the next decade is just over age 40; without AIDS, it would have been 70. In Namibia, the infant mortality rate is expected to reach 72 deaths per 1000, up from a non-AIDS rate of 45 per 1000.

The United States has a relatively small percentage of the world's children living with HIV/AIDS. From the beginning of the epidemic through the end of 1998, 5,237 American children under age 13 had been reported to the Centers for Disease Control and Prevention (CDC) as living with HIV/AIDS.[4] Three hundred eighty-two cases of pediatric AIDS were reported in 1998.[5] There are many more children who are infected with HIV but have not yet developed AIDS. Half of all new HIV infections reported to the CDC have been in people younger than 25.6. One encouraging fact is that the number of pediatric AIDS cases estimated by the CDC fell by two-thirds from 1992 to 1997 (947 to 310 cases).[7]

The U.S. cities that had the five highest rates of pediatric AIDS during 1998 were New York City; Miami, Florida; Newark, New Jersey; Washington, D.C.; and San Juan, Puerto Rico.[8] The disease disproportionately affects children in minority groups, especially African Americans.[9] Out of 8,461 cases in children under 13 reported to the CDC through December 1998, 58 percent were in blacks/not-Hispanic, 23 percent were in Hispanics, 17.5 percent were in whites/not-Hispanic, and 5.33 percent were in other minority groups.[10]

According to 1996 data, the latest available, HIV infection was the seventh leading cause of death for U.S. children through 14 years of age.[11] However, the CDC reported a drop of 56 percent from 1994 to 1997 in the estimated number of children who died from AIDS.[12] New anti-HIV drug therapies and promotion of voluntary testing are having a major impact.

Transmission

Almost all HIV-infected children acquire the virus from their mothers before or during birth or through breast-feeding. In the United States, approximately 25 percent of pregnant HIV-infected women not receiving AZT therapy have passed on the virus to their babies. The rate is higher in developing countries.

Most mother-to-child transmission, estimated to cause over 90 percent of infections worldwide in infants and children,[13,14] probably occurs late in pregnancy or during birth. Although the precise mechanisms are unknown, scientists think HIV may be transmitted when maternal blood enters the fetal circulation, or by mucosal exposure to virus during labor and delivery. The role of the placenta in maternal-fetal transmission is unclear and the focus of ongoing research.

The risk of maternal-infant transmission (MIT) is significantly increased if the mother has advanced HIV disease, increased levels of HIV in her bloodstream, or fewer numbers of the immune system cells—CD4+ T cells—that are the main targets of HIV.

Other factors that may increase the risk are maternal drug use, severe inflammation of fetal membranes, or a prolonged period between membrane rupture and delivery. A study sponsored by NIAID and others found that HIV-infected women who gave birth more than four hours after the rupture of the fetal membranes were nearly twice as likely to transmit HIV to their infants, as compared to women who delivered within four hours of membrane rupture.[15]

HIV also may be transmitted from a nursing mother to her infant. Studies have suggested that breast-feeding introduces an additional risk of HIV transmission of approximately 10 to 14 percent among women with chronic HIV infection.[16] In developing countries, an estimated one-third to one-half of all HIV infections are transmitted through breast-feeding.[17] The WHO recommends that all HIV-infected women be advised as to both the risks and benefits of breast-feeding of their infants so that they can make informed decisions. In countries where safe alternatives to breast-feeding are readily available and economically feasible, this alternative should be encouraged. In general, in developing countries where safe alternatives to breast-feeding are not readily available, the benefits of breast-feeding in terms of decreased illness and death due to other infectious diseases greatly outweigh the potential risk of HIV transmission.

Prior to 1985 when screening of the nation's blood supply for HIV began, some children were infected through transfusions with blood or blood products contaminated with HIV. A small number of children also have been infected through sexual or physical abuse by HIV-infected adults.

Preventing Maternal-Infant Transmission (MIT)

In 1994, a landmark study conducted by the Pediatric ACTG demonstrated that AZT, given to HIV-infected women who had very little or no prior antiretroviral therapy and CD4+ T cell counts above 200/mm3, reduced the risk of MIT by two-thirds, from 25 percent to 8 percent.[18] In the study, known as ACTG 076, AZT therapy was initiated in the second or third trimester and continued during labor, and infants were treated for six weeks following birth. AZT produced no serious side effects in mothers or infants. Long-term follow-up of the infants and mothers is ongoing. Pediatric ACTG protocol 185 tested an AZT regimen and was reported in 1999 to have lowered MIT to about 5 percent.[19] Combination therapies have been shown to be beneficial in the treatment of HIV-infected adults, and current guidelines have been designed accordingly.[20] In HIV-infected pregnant women, the safety and pharmacology of these potent drug combinations need to be better understood, and NIAID is conducting studies in this area.

Researchers have shown that this AZT regimen has reduced MIT in other populations in which it has been used. Observational studies in the past few years in the United States and Europe indicate that similar reductions can be achieved by using this regimen in regular clinical care settings. In the U.S., the number of MIT-acquired AIDS cases reported to the CDC fell 43 percent from 1992 to 1996, probably because of providing AZT to HIV-infected mothers, better guidelines for prenatal HIV counseling and testing, and changes in obstetrical management.[21,22]

Recent studies have shown that short regimens, too, of AZT can be beneficial in cutting back on MIT. In March 1999, researchers reported on a randomized study in Thailand on the short-term use of AZT during late pregnancy and labor in a group of non-breast-feeding women (the drug was not given to infants). They concluded that the treatment was safe and effective and can reduce the rate of MIT by 50 percent.[23] Another recent study using a short-term AZT regimen (including post-partum) in groups of women in Ivory Coast and Burkina Faso, Africa, while limited, supported this finding.[24]

Following up on the success of ACTG 076, the Pediatric ACTG has begun new HIV prevention trials that build on the AZT regimen. These trials include other antiviral agents and multidrug combinations in an attempt to reduce MIT even more than that achieved by AZT alone. Also, in early 1999, a study sponsored by UNAIDS of a combination regimen of AZT plus lamivudine (3TC) in three African countries showed promising results.[25]

The AZT regimen used in ACTG 076 is not available in much of the world because of its high cost (approximately $1000 per pregnancy, not counting counseling or testing) and logistical demands. The cost of a short-course AZT regimen is substantially lower, but is still prohibitive in many countries. International agencies are studying whether there may be innovative ways to provide AZT at lower cost, e.g., through reductions in drug prices to developing countries, partnerships with industry, etc. NIAID is pursuing a global strategy that assesses whether simpler and less costly regimens to prevent mother-to-infant HIV transmission can be effective in various settings.

In September 1999, an NIAID-funded study (HIVNET 012) demonstrated that short-course therapy with nevirapine lowered the risk of HIV-1 transmission during the first 14-16 weeks of life by nearly 50 percent compared to AZT in a breastfeeding population.[26] This simple, inexpensive regimen offers a potential cost-effective alternative for decreasing mother-to-child transmission in developing countries.[27]

The International Perinatal HIV Group reported in April 1999 that elective caesarean section delivery can help reduce vertical transmission of HIV, though it is not without risk to certain women.[28] When AZT treatment is combined with elective caesarean delivery, a transmission rate of 2 percent has been reported.[29]

Because a significant amount of MIT occurs around the time of birth, and the risk of maternal-fetal transmission depends, in part, on the amount of HIV in the mother's blood, it may be possible to reduce transmission using drug therapy only around the time of birth. NIAID has planned other studies that will assess the effectiveness of this approach as well as the role of new antiretrovirals, microbicides and other innovative strategies in reducing the risk of MIT of HIV.

Diagnosis

HIV infection is often difficult to diagnose in very young children. Infected babies, especially in the first few months of life, often appear normal and may exhibit no telltale signs that would allow a definitive diagnosis of HIV infection. Moreover, all children born to infected mothers have antibodies to HIV, made by the mother's immune system, that cross the placenta to the baby's bloodstream before birth and persist for up to 18 months. Because these maternal antibodies reflect the mother's but not the infant's infection status, the test is not useful in newborns or young infants.

In recent years, investigators have demonstrated the utility of highly accurate blood tests in diagnosing HIV infection in children 6 months of age and younger. One laboratory technique called polymerase chain reaction (PCR) can detect minute quantities of the virus in an infant's blood. Another procedure allows physicians to culture a sample of an infant's blood and test it for the presence of HIV.

Currently, PCR assays or HIV culture techniques can identify at birth about one-third of infants who are truly HIV-infected. With these techniques, approximately 90 percent of HIV-infected infants are identifiable by 2 months of age, and 95 percent by 3 months of age. One innovative new approach to both RNA and DNA PCR testing uses dried blood spot specimens, which should make it much simpler to gather and store specimens in field settings.

Progression of HIV Disease in Children

Researchers have observed two general patterns of illness in HIV-infected children. About 20 percent of children develop serious disease in the first year of life; most of these children die by age 4 years.

The remaining 80 percent of infected children have a slower rate of disease progression, many not developing the most serious symptoms of AIDS until school entry or even adolescence. A recent report from a large European registry of HIV-infected children indicated that half of the children with perinatally acquired HIV disease were alive at age 9. Another study, of 42 perinatally HIV-infected children who survived beyond 9 years of age, found about one-quarter of the children to be asymptomatic with relatively intact immune systems.

The factors responsible for the wide variation observed in the rate of disease progression in HIV-infected children are a major focus of the NIAID pediatric AIDS research effort. The Women and Infants Transmission Study, a multisite perinatal HIV study funded by NIH, has found that maternal factors including Vitamin A level and CD4 counts during pregnancy, as well as infant viral load and CD4 counts in the first several months of life, can help identify those infants at risk for rapid disease progression who may benefit from early aggressive therapy.

Signs and Symptoms of Pediatric HIV Disease

Many children with HIV infection do not gain weight or grow normally. HIV-infected children frequently are slow to reach important milestones in motor skills and mental development such as crawling, walking and speaking. As the disease progresses, many children develop neurologic problems such as difficulty walking, poor school performance, seizures, and other symptoms of HIV encephalopathy.

Like adults with HIV infection, children with HIV develop life-threatening opportunistic infections (OIs), although the incidence of various OIs differs in adults and children. For example, toxoplasmosis is seen less frequently in HIV-infected children than in HIV-infected adults, while serious bacterial infections occur more commonly in children than in adults. Also, as children with HIV become sicker, they may suffer from chronic diarrhea due to opportunistic pathogens.

Pneumocystis carinii pneumonia (PCP) is the leading cause of death in HIV-infected children with AIDS. PCP, as well as cytomegalovirus (CMV) disease, usually are primary infections in children, whereas in adults these diseases result from the reactivation of latent infections.

A lung disease called lymphocytic interstitial pneumonitis (LIP), rarely seen in adults, also occurs frequently in HIV-infected children. This condition, like PCP, can make breathing progressively more difficult and often results in hospitalization.

Children with HIV suffer the usual childhood bacterial infections—only more frequently and more severely than uninfected children. These bacterial infections can cause seizures, fever, pneumonia, recurrent colds, diarrhea, dehydration and other problems that often result in extended hospital stays and nutritional problems.

HIV-infected children frequently have severe candidiasis, a yeast infection that can cause unrelenting diaper rash and infections in the mouth and throat that make eating difficult.

Treatment of HIV-Infected Children

NIAID investigators are defining the best treatments for pediatric patients. Currently there are 16 drug products approved by the FDA for the treatment of adult HIV infection. Through major contributions by the Pediatric ACTG, 10 antiretroviral agents have pediatric label information, including 3 protease inhibitors.[28] While the basic principles that guide treatment of pediatric HIV infection are the same as for any HIV-infected person, there are a number of unique scientific and medical concerns that are important to consider in the treatment of children with HIV infection. These range from differences from adults in age-related issues such as CD4 lymphocyte counts and drug metabolism to requirements for special formulations and treatment regimens that are appropriate for infants through adolescents. As in adults, treatment of HIV-infected children today is a complex task of using potent combinations of antiretroviral agents to maximally suppress viral replication.

Researchers supported by NIAID are focusing not only on the development of new antiretroviral products but also on the critical question of how to best use the treatments that are currently available. Treatment strategy questions designed to identify what the best initial therapy is, when failing regimens should be switched and strategies for how to address the antiretroviral needs of children with advanced disease are examples. Long-term assessment of these children is also a high priority to assess sustained antiretroviral benefits as well as to monitor for potential adverse consequences of treatment.

Problems of Families

A mother and child with HIV usually are not the only family members with the disease. Often, the mother's sexual partner is infected, and other children in the family may be infected as well. Frequently, a parent with AIDS does not survive to care for his or her HIV-infected child.

In the countries hardest hit by the AIDS epidemic, some 8.2 million children under 15 around the world have been orphaned by AIDS—90 percent of them in sub-Saharan Africa alone.[31] The rate is expected to increase. One in three of these orphans is under age five.[32] Communities and extended families are struggling with and often overwhelmed by the vast number of AIDS orphans. Many orphans and other children from families devastated by AIDS face multiple risks, such as forced relocation, violence, living on the streets, drug use, and even commercial sex. Other children suffer because sex education and services are not available to them or do not communicate effectively to them. Living in a country undergoing political turmoil or where fathers migrate for work can also raise the risk of a child becoming HIV-infected.

In the U.S., most children living with HIV/AIDS live in inner cities, where poverty, illicit drug use, poor housing and limited access to and use of medical care and social services add to the challenges of HIV disease.

One encouraging note is that, according to UNAIDS, where information, training, and services to help prevent HIV infection are made available and affordable to young people, they are more likely to make use of them than their elders are.[33]

Management of the complex medical and social problems of families affected by HIV requires a multidisciplinary case management team, integrating medical, social, mental health and educational services. NIAID provides special funding to many of its clinical research sites to provide for services, such as transportation, day care, and the expertise of social workers, crucial to families devastated by HIV.

Resources

Note: The UNAIDS and CDC publications referenced in this article may be viewed on the World Wide Web at http://www.unaids.org/ and http://www.cdc.gov/.

AIDS Clinical Trials Information Service. For information about pediatric and adult AIDS clinical trials open to enrollment, call (800) TRIALS-A, 9 a.m. to 7 p.m. Eastern Time, Monday through Friday. Web: http://www.actis.org/ E-mail: actis@actis.org.

National AIDS Hotline. Staffed 24 hours a day, seven days a week. English Service: 1-800-342-AIDS. Spanish service: 1-800-344-7432. Deaf service (TDD): 1-800-243-7889.

The National Pediatric HIV Resource Center. A non-profit organization that serves professionals who care for children, adolescents and families with HIV infection and AIDS. Phone: 973-972-0410 or toll free: 1-800-362-0071. Web: http://pedhivaids.org/. E-mail: ortegaes@ umdnj.edu.

The Elizabeth Glaser Pediatric AIDS Foundation. A national non-profit organization dedicated exclusively to supporting research for AIDS in children. Phone: 310-314-1459. Web: http://www.pedaids.org/ E-mail: info@ pedaids.org.

The Pediatric Branch of the National Cancer Institute (NCI) conducts clinical trials for HIV-infected children on the NIH campus in Bethesda, Md. Phone: (888) NCI-1937. NCI webpage: http://bethesdatrials.nci. nih.gov.

References

1. Connor, E. et al. 1994. Reduction of maternal-infant transmission of human immunodeficiency virus type 1 with zidovudine treatment. *N Engl J Med* 311:1173-80.

2. UNAIDS. AIDS Epidemic Update (Dec., 1998):1, 2, 3, 7, 8., 9, 17.

3. UNAIDS. Report on the Global HIV/AIDS Epidemic (June, 1998):6, 8.

4. Centers for Disease Control and Prevention. *HIV/AIDS Surveillance Report* (Dec. 1998) 10(2):7.

5. Ibid., p. 26.

6. Rosenberg, P., et al. 1994. Declining age at HIV infection in the United States. *N Engl J Med* 330:789-90.

7. Centers for Disease Control and Prevention, op cit., p. 36.

8. Ibid., pp. 10-11.

9. UNAIDS, Update, p. 6.

10. Centers for Disease Control and Prevention, op. cit., p. 24.

11. Centers for Disease Control and Prevention. National Center for Health Statistics. 1998. *National Vital Statistics Report* 47 (9):26.

12. Centers for Disease Control and Prevention, *HIV/AIDS Surveillance Report*, p. 39.

13. NAIDS, Report.

14. Quinn, T. 1996. Global burden of the HIV pandemic. *Lancet*: 348:99-106.

15. Landesman, S., et al. 1996. Obstetrical factors and the transmission of human immunodeficiency virus type 1 from mother to child. *N Engl J Med* 334: 1617-23.

16. Monitoring the AIDS Pandemic (MAP) Network. 1998. The status and trends of the HIV/AIDS epidemics in the world:17.

17. UNAIDS, Report, p. 48.

18. Connor, E., et al., op. cit.

19. Stiehm, E., et al. 1999. Efficacy of zidovudine and human immunodeficiency virus (HIV) hyperimmune immunoglobulin for reducing perinatal HIV transmission from HIV-infected women with advanced disease: results of Pediatric ACTG protocol 185. *J Infect Dis* 179(3):567-75.

20. Centers for Disease Control and Prevention. 1998. Public Health Service Task Force recommendations for the use of antiretroviral drugs in pregnant women infected with HIV-1 for maternal health and for reducing perinatal HIV-1 transmission in the United States. *MMWR* Recommendations and Reports 47 (RR-2). May be viewed on the Web at http://www.hivatis.org/.

21. Wilfert, C., et al. 1999. Consensus statement: Science, ethics, and the future of research into maternal infant transmission of HIV-1. *Lancet* 353 (9155):832-35.

22. Centers for Disease Control and Prevention. 1997. Update: Perinatally acquired HIV/AIDS-United States, 1997. *MMWR* 46: 1086-92.

23. Shaffer, N., et al. 1999. Short-course zidovudine for perinatal HIV-1 transmission in Bangkok, Thailand: A randomized controlled trial. *Lancet* 353 (9155):773-79.

24. Dabis, F. et al. 1999. 6-month efficacy, tolerance, and acceptability of a short regimen of oral zidovudine to reduce vertical

transmission of HIV in breastfed children in Cote d'Ivoire and Burkina Faso. *Lancet* 353 (9155):786-92.

25. Saba, J., The PETRA Trial Study Team. 1999. Interim analysis of early efficacy of three short course ZDV/3TC combination regimens to prevent mother-to-child transmission of HIV-1. Presented at the Sixth Conference on Retroviruses and Opportunistic Infections. Chicago: February 1, 1999.

26. Guay, L, et al. 1999. Intrapartum and neonatal single-dose nevirapine compared with zidovudine for prevention of mother-to-child transmission of HIV-1 in Kampala, Uganda: HIVNET 012 randomized trial. *Lancet* 354:795-802.

27. Marseille, E., et al. 1999. Cost effectiveness of single-dose nevirapine regimen for mothers and babies to decrease vertical HIV-1 transmission in sub-Saharan Africa. *Lancet* 654:803-09.

28. Riley, L.E. and Green, M.F. Elective caesarean delivery to reduce the transmission of HIV. 1999. *N Engl J Med* 340:13, 1032.

29. Mofenson, L.M., Fowler, M.G. In press. Interruption of materno-fetal transmission. Reported in Shaffer, N., op. cit.

30. HIV/AIDS Treatment Information Service. 1999. Guidelines for the use of antiretroviral agents in pediatric HIV infection. May be viewed on the Web at http://www.hivatis.org/.

31. UNAIDS, Report, p. 9.

32. Centers for Disease Control and Prevention. National Center for HIV, STD, and TB Prevention. Divisions of HIV/AIDS. International Projections/Statistics. Web: http://www.cdc.gov/nchstp/hiv_aids/stats/internat.htm

33. UNAIDS, Update, p. 9.

Chapter 16

Human Papillomavirus (HPV)

Chapter Contents

Section 16.1

Human Papillomavirus Infection

1998 Centers for Disease Control (CDC), excerpted from
"1998 Guidelines for Treatment of Sexually Transmitted Disease,"
MMWR 1998, 47(NO.RR-1), 1-118.

Genital Warts

More than 20 types of HPV can infect the genital tract. Most HPV infections are asymptomatic, subclinical, or unrecognized. Visible genital warts usually are caused by HPV types 6 or 11. Other HPV types in the anogenital region (i.e., types 16, 18, 31, 33, and 35) have been strongly associated with cervical dysplasia. Diagnosis of genital warts can be confirmed by biopsy, although biopsy is rarely needed (e.g., if the diagnosis is uncertain; the lesions do not respond to standard therapy; the disease worsens during therapy; the patient is immunocompromised; or warts are pigmented, indurated, fixed, and ulcerated). No data support the use of type-specific HPV nucleic acid tests in the routine diagnosis or management of visible genital warts.

HPV types 6 and 11 also can cause warts on the uterine cervix and in the vagina, urethra, and anus; these warts are sometimes symptomatic. Intra-anal warts are seen predominately in patients who have had receptive anal intercourse; these warts are distinct from perianal warts, which can occur in men and women who do not have a history of anal sex. Other than the genital area, these HPV types have been associated with conjunctival, nasal, oral, and laryngeal warts. HPV types 6 and 11 are associated rarely with invasive squamous cell carcinoma of the external genitalia. Depending on the size and anatomic locations, genital warts can be painful, friable, and/or pruritic.

HPV types 16, 18, 31, 33, and 35 are found occasionally in visible genital warts and have been associated with external genital (i.e., vulvar, penile, and anal) squamous intraepithelial neoplasia (i.e., squamous cell carcinoma in situ, bowen-oid papulosis, Erythroplasia of Queyrat, or Bowen's disease of the genitalia). These HPV types have been associated with vaginal, anal, and cervical intraepithelial dysplasia and squamous cell carcinoma. Patients who have visible genital warts can be infected simultaneously with multiple HPV types.

Treatment

The primary goal of treating visible genital warts is the removal of symptomatic warts. Treatment can induce wart-free periods in most patients. Genital warts often are asymptomatic. No evidence indicates that currently available treatments eradicate or affect the natural history of HPV infection. The removal of warts may or may not decrease infectivity. If left untreated, visible genital warts may resolve on their own, remain unchanged, or increase in size or number. No evidence indicates that treatment of visible warts affects the development of cervical cancer.

Regimens

Treatment of genital warts should be guided by the preference of the patient, the available resources, and the experience of the health-care provider. None of the available treatments is superior to other treatments, and no single treatment is ideal for all patients or all warts.

The available treatments for visible genital warts are patient-applied therapies (i.e., podofilox and imiquimod) and provider-administered therapies (i.e., cryotherapy, podophyllin resin, trichloroacetic acid {TCA}, bichloroacetic acid {BCA}, interferon, and surgery). Most patients have from one to 10 genital warts, with a total wart area of 0.5-1.0 cm2, that are responsive to most treatment modalities. Factors that might influence selection of treatment include wart size, wart number, anatomic site of wart, wart morphology, patient preference, cost of treatment, convenience, adverse effects, and provider experience. Having a treatment plan or protocol is important, because many patients will require a course of therapy rather than a single treatment. In general, warts located on moist surfaces and/or in intertriginous areas respond better to topical treatment (e.g., TCA, podophyllin, podofilox, and imiquimod) than do warts on drier surfaces.

The treatment modality should be changed if a patient has not improved substantially after three provider-administered treatments or if warts have not completely cleared after six treatments. The risk-benefit ratio of treatment should be evaluated throughout the course of therapy to avoid overtreatment. Providers should be knowledgeable about, and have available to them, at least one patient-applied and one provider-administered treatment.

Complications rarely occur if treatments for warts are employed properly. Patients should be warned that scarring in the form of persistent hypopigmentation or hyperpigmentation is common with ablative modalities. Depressed or hypertrophic scars are rare but can occur, especially if the patient has had insufficient time to heal between treatments. Treatment can result rarely in disabling chronic pain syndromes (e.g., vulvodynia or hyperesthesia of the treatment site).

External Genital Warts, Recommended Treatments

Patient-Applied

Podofilox 0.5% solution or gel. Patients may apply podofilox solution with a cotton swab, or podofilox gel with a finger, to visible genital warts twice a day for 3 days, followed by 4 days of no therapy. This cycle may be repeated as necessary for a total of four cycles. The total wart area treated should not exceed 10 cm2, and a total volume of podofilox should not exceed 0.5 mL per day. If possible, the healthcare provider should apply the initial treatment to demonstrate the proper application technique and identify which warts should be treated. The safety of podofilox during pregnancy has not been established.

OR

Imiquimod 5% cream. Patients should apply imiquimod cream with a finger at bedtime, three times a week for as long as 16 weeks. The treatment area should be washed with mild soap and water 6-10 hours after the application. Many patients may be clear of warts by 8-10 weeks or sooner. The safety of imiquimod during pregnancy has not been established.

Provider-Administered

Cryotherapy with liquid nitrogen or cryoprobe. Repeat applications every 1 to 2 weeks.

OR

Podophyllin resin 10%-25% in compound tincture of benzoin. A small amount should be applied to each wart and allowed to air dry. To avoid the possibility of complications associated with systemic absorption and toxicity, some experts recommend that application be limited to less than or equal to 0.5 mL of podophyllin or less than or equal to 10 cm2 of warts per session. Some experts suggest that the preparation should be thoroughly washed off 1-4 hours after application to reduce local irritation. Repeat weekly if necessary. The safety of podophyllin during pregnancy has not been established.

OR

TCA or BCA 80%-90%. Apply a small amount only to warts and allow to dry, at which time a white "frosting" develops; powder with talc or sodium bicarbonate (i.e., baking soda) to remove unreacted acid if an excess amount is applied. Repeat weekly if necessary.

OR

Surgical removal either by tangential scissor excision, tangential shave excision, curettage, or electrosurgery.

External Genital Warts, Alternative Treatments

Intralesional interferon or laser surgery. For patient-applied treatments, patients must be able to identify and reach warts to be treated. Podofilox 0.5% solution or gel is relatively inexpensive, easy to use, safe, and self-applied by patients. Podofilox is an antimitotic drug that results in destruction of warts. Most patients experience mild/moderate pain or local irritation after treatment. Imiquimod is a topically active immune enhancer that stimulates production of interferon and other cytokines. Before wart resolution, local inflammatory reactions are common; these reactions usually are mild to moderate.

Cryotherapy, which requires the use of basic equipment, destroys warts by thermal-induced cytolysis. Its major drawback is that proper use requires substantial training, without which warts are frequently overtreated or undertreated, resulting in poor efficacy or increased likelihood of complications. Pain after application of the liquid nitrogen, followed by necrosis and sometimes blistering, are not unusual. Although local anesthesia (topical or injected) is not used routinely, its use facilitates treatment if there are many warts or if the area of warts is large.

Podophyllin resin contains a number of compounds, including the podophyllin lignans that are antimitotic. The resin is most frequently compounded at 10%-25% in tincture of benzoin. However, podophyllin resin preparations differ in the concentration of active components and contaminants. The shelf life and stability of podophyllin preparations are unknown. It is important to apply a thin layer of podophyllin resin to the warts and allow it to air dry before the treated area comes into contact with clothing. Overapplication or failure to air dry can result in local irritation caused by spread of the compound to adjacent areas.

Both TCA and BCA are caustic agents that destroy warts by chemical coagulation of the proteins. Although these preparations are widely used, they have not been investigated thoroughly. TCA solutions have a low viscosity comparable to water and can spread rapidly if applied excessively, thus damaging adjacent normal tissue. Both TCA and BCA should be applied sparingly and allowed to dry before the patient sits or stands. If pain is intense, the acid can be neutralized with soap or sodium bicarbonate (i.e., baking soda).

Surgical removal of warts has an advantage over other treatment modalities in that it renders the patient wart-free, usually with a single visit. However, substantial clinical training, additional equipment, and a longer office visit are required. Once local anesthesia is achieved, the visible genital warts can be physically destroyed by electrosurgery, in which case no additional hemostasis is required. Alternatively, the warts can be removed either by tangential excision with a pair of fine scissors or a scalpel or by curettage. Because most warts are exophytic, this can be accomplished with a resulting wound that only extends into the upper dermis. Hemostasis can be achieved with an electrosurgical unit or a chemical styptic (e.g., an aluminum chloride solution). Suturing is neither required nor indicated in most cases when surgical removal is done properly. Surgery is most beneficial for patients who have a large number or area of genital warts. Carbon dioxide laser and surgery may be useful in the management of extensive warts or intraurethral warts, particularly for those patients who have not responded to other treatments.

Interferons, either natural or recombinant, used for the treatment of genital warts have been administered systemically (i.e., subcutaneously at a distant site or IM) and intralesionally (i.e., injected into the warts). Systemic interferon is not effective. The efficacy and recurrence rates of intralesional interferon are comparable to other treatment modalities. Interferon is believed to be effective because of antiviral and/or immunostimulating effects. However, interferon therapy is not recommended for routine use because of inconvenient routes of administration, frequent office visits, and the association between its use and a high frequency of systemic adverse effects.

Because of the shortcomings of available treatments, some clinics employ combination therapy (i.e., the simultaneous use of two or more modalities on the same wart at the same time). Most experts believe that combining modalities does not increase efficacy but may increase complications.

Cervical Warts

For women who have exophytic cervical warts, high-grade squamous intraepithelial lesions (SIL) must be excluded before treatment is begun. Management of exophytic cervical warts should include consultation with an expert.

Vaginal Warts

Cryotherapy with liquid nitrogen. The use of a cryoprobe in the vagina is not recommended because of the risk for vaginal perforation and fistula formation.

OR

TCA or BCA 80%-90% applied only to warts. Apply a small amount only to warts and allow to dry, at which time a white "frosting" develops; powder with talc or sodium bicarbonate (i.e., baking soda) to remove unreacted acid if an excess amount is applied. Repeat weekly if necessary.

OR

Podophyllin 10%-25% in compound tincture of benzoin applied to a treated area that must be dry before the speculum is removed. Treat with less than or equal to 2 cm2 per session. Repeat application at weekly intervals. Because of concern about potential systemic absorption, some experts caution against vaginal application of podophyllin. The safety of podophyllin during pregnancy has not been established.

Urethral Meatus Warts

Cryotherapy with liquid nitrogen.

OR

Podophyllin 10%-25% in compound tincture of benzoin. The treatment area must be dry before contact with normal mucosa. Podophyllin must be applied weekly if necessary. The safety of podophyllin during pregnancy has not been established.

Anal Warts

Cryotherapy with liquid nitrogen.

OR

TCA or BCA 80%-90% applied to warts. Apply a small amount only to warts and allow to dry, at which time a white "frosting" develops; powder with talc or sodium bicarbonate (i.e., baking soda) to remove unreacted acid if an excess amount is applied. Repeat weekly if necessary.

OR

Surgical removal.
Note: Management of warts on rectal mucosa should be referred to an expert.

Oral Warts

Cryotherapy with liquid nitrogen.

OR

Surgical removal.

Follow-Up

After visible genital warts have cleared, a follow-up evaluation is not mandatory. Patients should be cautioned to watch for recurrences, which occur most frequently during the first 3 months. Because the sensitivity and specificity of self-diagnosis of genital warts is unknown, patients concerned about recurrences should be offered a follow-up evaluation 3 months after treatment. Earlier follow-up visits also may be useful a) to document a wart-free state, b) to monitor for or treat complications of therapy, and c) to provide the opportunity for patient education and counseling. Women should be counseled regarding the need for regular cytologic screening as recommended for women without genital warts. The presence of genital warts is not an indication for cervical colposcopy.

Management of Sex Partners

Examination of sex partners is not necessary for the management of genital warts because the role of reinfection is probably minimal and, in the absence of curative therapy, treatment to reduce transmission is not realistic. However, because self- or partner-examination has not been evaluated as a diagnostic method for genital warts, sex partners of patients who have genital warts may benefit from examination to assess the presence of genital warts and other STDs. Sex partners also might benefit from counseling about the implications of having a partner who has genital warts.

Because treatment of genital warts probably does not eliminate the HPV infection, patients and sex partners should be cautioned that the patient might remain infectious even though the warts are gone. The use of condoms may reduce, but does not eliminate, the risk for transmission to uninfected partners. Female sex partners of patients who have genital warts should be reminded that cytologic screening for cervical cancer is recommended for all sexually active women.

Special Considerations

Pregnancy

Imiquimod, podophyllin, and podofilox should not be used during pregnancy. Because genital warts can proliferate and become friable during pregnancy, many experts advocate their removal during pregnancy. HPV types 6 and 11 can cause laryngeal papillomatosis in infants and children. The route of transmission (i.e., transplacental, perinatal, or postnatal) is not completely understood.

The preventive value of cesarean section is unknown; thus, cesarean delivery should not be performed solely to prevent transmission of HPV infection to the newborn. In rare instances, cesarean delivery may be indicated for women with genital warts if the pelvic outlet is obstructed or if vaginal delivery would result in excessive bleeding.

Immunosuppressed Patients

Persons who are immunosuppressed because of HIV or other reasons may not respond as well as immunocompetent persons to therapy for genital warts, and they may have more frequent recurrences after treatment. Squamous cell carcinomas arising in or resembling genital warts might occur more frequently among immunosuppressed persons, requiring more frequent biopsy for confirmation of diagnosis.

Squamous Cell Carcinoma In Situ

Patients in whom squamous cell carcinoma in situ of the genitalia is diagnosed should be referred to an expert for treatment. Ablative modalities usually are effective, but careful follow-up is important. The risk for these lesions leading to invasive squamous cell carcinoma of the external genitalia in immunocompetent patients is unknown but is probably low. Female partners of patients who have squamous cell carcinoma in situ are at high risk for cervical abnormalities.

Subclinical Genital HPV Infection (Without Exophytic Warts)

Subclinical genital HPV infection occurs more frequently than visible genital warts among both men and women. Infection often is indirectly diagnosed on the cervix by Pap smear, colposcopy, or biopsy and on the penis, vulva, and other genital skin by the appearance of white areas after application of acetic acid. However, the routine use of acetic acid soaks and examination with light and magnification, as a screening test, to detect "subclinical" or "acetowhite" genital warts is not recommended. Acetowhitening is not a specific test for HPV infection. Thus, in populations at low risk for this infection, many false-positives may be detected when this test is used for screening. The specificity and sensitivity of this procedure has not been defined. In special situations, experienced clinicians find this test useful for identification of flat genital warts.

A definitive diagnosis of HPV infection depends on detection of viral nucleic acid (DNA or RNA) or capsid protein. Pap smear diagnosis of HPV does not always correlate with detection of HPV DNA in cervical cells. Cell changes attributed to HPV in the cervix are similar to those of mild dysplasia and often regress spontaneously without treatment. Tests that detect several types of HPV DNA or RNA in cells scraped from the cervix are available, but the clinical utility of these tests for managing patients is unclear. Management decisions should not be made on the basis of HPV tests. Screening for subclinical genital HPV infection using DNA or RNA tests or acetic acid is not recommended.

Treatment

In the absence of coexistent dysplasia, treatment is not recommended for subclinical genital HPV infection diagnosed by Pap smear, colposcopy, biopsy, acetic acid soaking of genital skin or mucous membranes, or the detection of HPV (DNA or RNA). The diagnosis of subclinical genital HPV infection is often questionable, and no therapy has been identified to eradicate infection. HPV has been demonstrated in adjacent tissue after laser treatment of HPV-associated dysplasia and after attempts to eliminate subclinical HPV by extensive laser vaporization of the anogenital area. In the presence of coexistent dysplasia, management should be based on the grade of dysplasia.

Management of Sex Partners

Examination of sex partners is unnecessary. Most sex partners of infected patients probably are already infected subclinically with HPV. No practical screening tests for subclinical infection are available. The use of condoms may reduce transmission to sex partners who are likely to be uninfected (e.g., new partners); however, the period of communicability is unknown. Whether patients who have subclinical HPV infection are as contagious as patients who have exophytic warts is unknown.

Section 16.2

The Impact of HPV on Women's Health

© 1997 Springhouse Corp., http://www.springnet.com, from
The Nurse Practitioner, April 1997, Vol.22, No.4, Pg.24(7),
by Sylvia Carson; reprinted with permission.

Sexually transmitted diseases (STDs), rampant throughout American society, are a major health problem costing more than $3.5 billion each year.[1] STDs affect people of all ages and from all socioeconomic levels. There are an estimated 12 million new cases of STDs each year, with two-thirds of cases affecting people under the age of 25. Half of all Americans will acquire an STD at least once by the age of 30.[1,2] Human papilloma virus (HPV) is one STD that has long-term consequences. HPV, the most prevalent viral STD, causes genital warts or condyloma acuminate and can lead to cervical neoplasia. It is estimated that 40 million Americans have HPV, and each year 1 million more are infected.[3]

Today there is much concern about HPV preceding cervical cancer. More than 60 HPV types have been identified, and 20 are known to cause genital warts. Most HPV infections are subclinical and are recognized as a precursor to malignancy.

Types 6 and 11 are most often associated with genital warts. They have a low oncogenic potential and do not usually progress to cancer. The virus infects the top layers of the skin and can remain inactive, or latent, for months or years before there is any sign of a wart. Most of the time a wart will appear within 3 to 6 months after exposure.[4]

Genital HPV is most commonly spread through sexual contact; studies show that about two-thirds of people with HPV are infected in this way. Fifty percent will have clinically visible lesions, with 25% having subclinical lesions. However, recent studies have shown that HPV can also be transmitted nonsexually by HPV fomites on underwear and medical instruments.[5,6] Recurrences of HPV warts are most likely due to latent infection rather than reinfection. Treatment of the partner is not a significant factor in the recovery of the woman as it is in other STDs.[4,7]

Types 16, 18, 31, and 33 have the most oncogenic potential and are most often found in severe dysplasia and cancerous cervical lesions.[4] A recent study found that women who had a low-grade cervical disease were more likely to progress to more severe disease than those without evidence of cervical abnormality. It was concluded that evidence of low-grade cervical disease was a better predictor of disease progression than HPV 16 positivity.[8]

During pregnancy the genital warts may grow rapidly and become macerated with development of a secondary infection. The lesions may block the vaginal canal and cause profuse bleeding. The rapid growth of warts during pregnancy is thought to be related to a suppressed immune system. Genital warts should be closely monitored during pregnancy, treated as indicated, and then treated definitively after delivery.[4]

The risk of exposure of the neonate to HPV by the mother during delivery raises some concerns. Although laryngeal papillomas can be life-threatening and often appear within the first 5 years of life, only 2% to 5% of all births are at risk for this problem. Vaginal delivery carries only a 0.04% risk of laryngeal infection in the neonate. Therefore, experts feel the risk to the newborn is not high enough to warrant routine cesarean section in the mother. Each case needs to be examined individually. Cesarean section may be indicated when the genital warts are so large that they obstruct the vagina or interfere with the course of labor and delivery or complicate the immediate postpartum period.[4,7]

Risk of HPV and Cervical Dysplasia

Unsafe sex practices can contribute to infection with HPV. Cofactors in the development of cervical disease with HPV include oral contraceptive use, pregnancy and parity, nutrition, cigarette smoking, and immunosuppression. A study was done assessing high-risk factors for cervical dysplasia among Latino and white women. Interviews of the subjects were done focusing on history of STDs, sexual practices, reproductive history, contraceptive use, cigarette smoking, diet, and hygienic practices. Lab tests were done to identify HPV. It was concluded that the strongest risk factor for the development of cervical dysplasia was the presence of HPV infection. Other risk factors included smoking, low income, low educational level, history of STDs, and positive hepatitis B antibodies.[9]

Research on oral contraceptives (OC) as a factor in the development of cervical cancer is conflicting. The risk of cervical dysplasia in OC users is greatest in those who have used OCs for 10 years or more. One theory states that these women may be more sexually active and therefore are more likely to be exposed to HPV through multiple partners. Contraceptive steroids have direct and indirect effects on microorganisms, physiologic changes in the reproductive tract, and host immunologic responses. The increased cervical ectopy caused by OCs provides a larger surface area susceptible to potential infection. OCs may increase-risk of cervical dysplasia by causing folate deficiencies or reducing metabolism of mutagens.[10] Other studies do not support OCs as a risk factor.

Poor nutrition is associated with cervical dysplasia. A correlation was found between cervical dysplasia and low levels of vitamin A, beta-carotene, vitamin C, and folic acid. Poor nutrition is often correlated with alcohol consumption, and studies have shown a correlation between alcohol consumption and increased risk for cervical dysplasia.[11] Low socioeconomic class may also be a predisposing factor in the development of cervical dysplasia, possibly because of poor nutritional habits and lack of health care.

Cigarette smokers have a twofold increase in risk for cervical dysplasia compared to nonsmokers. This is dose related. Nicotine and cotinine have been found in the cervix of smokers. Nicotine was also found in the cervix of women who are exposed to passive smoke.[12] A relationship has also been found between smoking and vitamin C. Smoking decreases plasma vitamin C, which is involved in the detoxification of tobacco nitrosamines. It was speculated that smoking affects cervical dysplasia by reducing plasma vitamin C.[13] Previous studies have shown a decrease in the Langerhans' antigen-presenting cells in immunocompromised women, which leads to development of cervical neoplasia. HPV and cigarette smoking were found to reduce the protective Langerhans' cells, which may explain the increased risk of cervical neoplasia in smokers.[14]

Women who have compromised immune systems, such as those who have had transplants, those with HIV, those on chemotherapy, and those that are pregnant, have been found to have a higher incidence of cervical dysplasia.[15]

Sexual habits may increase the risk for cervical dysplasia. Multiple partners has been positively correlated with increased cervical dysplasia.[4] Being married more than once, separated, or divorced also increases the risk. Sexarche, the onset of sexual activity, at age 17 or earlier has been shown to be a risk factor for cervical dysplasia. In women with HPV, the number of partners has been found to be directly related to age. Physiologic evidence implies that adolescent sexual activity may prolong the normal cervical maturation process, increasing the time which immature metaplastic tissue can come into proximity with causative agents.[16]

Treatment of HPV Infections

Because HPV is associated with precancerous changes on the cervix, a thorough assessment must be done before treatment is initiated. When a Pap smear shows HPV, a colposcopy with biopsies is performed to deter mine if dysplasia is present. The goal of treatment is to control the HPV. Because many HPV infections are subclinical, complete eradication of the virus is impossible. When the only finding is HPV during colposcopy and no warts are present, recommendations are usually to repeat the Pap smear in 3 to 6 months with an annual colposcopy and vulvar examination.[4,7,17]

A recent survey of college health providers found that there were many different management strategies for treating women with HPV infections. Most providers did not follow the CDC treatment guidelines.[18]

The goal of treating genital warts is to destroy the visible lesions and then wait for the host immune response to control viral replication. The first treatment choice is topical therapy because of simplicity and cost-effectiveness. Trichloroacetic acid (TCA) is a desiccant acid that works best on moist mucosal warts and causes a visible whitening of the skin. TCA may be applied as often as three times a week, but it is usually used only once a week to decrease the irritation of the surrounding skin. Xylocaine jelly can be applied to the skin around the warts to decrease discomfort. The client will experience intense burning for about 10 minutes after the TCA is applied. TCA is nontoxic and can be used on the external genitalia, the vagina, and the cervix. TCA is safe to use during pregnancy.[4,7,17]

Podophyllum resin, an extract from the root of the mandrake plant, has been used often in the past for the treatment of genital warts. However, it is not used as much today due to the potential side effects of myelotoxicity and neurotoxicity. It cannot be used on the cervix, in the vagina, or during pregnancy.[4,7] It must be washed off the vulva after 4 to 6 hours. Podofilox is a purified form of podophyllum that does not have the unwanted side effects of podophyllum resin. It can be self-administered and used on the vulva and perianal tissues. Clients need detailed instruction on use, including the importance of maintaining separation of the labia until completely dry. It may be used twice a day, 3 days a week, for up to 4 weeks.[7,17]

Topical 5-fluorouracil has been used to treat persistent recurrent vaginal and vulvar warts. It is very caustic, and the patient must receive thorough instruction in its use and be observed weekly.[4] The client is instructed to insert a vaginal applicator one-third full into her vagina and then insert a tampon before bedtime. Zinc oxide or hydrocortisone ointment is applied to the vulvar skin to prevent irritation. The genital area must be thoroughly washed off the next morning. The CDC does not feel that 5-fluorouracil has been studied enough to recommend it for treatment of genital warts.[7]

Laser vaporization is often used when the warts do not respond to acid treatment. Laser therapy is not recommended in patients who are in the proliferative phase of rapid condyloma growth. The best response is seen on thick keratotic lesions. The goal of laser therapy is to vaporize the thick epidermal growth without damaging the papillary dermis below.[7,19]

Simple excision, cryocautery, liquid nitrogen, or electrocautery are also used to remove genital warts. Cryocautery is often used to treat cervical intracpithelial neoplasia (CIN) lesions of the cervix. Cryocautery is a cytodestructive freezing technique that causes thermal damage and necrosis of the epithelium. The loop electrode excision procedure (LEEP) is a newer procedure used to treat CIN lesions of the cervix. A thin layer of tissue is removed by the LEEP. This is advantageous because tissue is removed rather than destroyed, which enables the pathologist to identify the tissue margins.[20] The client may experience cramping during either procedure and may have a heavy watery vaginal discharge for 3 to 4 weeks. The client should be given instructions to place nothing in the vagina for 3 weeks, which precludes intercourse, douching, or tampons. A Pap smear is repeated 3 months after the cryocautery.[4,17] Warts that are thick and appear keratinized and do not respond to treatment should be biopsied to rule out a cancerous lesion.[4]

Interferon injections have also been used to treat persistent recurrent genital warts. Interferon has been used in clients who have not responded to laser therapy. In one of the first studies on Interferon as a treatment for genital warts, 53% in the experimental group had complete clearing of warts compared to 17% in the control group. The therapy lasted 3 weeks, with the response not seen until 4 to 9 weeks.[19] Interferon is most often injected intralesionaly with a fine-gauge needle. Client instructions should include the possibility of flu-like symptoms that may diminish after the initial injection.[4,19] The CDC does not recommend Interferon for treatment of genital warts because of its high cost and the high incidence of side effects, and also because its efficacy is no better than other treatment modalities.[7]

Self-Care Management of HPV

Health care providers have an important role in educating and counseling women about HPV infections. It is important to establish a nonjudgmental, trusting, and caring relationship so that the client will be comfortable in discussing her sexual behaviors, activities, and concerns. There is social stigma associated with any STD, including HPV. Women may feel unclean and describe themselves in demeaning ways. Psychosocial as well as sexual trauma occurs with HPV infection. Interpersonal relationships can become strained, resulting in feelings of shame and/or denial of the problem. Many times women with HPV feel that they cannot get the answers they need from health care providers to understand what has happened to them. Partners will often blame the woman for the HPV infection.[21] Health care providers must educate clients about risk factors, prevention, and signs and symptoms of STDs, including HPV, using verbal and written teaching methods.

All women should begin Pap smears at age 18 or at sexarche and then have them annually unless the client and the health care provider have determined that this is not needed.[4] Women with genital warts should be instructed to perform regular vulvar self-examination to detect the presence of recurrent lesions. Women with HPV should be informed that their immune status is the most important factor in decreasing their cancer risk. It is important to discuss lifestyle factors that affect the immune response such as diet, smoking, sleep, exercise, and stress. Other risk factors include early age of sexual activity, infections with other STDs, number of sexual partners, and alcohol consumption. Testing for HIV should be offered to women with HPV infection. Nutritional instruction, use of a daily multiple vitamin, and smoking cessation should be provided by the health care provider for women with HPV infections. Health care providers should encourage women to practice risk-reduction measures during periods of marital discord, pregnancy, or when involved with a high-risk partner. It is important that the health care provider provide the client with both verbal and written material about coping and stress reduction.

Empowerment of Women and Prevention of HPV

The primary goal of HPV management should be prevention. Safe sex means protecting oneself from exposure to STDs, whether that means abstinence, monogamy, or use of condoms. Self-esteem has been identified as a factor in condom use among single women. Fear of losing a sexual partner was identified as a greater concern than infection with an STD. When questioned about ability to protect themselves from infection with an STD, 107 women believed that they could protect themselves. Eighteen women did not feel they could protect themselves. It could not be determined if this was due to lack of information or inability to empower themselves.[22]

It is important to examine self-attitudes about sexuality. STDs must be viewed in the context of interpersonal relationships. Couples should discuss safe sex before becoming sexually active. Safe sexual practices need to be emphasized to minimize the spread of HPV. Knowing that women who did not use condoms had lower self-esteem provides a focus for intervention. Although condom use should be encouraged in all sexually active people, condom use may not totally prevent transmission of HPV infection. The condom covers the penis, but it does not prevent skin-to-skin contact in the external genital area, allowing exposure to HPV. The female condom may be a good choice for some women. The mechanism of action is the same as the male condom. The female condom covers the vagina, cervix, and some of the external vulvar area thus preventing skin to skin contact in the covered areas. Safe sex should be discussed with all sexually active women seeking care. Women need to be empowered to protect themselves from the epidemic of STDs, including HPV. The ideal prevention would be to educate women about STDs before they become sexually active so that preventive measures could be taken prior to sexarche.

Women who discover that they have an STD, including HPV, often feel embarrassed, ashamed, betrayed, and angry.[21] It may be difficult for some women to abstain from intercourse during the treatment interval. Pregnant women must deal with the guilt and responsibilities of caring for an infected infant.

Empowerment is a concept that can serve as intervention strategy for clinicians working with women who have HPV. Because HPV can have adverse outcomes for women, clinicians can help empower women to act on the information provided to them. Empowerment has been defined as a process by which a person gains mastery over her own life. Women often feel they are in a situation in which they are powerless. Sense of self may be lost. Only the woman can empower herself, so the clinician's role is to support and help identify obstacles to empowerment.[23]

Empowerment is a process of helping individuals develop an awareness of the root causes of problems and a readiness to act on this awareness. It is a process enabling the woman to master her environment and achieve self-determination through changes in self.[23] Many women who have HPV feel a loss of power, a sense of distrust, alienation, a sense of hopelessness, and an attitude of self-blame. Clinicians have an important role helping women to understand that they do have control over their own bodies; they must help women take a positive approach to the problem.

Empowerment is a long-term process that involves the development of participatory skills. The individual has the option and freedom to choose, which includes self-control by assuming responsibility for one's own actions, such as safe sex practices.[23] Health care providers can encourage the woman to choose to become an active participant during the pelvic examination. Use a mirror to show the woman her genital area. Show her how to perform a genital self-examination. This will facilitate understanding of her body and sexuality. Empowerment also involves supporting, which includes caring, relating, accepting, coaching, and sharing.[23] The health care provider should offer support to the woman by listening to her concerns using active listening skills. The use of role playing can help support the woman by working through possible scenarios when discussing HPV with her partner. She can practice what she will say and do during the encounter. Negotiating is another aspect of empowerment and involves taking and relinquishing of power by those involved. By negotiating, the woman feels equal in the relationship with certain rights and feels more at ease in asking questions, volunteering information, and discussing her concerns.[23] The outcomes of empowerment are recognition by the woman that she must be a willing participant in any sexual encounter and that she has the right to protect herself from STDs, including HPV. She can embrace the notion that her body is her own domain and she has responsibility for keeping it healthy.

Conclusion

The high incidence of HPV infections in women under the age of 24, the progressive nature of HPV, and the cost to the woman and the health care system indicate that early intervention to detect HPV infection is of the utmost importance. Health care providers need to focus on educating women about the serious, long-lasting, and lifelong consequences of HPV infection. Prevention of all STDs, including HPV, must be a goal of all health care providers working with women.

There are an estimated 12 million new cases of STDs each year, with two-thirds of cases affecting people under the age of 25. Americans will acquire an STD at least once by the age of 30. HPV, the most prevalent viral STD, causes genital warts or condyloma acuminata and can lead to cervical neoplasia. More than 60 HPV types have been identified, and 20 are known to cause genital warts. More HPV infections are subclinical and are recognized as a precursor to malignancy. Types 6 and 11 are most often associated with genital warts. They have a low oncogenic potential and do not usually progress to cancer. Genital HPV is most commonly spread through sexual contact; studies show that about two-thirds of people with HPV are infected in this way.

Treatment of the partner is not a significant factor in the recovery of the woman as it is in other STDs. Types 16, 18, 31, and 33 have the most oncogenic potential and are most often found in severe dysplasia and cancerous cervical lesions. During pregnancy the genital warts may grow rapidly and become macerated with development of a secondary infection. The risk of exposure of the neonate to HPV by the mother during delivery raises some concerns. Vaginal delivery carries only a 0.04% risk of laryngeal infection in the neonate. Therefore, experts feel the risk to the newborn is not high enough to warrant routine cesarean section in the mother.

Cofactors in the development of cervical disease with HPV include oral contraceptive use, pregnancy and parity, nutrition, cigarette smoking, and immunosuppression. The strongest risk factor for the development of cervical dysplasia is the presence of HPV infection. Other risk factors included smoking, low income, low educational level, history of STDs, and positive hepatitis B antibodies. Poor nutrition is associated with cervical dysplasia.

Women who have compromised immune systems, such as those who have had transplants, those with HIV, those on chemotherapy, and those that are pregnant, have been found to have a higher incidence of cervical dysplasia. Sexual habits may increase the risk for cervical dysplasia. Multiple partners has been positively correlated with increased cervical dysplasia

When a Pap smear shows HPV, a colposcopy with biopsies is performed to determine if dysplasia is present. When the only finding is HPV during colposcopy and no warts are present, recommendations are usually to repeat the Pap smear in 3 to 6 months with an annual colposcopy and vulvar examination. The goal of treating genital warts is to destroy the visible lesions and then wait for the host immune response to control viral replication. The first treatment choice is topical therapy because of simplicity and cost-effectiveness. Trichloroacetic acid (TCA) is a desiccant acid that works best on moist mucosal warts and causes a visible whitening of the skin.

Podofilox is a purified form of podophyllum that does not have the unwanted side effects of podophyllum resin. It can be self-administered and used on the vulva and perianal tissues. Laser vaporization is often used when the warts do not respond to acid treatment. Simple excision, cryocautery, liquid nitrogen, or electrocautery are also used to remove genital warts. Interferon injections have also been used to treat persistent recurrent genital warts.

Health care providers have an important role in educating and counseling women about HPV infections. It is important to establish a nonjudgmental, trusting, and caring relationship so that the client will be comfortable in discussing her sexual behaviors, activities, and concerns. Women with genital warts should be instructed to perform regular vulvar self-examination to detect the presence of recurrent lesions. Women with HPV should be informed that their immune status is the most important factor in decreasing their cancer risk.

The primary goal of HPV management should be prevention. Safe sex means protecting oneself from exposure to STDs, whether that means abstinence, monogamy, or use of condoms. Self-esteem has been identified as a factor in condom use among single women. The female condom may be a good choice for some women. The mechanism of action is the same as the male condom. The female condom covers the vagina, cervix, and some of the external vulvar area thus preventing skin-to-skin contact in the covered areas. Women who discover that they have an STD, including HPV, often feel embarrassed, ashamed, betrayed, and angry. Empowerment is a concept that can serve as intervention strategy for clinicians working with women who have HPV.

Empowerment is a concept that can serve as intervention strategy for clinicians working with women who have HPV. Empowerment has been defined as a process by which a person gains mastery over her own life. Only the woman can empower herself, so the clinician's role is to support and help identify obstacles to empowerment. Empowerment is a long-term process that involves the development of participatory skills. Empowerment also involves supporting, which includes caring, relating, accepting, coaching, and sharing. Negotiating is another aspect of empowerment and involves taking and relinquishing of power by those involved. The outcomes of empowerment are recognition by the woman that she must be a willing participant in any sexual encounter and that she has the right to protect herself from STDs. She can embrace the notion that her body is her own domain and she has responsibility for keeping it healthy.

References

1. Public Health Service, Department of Health and Human Services Healthy People 2000: National Health Promotion and Disease Prevention Objectives. Washington, D.C.: U.S. Government Printing Office, 1991;496-501.

2. Horton, JA: *The Women's Health Data Book: A Profile of Health in the United States*. New York: Elsevier, 1992;27-35.

3. HPV News: HPV Perspective. Research Triangle Park N.C.: *ASHA* 1991: 1(1);4-7.

4. ACOG Technical Bulletin. Genital Human Papillomavirus Infections. Number 193. Washington, D.C.: *ACOG*, 1994.

5. Bergeron, C; Ferenczy, A; Richart, R. Underwear: Contamination by human papillomaviruses. *Am J Obstet Gynecol* 1990; 162(1):25-29.

6. Ferenczy, A; Bergeron, C; Richart, RM, Human papillomavirus DNA in fomites on objects used for the management of patients with genital human papillomavirus infections. *Obstet Gynecol* 1989;74(6):950-54.

7. Centers for Disease Control and Prevention: 1993 Sexually Transmitted Disease Treatment Guidelines. U.S. Department of Health and Human Services.

8. Downey, GP; Bavin, PJ; Deery, ARS, et al: Relation between human papillomavirus type 16 and potential for progression of minor-grade cervical disease. *Lancet* 1994;344(8): 432-35.

9. Becker, TM; Wheeler, CM; McGough, NS, et al: Sexually transmitted diseases and other risk factors for cervical dysplasia among southwestern Hispanic and non-Hispanic white women. *JAMA* 1994;271(15)1181-88.

10. McGregor, JA; Hammill, HA, Contraception and sexually transmitted diseases: Interactions and opportunities. *Am J Obstet Gynecol* 1993;168(6): 2033-41.

11. Schneider, A; Shah, K, The role of vitamins in the etiology of cervical neoplasia: An epidemiological review. *Archives Gynecol Obstet* 1989;246:1-13.

12. Jones, CJ; Schiffman, MH; Kuman, R, et al, Elevated nicotine levels in cervical ravages from passive smokers. *Am J Pub Heal* 1991;81(3):378-79.

13. Basu, J; Palan, P; Vermund, S, et al, Plasma ascorbic acid and beta-carotene levels in women evaluated for HPV infection, smoking, and cervix dysplasia. *Cancer Detect Preven* 1991;15(3):165-70.

14. Barton, SE; Hollingworth, A; Maddox, PH, et al, Possible cofactors in the etiology of cervical intraepithelial neoplasia: An immunopathologic study. *J Reprod Med* 1989;34(9):613-16.

15. Vermund, S; Kelley, K; Klein, R, et al, High risk of human papillomavirus infection and cervical squamous intraepithelial lesions among women with symptomatic human immunodeficiency virus infection. *Am J Obstet Gynecol* 1991;165(2):392-400.

16. Gottardi, G; Gritti, P; Marzi, MM, et al, Colposcopic findings in virgin and sexually active teenagers. *Obstet Gynecol* 1984;63:613-15.

17. Brucks, JA; Jacobs, EW, Practical tips for assessment and management of vulvar and vaginal human papillomavirus. *Nurse Pract Forum* 1992; 3(3):169-76.

18. Linnehan, MJ; Andrews, S; Groce, NE, College health providers' knowledge, attitudes and management practices of genital HPV infection. *Nurse Pract* 1996;21(5):122-28.

19. Hatch, KD, Vulvovaginal human papillomavirus infections: Clinical implications and management. *Am Obstet Gynecol* 1991;165(4):1183-88.

20. Mayeaux, EJ; Harper, MB, Loop electrosurgical excision procedure. *J Fam Prac* 1993;36(2):214-19.

21. Lehr, ST; Lee, ME, The psychosocial and sexual trauma of a genital HPV infection. *Nurse Pract Forum* 1990;1(1):25-30.

22. Able, E; Hilton, P; Miller, I, Sexual risk behavior among urban women of childbearing age Implications for clinical practice. *J Am Acad Nurse Pract* 1996;8(3):115-24.

23. Connely, LM; Keele, BS; Kleinbeck, SV, et al, A place to be yourself: Empowerment from the client's perspective. *IMAGE: J Nurs Scholar* 1993; 25(4):297-303.

Section 16.3

Advice from Affected Persons about Living with HPV

Human papillomavirus (HPV) infection is responsible for genital warts, also known as venereal warts and condylomata acuminate. Approximately 24 million Americans are infected with HPV (Noegel, Kirby, Schrader, & Wasserheit, 1993) and one million new infections occur annually (Becker, Stone, & Alexander, 1987; Carlone & Schenk, 1990; Koutsky & Wolner-Hanssen, 1989). These figures represent an increase of over 500% during the past 20 years (Carlone & Schenk, 1990; Lucas, 1988). Most commonly, HPV is transmitted through sexual contact; it is highly contagious and probably incurable. There is a growing body of evidence linking certain viral strains to anogenital cancer, particularly cervical cancer (Alvey, 1990; Richart & Wright, 1993). Thus, persons who have HPV are faced with a disease that has significant implications for their psychological and physical health.

Research on HPV has focused on the pathogenesis of various strains as well as treatment. Very little attention has been paid to how people live with and adapt to this stressful disease. Because they "speak from experience," individuals who have lived with HPV may offer important advice to the newly diagnosed. Furthermore, their advice can provide clinicians with insight about possible interventions. Therefore, the purpose of this study was to identify the "advice or information" individuals who have had HPV for 1 year would give to newly diagnosed persons. In addition, gender differences in advice and information were examined.

Background

Characteristics, Transmission, and Treatment of HPV

Seventy types of HPV have been identified; approximately 20 types are associated with the genital tract and found to cause genital warts (Richart & Wright, 1993). HPV infection is commonly found on the vulva, cervix, penis, or rectum, but has been identified in all mucous membranes including the urethra, bladder, and ocular and oral mucosas (Enterline & Leonardo, 1989).

If visible warts are present, the infection can be diagnosed on physical examination. However, subclinical HPV infections are common and not apparent on routine clinical inspection (Bourcier & Seidler, 1987; Enterline & Leonardo, 1989; Kelley, Galbraith, & Vermund, 1992; Rapini, 1990; Spitzer & Krumholz, 1992; Tinkle, 1990). Some investigators estimate that there are two cases of subclinical HPV for every case of clinically visible external genital warts (Spitzer & Krumholz, 1992).

Between 60% and 90% of the sexual partners of persons who have warts will also develop warts. This usually occurs within 3 months of sexual contact; however, the incubation period may be much longer (Becker et al., 1987; Bourcier & Seidler, 1987; King, 1990; Lucas, 1988; Tinkle, 1990). Genital sexual contact is probably the primary route of HPV transmission, however it can be transmitted to or from the mouth, throat, and anus; and from mother to fetus (Becker et al., 1987; Enterline & Leonardo, 1989; Kelley et al, 1992; King, 1990; Tinkle, 1990). Infection generally occurs in areas that are traumatized during sexual intercourse, but the virus may spread to adjacent areas of the genital tract (Enterline & Leonardo, 1989; Kelley et al., 1992).

A number of treatment modalities are used for HPV. Treatment depends on the site of infection and extent of disease. The goal of therapy is removal of exophytic warts and the amelioration of signs and symptoms, not eradication of HPV (Centers for Disease Control [CDC] STD Treatment Guidelines, 1993). No therapy has been shown to eradicate the virus (Kraus & Stone, 1990). Some cases of HPV respond well to treatment. Other cases have been known to regress spontaneously, or progress independently (Nash, Burke, & Hoskins, 1987). Treatment may be complex, requiring a combination of modalities. It can also be lengthy, costly, painful, and might produce scarring (Enterline & Leonardo, 1989; Kelley, Galbraith, & Vermund, 1992).

Recurrences of warts are common but their origins can be difficult to pinpoint. A recurrence may be due to regrowth of HPV infected cells or transmission from a partner (Kelley et al., 1992). Treatment success depends on many factors, including the anatomic site involved, the severity of lesions, the specific HPV type and the immunocompetence of the infected person (Tinkle, 1990). There is strong evidence linking HPV to anogenital cancer, particularly cervical cancer (Deitch & Smith, 1983; Kelley et al., 1992; King, 1990; Koutsky & Wolner-Hanssen, 1989; Richart & Wright, 1993; Tinkle, 1990). Although some viral types are probably harmless and self-limiting, others progress to advanced cervical lesions. In a recent study, Richart and Wright (1993) reported that high grade lesions of cervical intraepithelial neoplasia were more likely to be homogenous for HPV viral type and that 89% of high grade lesions contained either HPV types 16, 18, or 33. After an extensive review of the research literature, Alvey (1990) warned of a coming epidemic of cervical cancer related to HPV. Although HPV infection can be dangerous to both genders, it is of particular concern to women. Because the course and severity of HPV infection is so unpredictable, patients often experience a significant amount of anxiety about their health. Their distress may be compounded by the fact that sexually transmitted diseases carry a social stigma.

Psychosocial Aspects of HPV Infection

Clinicians have observed that HPV may cause significant emotional distress and have recommended that nurses provide emotional support (Bourcier & Seidler, 1987; Enterline & Leonardo, 1989). Tinkle (1990) noted that HPV might produce anxiety about treatment, confusion and anger regarding sexual transmission, and feelings of guilt, blame, and fear. Extensive, visible warts can also have negative effects on body image and self-esteem (Enterline & Leonardo, 1989; Tinkle, 1990). Lehr and Lee (1990) described a variety of responses by women following the diagnosis of HPV infection including fear, embarrassment, shame, anxiety, and frustration.

A 1994 study focusing on stressors associated with HPV at time of diagnosis indicated that many women have psychosocial difficulties. Stressors included fear of telling a partner about the disease, inability to trust partners, and loss of sexual spontaneity (Mime, Keller, & Egan, 1994). Furthermore, even 1 year after diagnosis, 40% of a sample of men and women with HPV reported that the disease had a negative effect on their perceptions of themselves. They identified feeling "guilty," "dirty," "contaminated," and "impure" (Keller & Egan, 1994).

Recently, Redfern and Hutchinson (1994) stated that women and men may respond differently to sexually transmitted diseases (STDs). Using a qualitative approach, these researchers found that women reported feeling a sense of inevitability about contracting STDs and saw themselves as powerless to prevent them.

In summary, HPV infection can produce serious physical and psychosocial sequelae. To provide comprehensive care, practitioners must be aware of the broad array of consequences. People who have lived with HPV for an extended period are an important source of information about interventions that may be helpful at the time of diagnosis. This descriptive study addressed two research questions: One year after diagnosis with HPV, what advice and information do affected persons give to newly diagnosed individuals? Are there gender differences in the advice and information given by affected persons?

Methods

Sample and Setting

Eligible persons were those who had a documented first-time diagnosis of HPV, were 18 years of age or older, and could read and write English. They were recruited between 1990 and 1993 from university-affiliated outpatient internal medicine and dermatology clinics, a university student women's health clinic, and a community sexually transmitted disease clinic. All four sites were located in one midwestern community. Although it was not possible to keep precise records, clinicians estimated that over 75% of persons who were invited to participate in the study actually did so.

A total of 88 persons, 61 women and 27 men, completed the questionnaire. Their average age was 23.75 years (SD = 4.82). The majority were single (93.2%), White (96.6%), students (66.3%). Fifty-four percent were employed; 72% reported an annual income of less than $10,000. Potential participants were identified by clinicians at the time of diagnosis. The clinician verbally described the study and also provided a brief, written description. Individuals interested in learning more about the study gave written permission for an investigator to contact them. During this contact, the study was discussed thoroughly, and a data collection session was scheduled at which time any remaining questions were answered and informed consent was obtained. The identity of participants was known only to the researchers and all data were confidential. Participants completed a set of questionnaires at the time of diagnosis, 6 months after diagnosis, and

1 year after diagnosis. Because of unexpected relocations during the year, 20 participants completed the final questionnaires by mail. Over 1 year, the dropout rate for the study was 9%. Persons who completed the entire study received U.S. $50.

Data Collection and Analysis

At the 1-year follow-up, the set of questionnaires completed by respondents included an open-ended item focusing on their ideas about information that might be helpful for people newly diagnosed with HPV. It asked, "Now that you have lived with genital warts for a year, if you had the opportunity to give advice or information to others who have just found out they have genital warts, what would you tell them?" Content analysis was used to analyze responses to this open-ended question. This procedure had a number of steps. First, one rater wrote each response on an index card, examined all responses, and sorted the cards into categories that shared a common theme. Second, categories were named and definitions were developed for each category. Third, cards were sorted into the named categories by a second rater. Definitions of some categories were then refined and the cards were resorted by each rater independently. Using percentage agreement, inter-rater reliability was 95.6% after the second sorting. Discrepancies between raters were then resolved through discussion.

Results

The first research question focused on the advice and information persons with HPV would give to others at time of diagnosis. A total of 19 advice and information categories in six general areas were identified: maintaining a balanced perspective; treatment; sexual behavior; knowledge; self care; and other.

Under the general area titled "maintain a balanced perspective" were four categories. The first concerned advice to avoid blaming oneself for getting HPV and to guard against letting HPV affect self-esteem. For example, one woman said, "Avoid negative feelings about yourself." Others advised, "Don't feel badly about yourself or blame yourself." The second category included responses advising newly diagnosed persons to recognize that their disease and their feelings will improve over time. One stated, "Initially you may have negative feelings about genital warts, but over time, the feelings improve." A third category contained responses advising newly diagnosed persons to maintain a positive outlook and move forward with their lives. One individual stated: "Having genital warts is really not that bad... it's not the end of the world". The final category included responses advising newly diagnosed persons to remember that they are not alone and that millions of other people have HPV also. For example, one woman said, "There is comfort in knowing that genital warts are very common and affect many people."

A second major area of advice to the newly diagnosed focused on treatment. Six categories emerged. The first contained responses advising newly diagnosed persons to seek treatment and appropriate follow-up for HPV and to follow prescribed regimens. One respondent said, "Have regular medical exams and follow medical advice." Another stated, "Have recurrences checked and treated." A second category included responses encouraging the newly diagnosed to seek evaluation and treatment of their partners. A third category contained responses advising others to find a health care provider who can be trusted and who communicates well. For example, one participant stated, "Find a care provider you can trust." Another said, "Find a care provider who is understanding and nonjudgmental." The fourth category included advice reminding newly diagnosed persons that HPV is treatable and obvious warts will usually go away. One stated, "Be aware that eventually the obvious warts will go away and no longer be a problem or nuisance." Respondents also advised others to be realistic about the chronic nature of this viral infection. Thus, the fifth category contained statements warning newly diagnosed persons to develop a realistic perception of HPV. The final category included responses advising newly diagnosed persons to monitor themselves for recurrences. One said, "Be aware of changes in your body or signs that warts have come back."

A third general area of advice focused on sexual behavior. There were two themes in this area. The first contained responses advising newly diagnosed persons to tell all partners about the HPV. One wrote, "Tell past and present sexual partners they may have been exposed to genital warts." The second category contained advice to practice safer sex to prevent future transmission of HPV and to protect against other sexually transmitted diseases. For example, one man wrote, "Protect yourself from transmitting the virus or contracting sexually transmitted diseases by changing your sexual behaviors, using condoms, abstinence, monogamy."

A fourth general area of advice concerned development of knowledge about HPV. In this area, the first category contained responses advising newly diagnosed persons to seek information from a number of sources including health care providers and to develop their knowledge about HPV. One wrote, "Learn as much as you can about the disease process by asking questions, talking to health care providers, or talking to others who are knowledgeable about the disease." Interestingly, newly diagnosed persons were also advised to expect inconsistent information. Hence, the second category in this area contained responses advising the newly diagnosed that they will receive, and should expect, inconsistent or incomplete information about HPV. Several made statements such as, "You may feel frustrated about the lack of information given on genital warts" or "You'll get conflicting information from health care providers" or "Information is constantly changing." The fifth general area of advice concerned self-care and there were two categories. The first contained responses advising the newly diagnosed to develop a source of emotional support related to the HPV. Respondents wrote, "Find someone you can talk to, share your feelings with" and "someone who will provide you with emotional support." The second category included advice about maintaining a healthy lifestyle both physically and emotionally. Typical responses were, "Maintain a proper diet," "Get plenty of sleep," "Exercise," "No smoking," and "Be aware of changes in emotion and mood."

The final area of advice contained a variety of other responses. Within this general area, was a category called "no effect" which contained responses advising newly diagnosed persons that HPV will have no effect at all. One person said, "Having genital warts did not affect my life in any way." A second category contained responses indicating that the participant did not know what advice or information might be helpful. For example, one woman wrote, "I don't know what advice to give someone."

Participants gave a range of one to four responses; all were coded. The general area of advice given most frequently focused on maintaining a balanced perspective about living with HPV. Many respondents advised newly diagnosed people to maintain a positive outlook and move forward with life, to remember that they are not alone, and to avoid self-blame. Advice related to treatment was also given frequently. Most often, this advice focused on seeking treatment and monitoring self. Fewer respondents advised newly diagnosed persons to remember that warts are treatable and to establish a positive relationship with their health care providers.

Many participants gave advice in the general area of sexual behavior. They advised newly diagnosed persons to practice safer sex. Surprisingly few respondents stated that newly diagnosed persons should inform their sexual partners about the HPV. The importance of developing knowledge about HPV was also emphasized. This advice generally focused on educating oneself and asking questions about HPV. A small percentage of participants noted that newly diagnosed persons should expect inconsistent information. Finally, some of the participants emphasized self-care.

The second research question addressed gender differences in the advice and information affected persons would give to newly diagnosed persons. Statistical tests of the gender differences were not possible because of the small number of men in the sample. However, examination of the percentages suggests a number of interesting similarities and differences. First, in the general area of maintaining a balanced perspective, an equal percentage of men and women emphasized the importance of a positive outlook on life and remembering that many people are infected with HPV. On the other hand, 28% of women as compared to 4% of men thought newly diagnosed persons should avoid self-blame and negative self evaluations as a result of HPV. In the general area of treatment, the percentages were quite similar by gender. For example, about half of both men and women advised people to seek treatment and monitoring for themselves. Some gender differences are apparent in the category of sexual behavior. More than half of the men advised newly diagnosed persons to practice safer sex compared to one third of the women. Also, 18% of the women recommended informing sexual partners about the HPV as compared to 11% of the men. In the area of self-care, another gender difference was found; 18% of the women advised the newly diagnosed to seek emotional support but none of the male participants gave this advice.

Discussion

Many participants gave advice in the general area of "keeping a balanced perspective on life." Newly diagnosed persons were encouraged to maintain a positive outlook, remember that many others are affected by the virus, and avoid letting HPV influence their self-evaluations. Such responses demonstrate a belief that this virus can have a powerful effect on one's self-concept and self-definition. Hence, participants were warning others to keep the disease in perspective. Half the participants also advised newly diagnosed persons to obtain treatment and monitoring of their infection. One might expect that all of the respondents would advise people to seek treatment and monitoring. However, treatment of HPV can be frustrating and warts often recur despite many efforts to control them. Participants who did not advise people to seek treatment might have been expressing their frustration about the lack of effective interventions and pessimism about the extent to which treatment and monitoring is helpful.

Only 2% of participants recommended that partners be evaluated for HPV and only 16% advised newly diagnosed persons to inform their partners. Although examination and treatment of partners is not mandatory, it is often recommended so that partners can be educated and treated if appropriate. The failure to recommend disclosure may indicate a lack of knowledge about disease transmission and the infectious nature of HPV. However, it is more likely to be a reflection of the embarrassment and shame attached to telling a partner that one has an infectious STD.

Another area of concern was the fact that only about one-third of participants advised practicing safer sex. Models of health behavior (e.g., The Health Belief Model) suggest that acquiring an STD should increase one's perceived susceptibility to other STDs, and be an impetus for adopting protective sexual behaviors. Thus, it seemed reasonable to expect that a majority of respondents would recommend safer sex to newly diagnosed persons. However, it is possible that respondents remembered their own emotional distress at hearing the diagnosis and thought it was more important to give advice related to coping with emotional responses. Interestingly, a greater percentage of men than women gave advice about practicing safer sex. Perhaps, this gender difference is because of the perception that decisions about use of safer sexual practices still rest with men (Stein, 1990). Thus, it may be not be helpful (from a woman's point of view) to suggest use of safer sex.

Implications for Practice

The variety of advice given indicates that responses to HPV can range from feelings of complete devastation to the rare perception that the diagnosis has no effect at all. In working with clients, practitioners can make no assumptions about the impact of HPV. Instead, a careful exploration of the client's reaction to this diagnosis is needed. It is critical for practitioners to pay attention to clients' self-evaluations and self-esteem. For some, the disease may begin to define the person. Social isolation, avoidance of intimacy, and depression can occur. The sense of isolation and stigma might be eased if clients are given information about the HPV newsletter of the American Social Health Association. This newsletter contains valuable information about treatment of HPV and psychosocial issues.

Obviously, newly diagnosed persons need factual information about HPV including the nature and incurability of the virus, possible consequences of HPV, and modes of transmission. Our data suggest that practitioners also need to discuss treatment and the benefits of follow-up. Various methods for managing HPV infections should be thoroughly explained. It may be helpful to discuss the possible need for repeated treatments to remove the obvious warts. In addition, affected women need to be aware of the fact that HPV can infect the cervix even if external visible warts are gone. Practitioners can emphasize that HPV is treatable and clients can benefit from regular monitoring because new lesions may be discovered and new treatments may become available.

Sexual behavior and safer sex practices should also be a part of our discussions with clients. It is important to emphasize both the benefits and risks of various sexual practices. For example, clients need to know that scrotal and vulvar tissue can be widely colonized with HPV and condoms provide only limited protection. However, at time of diagnosis, a discussion of the need to practice safer sex might be perceived as "rubbing salt in the wound." It may be more helpful to discuss sexual practices at a follow-up visit. Disclosing the disease to partners and encouraging evaluation of partners is important and should not be overlooked. Because it is often embarrassing and difficult to inform sexual partners, practitioners can offer suggestions about how to notify partners. Self-care issues should be addressed, because many individuals gave advice to seek emotional support and maintain a healthy lifestyle. Nurses can evaluate the support available to each client, and offer additional counseling and support as needed to those clients without a strong support system. Suggestions about how to maintain a healthy lifestyle, such as information about smoking cessation, stress management, daily exercise, and proper diet may also be helpful.

Throughout the course of treatment, practitioners should continue to address the sensitive, emotional elements of the disease and provide emotional support and positive reassurance. Additional support may be particularly helpful for individuals undergoing lengthy and complex treatment, having difficulty coping with having an STD, or experiencing stress in intimate relationships. A clinic appointment for discussing psychosocial matters is appropriate for some.

Summary and Limitations

Because of the nature of the sample, the findings should be interpreted with caution. Respondents were two-thirds women and mostly

White, young adults who were fairly well educated. The low average income of the sample is probably a reflection of the large number of college students and not a true indication of economic status. All of these factors limit generalizability of findings. As with any open-ended questions, there is the possibility of memory bias and researcher bias in conducting the content analysis. Despite these limitations, the study provides important information about clients' perspectives about the advice and information needed by persons newly diagnosed with HPV.

References

Alvey, J. (1990). Genital warts and contagious cancers. Jefferson, NC: McFarland & Co.

Becker, T., Stone, K., & Alexander, E. (1987). Genital human papillomavirus infection: A growing concern. Obstetrics and Gynecology Clinics of North America, 14, 389-395.

Bourcier, K., & Seidler, A. (1987). Chlamydia and condylomata acuminate: An update for the nurse practitioner. *Journal of Obstetric, Gynecologic, and Neonatal Nursing*, 16, 17-22.

Carlone, J., & Schenk, C. (1990). Genital HPV infection in the nonpregnant woman: Diagnosis and management options. *Nurse Practitioner Forum*, 1, 16-24.

Centers for Disease Control. (1993). 1993 STD treatment guidelines. *Morbidity and Mortality Reports Weekly*, 42, RR-14.

Deitch, K., & Smith, J. (1983). Cervical dysplasia and condylomata acuminata in young women. *Journal of Obstetric, Gynecologic, and Neonatal Nursing*, 12, 155-158.

Enterline, J., & Leonardo, J. (1989). Condylomata acuminate. *Nurse Practitioner*, 14, 8-16.

Keller, M.L., & Egan, J. (1994, April). Living with HPV: Impact on perceptions of self one year after diagnosis. Paper presented at the 18th Annual Research Conference of the Midwest Nursing Research Society, Milwaukee, WI.

Kelley, K., Galbraith, M., & Vermund, S. (1992). Genital human papillomavirus infection in women. *Journal of Obstetric, Gynecologic, and Neonatal Nursing*, 21, 503-515.

King, J. (1990). Epidemiology and pathophysiology of the human papillomavirus. *Nurse Practitioner Forum*, 1, 11-15.

Koutsky, L, & Wolner-Hanssen, P. (1989). Genital papillomavirus infections: Current knowledge and future prospects. *Obstetrics and Gynecology Clinics of North America*, 16, 541-557.

Kraus, S., & Stone, K. (1990). Management of genital infection caused by human papillomavirus infection. *Reviews of Infectious Diseases*, 12 (Suppl. 6), 620-632.

Lehr, S., & Lee, M. (1990). The psychosocial and sexual trauma of a genital HPV infection. *Nurse Practitioner Forum*, 1, 25-30.

Lucas, V. (1988). Human papillomavirus infection: A potentially carcinogenic sexually transmitted disease. *Nursing Clinics of North America*, 23, 917-935.

Mims, L.F., Keller, M.L., & Egan, J. (in press). Stressors and needs of women newly diagnosed with genital human papillomavirus infection.

Nash, J., Burke, T., & Hoskins, W. (1987). Biologic course of cervical human papillomavirus infection. *Obstetrics and Gynecology*, 69, 160-162.

Noegel, R., Kirby, J., Schrader, M., & Wasserheit, J. (1993). Sexually transmitted disease accelerated prevention campaigns. *Sexually Transmitted Diseases*, 20, 118-119.

Rapini, R. (1990). Venereal warts. *Primary Care*, 17, 127-143.

Redfern, N., & Hutchinson, S. (1994). Women's experiences of repetitively contracting sexually transmitted diseases. *Health Care for Women International*, 15, 423-433.

Richart, R., & Wright, J. (1993). Controversies in the management of low-grade cervical intraepithelial neoplasia. *Cancer*, 15, 1413-1421.

Spitzer, M., & Krumholz, B. (1992). Human papillomavirus-related diseases in the female patient. *Urologic Clinics of North America*, 19, 71-82

Stein, Z.A. (1990). HIV prevention: The need for methods women can use. *American Journal of Public Health*, 80, 460-462.

Tinkle, M. (1990). Genital human papillomavirus infection: A growing health risk. *Journal of Obstetric, Gynecologic, and Neonatal Nursing*, 19, 501-507.

Chapter 17

Lymphogranuloma Venereum

Lymphogranuloma venereum (LGV), a rare disease in the United States, is caused by the invasive serovars L1, L2, or L3 of *C. trachomatis*. The most frequent clinical manifestation of LGV among heterosexual men is tender inguinal and/or femoral lymphadenopathy that is usually unilateral. Women and homosexually active men might have proctocolitis or inflammatory involvement of perirectal or perianal lymphatic tissues that can result in fistulas and strictures. When most patients seek medical care, they no longer have the self-limited genital ulcer that sometimes occurs at the inoculation site. The diagnosis usually is made serologically and by exclusion of other causes of inguinal lymphadenopathy or genital ulcers.

Treatment

Treatment cures infection and prevents ongoing tissue damage, although tissue reaction can result in scarring. Buboes may require aspiration through intact skin or incision and drainage to prevent the formation of inguinal/femoral ulcerations. Doxycycline is the preferred treatment.

Recommended Regimens

Doxycycline 100 mg orally twice a day for 21 days.

Centers for Disease Control and Prevention (CDC), 1998 Guidelines for Treatment of Sexually Transmitted Diseases, *MMWR* 1998;47(No. RR-1).

Alternative Regimens

Erythromycin base 500 mg orally four times a day for 21 days.

The activity of azithromycin against *C. trachomatis* suggests that it may be effective in multiple doses over 2-3 weeks, but clinical data regarding its use are lacking.

Follow-Up

Patients should be followed clinically until signs and symptoms have resolved.

Management of Sex Partners

Sex partners of patients who have LGV should be examined, tested for urethral or cervical chlamydial infection, and treated if they had sexual contact with the patient during the 30 days preceding onset of symptoms in the patient.

Special Considerations

Pregnancy

Pregnant women should be treated with the erythromycin regimen.

HIV Infection

HIV-infected persons who have LGV should be treated according to the regimens cited previously. Anecdotal evidence suggests that LGV infection in HIV-positive patients may require prolonged therapy and that resolution might be delayed.

Chapter 18

Molluscum Contagiosum

Description

This common viral infection most often affects young children, who pass it to each other through saliva. In adults, however, the virus is transmitted sexually, resulting in lesions on the genitals, lower abdomen, buttocks, or inner thighs. Most people with the infection do not have noticeable symptoms, although sometimes the lesions, which are painless wart-like bumps, may itch or become irritated. The lesions often heal without treatment, although physicians may sometimes scrape them off or treat them with chemical irritants.

The symptoms of molluscum contagiosum are:

- raised, round, smooth-surfaced bumps on the skin that look like thick-walled pimples
- waxy or skin-colored surface on bumps
- dimple (indent) in center of bumps
- firm, white material rather than pus in cores of bumps
- found on just one area of body
- usually many different sizes, from pinhead to 1/4 inch across
- not painful, but occasionally itchy.

This diagnosis usually requires that the child be examined by a physician.

Cause

Molluscum is caused by a poxvirus. It is transmitted by skin-to-skin contact (close contact) with an infected person. Children 2 to 12 years old are most likely to be infected by this virus. Molluscum can spread to other parts of the body if a child picks at a bump and then scratches elsewhere (this process is called auto-inoculation).

Expected Course

Most molluscum disappear without treatment in 6 to 18 months. Molluscum can spread rapidly and last longer in children who also have atopic dermatitis. If repeatedly picked at, molluscum can become infected with bacteria and change into crusty sores (impetigo). Most children develop only five to ten molluscum, but some acquire more. Regardless of the number, they are a temporary condition.

Treatment

To Treat or Not to Treat?

Because molluscum are harmless, painless, and have a natural tendency to heal and disappear, some physicians recommend not treating them. The treatment itself may be painful and frightening, especially to younger children. In addition, treatment may be unsuccessful or need to be repeated. Treatment doesn't leave scars.

Treatment of molluscum will be considered if your child picks at them, the molluscum are in areas of friction (for example, the armpit), you feel they are a cosmetic problem, or the molluscum appear to be spreading rapidly.

Removal Techniques

There is no successful home treatment for molluscum. The following techniques must be performed in a physician's office. The molluscum can be destroyed with freezing (cryotherapy) or burning with a mild acid. Another type of treatment involves piercing the center of the molluscum with a needle or scalpel and scraping out the core. Newer techniques may become available.

Preventing the Spread of Molluscum to Other Areas

Every time your child picks at a molluscum and then scratches another area of skin with the same finger, a new site of molluscum can form. To prevent this spread of molluscum, discourage your child from picking at the molluscum. Use distractions to stop younger children from picking. Chewing or sucking on molluscum can lead to similar bumps on the lips or face. If your child is doing this, cover the molluscum with a Band-Aid. Keep your child's fingernails cut short and wash your child's hands more frequently.

Contagiousness

Molluscum is only mildly contagious to other people. (The incubation period is 4 to 8 weeks.) Your child can attend childcare, preschool, and school without undue concern about spread.

Call your child's physician during office hours if:

- A molluscum becomes open and looks infected.
- Your child continues to pick at the molluscum.
- The molluscum are spreading rapidly.
- You have other questions or concerns.

Chapter 19

Mononucleosis

Chapter Contents

Section 19.1

Infectious Mononucleosis

1999 National Institute of Allergy and Infectious Disease (NIAID).

Infectious mononucleosis—known popularly as "mono" or "the kissing disease"—has been recognized for more than a century. An estimated 90 percent of mononucleosis cases are caused by the Epstein-Barr virus (EBV), a member of the herpesvirus group. Most of the remaining cases are caused by certain other herpesviruses, particularly cytomegalovirus. This section focuses on mononucleosis caused by EBV.

EBV is a common virus that scientists estimate has infected over 90 percent of people aged 40 or older sometime during their lives. These infections can occur with no symptoms of disease. Like all herpesviruses, EBV remains in the body for life after infection, usually kept under control by a healthy immune system.

Almost anyone at any age can get mononucleosis. Seventy to 80 percent of all documented cases, however, involve persons between the ages of 15 and 30. Both men and women are affected, but studies suggest that the disease occurs slightly more often in men than in women. Doctors estimate that each year 50 out of every 100,000 Americans have mononucleosis symptoms. Among college students, the rate is several times higher.

Mononucleosis does not occur in any particular "season," although authorities in colleges and schools, where the disease has been well studied, report that they see most patients in the fall and early spring. Epidemics do not occur, but doctors have reported clustering of cases.

Transmission

EBV, the virus that causes most cases of mononucleosis, infects and reproduces in the salivary glands. It also infects white blood cells called B cells. Direct contact with virus-infected saliva, such as through kissing, can transmit the virus and result in mononucleosis. Someone with mononucleosis, however, does not need to be isolated.

Household members or college roommates have only a slight risk of being infected unless they come into direct contact with the patient's saliva.

A person is infectious several days before symptoms appear and for some time after acute infection. No one knows how long this period of infectiousness lasts, although the virus can be found routinely in the saliva of most people with mononucleosis for at least six months after the acute infection has subsided. It can be detected in the saliva of about 15 percent of people for years after first infection.

Symptoms

Symptoms may take between two and seven weeks to develop after exposure to the virus and can last a few days or as long as several months. In most cases, however, they disappear in one to three weeks. In fact, mononucleosis symptoms may be nonexistent or so mild that most people are not even aware of their illness.

In adolescents and young adults, the illness usually develops slowly and early symptoms are vague. Symptoms may include a general complaint of "not feeling well," headache, fatigue, chilliness, puffy eyelids, and loss of appetite. Later, the familiar triad of symptoms appears: fever, sore throat, and swollen lymph glands, especially at the side and back of the neck, but also under the arm and in the groin. A fever of 101°F to 105°F lasts for a few days and sometimes continues intermittently for one to three weeks. (High fever late in the illness suggests bacterial complications.) The swollen lymph glands, varying in size from that of a bean to a small egg, are tender and firm. Swelling gradually disappears over a few days or weeks. The spleen is enlarged in 50 percent of mononucleosis patients, and the liver is enlarged in 20 percent. Tonsillitis, difficulty in swallowing, and bleeding gums may accompany these symptoms. Rarely, jaundice or a rash that lasts one or two days is present.

In young children and older adults (more than 35 years old), mononucleosis may be difficult to diagnose because the typical mononucleosis symptoms are not present. A doctor may suspect mononucleosis in older adults, however, if the patient has had a high fever for at least a week, has an enlarged liver, has abnormal liver function studies, or has neurologic symptoms. In children, EBV infection can produce a different picture. A child may have a mild sore throat or tonsillitis or have no symptoms at all, and the illness often goes unrecognized by the parent or teacher.

Diagnosis

As mononucleosis symptoms appear, the body reacts to the virus in certain distinctive ways that can be detected through laboratory tests. White blood cells called lymphocytes increase in number (a process known as lymphocytosis), and atypical-looking (activated) lymphocytes involved in fighting the virus infection are commonly seen in blood samples. The body produces antibodies, or specific proteins, that protect against EBV. Blood tests that measure lymphocytes and antibodies aid in the diagnosis of mononucleosis.

In EBV infection, the body's immune system also produces more of substances called heterophil antibodies (Paul-Bunnell antibodies). These antibodies indicate that an EBV infection is present in the body, but they are not directed against the virus itself and do not serve a protective function. Because other types of infections and immunologic reactions also induce heterophil antibodies, their presence suggests, but does not indicate specifically, an EBV infection.

Symptoms play an important role in the diagnosis of mononucleosis. But because this disease can masquerade as other diseases, symptoms can be misleading. They may resemble, for instance, the sore throat of a "strep" infection, the painful stiff neck of meningitis, the abdominal pains of acute appendicitis, the cough and throat lesions of diphtheria, the rash of rubella or measles, or the swollen lymph glands seen in certain forms of cancer.

Rapid and inexpensive blood tests can detect heterophil antibodies in about 80 percent of persons with a current or recent infection. These antibodies can appear in sufficient strength to give a positive diagnosis as early as the fourth day and generally by the 21st day of illness. Heterophil antibodies can persist for months, however, so their appearance does not prove current infection. Furthermore, the level of heterophil antibodies in the blood does not correlate with the severity of symptoms.

The slide agglutination mono "spot test," which is widely used to screen for heterophil antibodies, is inexpensive, requires less than three minutes, and can be performed in a physician's office. Spot tests are generally accurate, but they can give false positive or false negative results. Sometimes, appearance of heterophil antibodies is delayed, and a repeat test may be necessary to establish a diagnosis. Moreover, young children, older adults, and individuals with EBV infections that do not resemble classic mononucleosis are less likely to develop heterophil antibodies.

If a patient with negative spot test results is seriously ill or has unusual symptoms, the doctor should conduct additional tests to rule out other illnesses or infections (such as HIV infection, toxoplasmosis or rubella). An EBV serologic profile is a series of blood tests that, if done and interpreted correctly, will provide a definite diagnosis of mononucleosis that is caused by EBV. Appearance of the antibodies specific for EBV proteins correlates with the stages of infection. The profile is highly accurate, but it is expensive. All physicians have access to laboratories that can perform these tests if they are necessary.

The single most meaningful test result to confirm a recent EBV infection is the demonstration of immunoglobulin M (IgM) antibodies to an EBV protein called the viral capsid antigen (VCA). This assay can be done several ways, but unfortunately some of the commercial test kits are overly sensitive and give false positive results.

Another way to prove recent EBV infection is to have blood collected at two separate time points, preferably at the first sign of symptoms and again three to four weeks later. The doctor will send both blood samples together to a lab for testing. A more than four-fold increase in immunoglobulin G (IgG) antibodies to several of the EBV-VCA proteins indicates recent infection.

Treatment and Recovery

Usually, mononucleosis is an acute, self-limited infection for which there is no specific therapy. For years, standard treatment was bed rest for four to six weeks, with limited activity for three months after all symptoms had disappeared. Today, doctors usually only recommend avoiding strenuous exercise. One real hazard of uncomplicated mononucleosis is the possibility of damaging one's enlarged spleen. Therefore, the patient should avoid lifting, straining, and competitive sports until recovery is complete. A person should limit other activity according to symptoms and how he or she feels.

Treatment of the acute phase of the illness is symptomatic and nonspecific because there is no specific drug treatment for mononucleosis. Rest, plenty of fluids to guard against dehydration, and a well-balanced diet are recommended. Doctors usually recommend acetaminophen or ibuprofen for headache, muscle pains, and chills, and salt gargles for sore throats. (Children and adolescents with a fever should not take aspirin because it can increase the risk of Reye syndrome.) Oral steroid drugs such as prednisone can help lessen some of the symptoms of mononucleosis, but because of their potential toxicity, these drugs are best reserved for treating severe complications.

Antibiotics are ineffective against viruses, and they should not be prescribed for mononucleosis itself. Some patients with mononucleosis also develop streptococcal (bacterial) throat infections, which should be treated with penicillin or erythromycin. Ampicillin (a form of penicillin) should not be used. When mononucleosis patients take ampicillin, 70 to 80 percent develop a rash for unknown reasons. Although not a true allergic reaction, the rash may be diagnosed as such, and the patient may be instructed unnecessarily to avoid penicillins in the future.

More than 90 percent of mononucleosis infections are benign and uncomplicated, but fatigue and weakness that continue for a month or more are not uncommon. The illness may be more severe and last longer in adults over the age of 30. Airway obstruction, rupture of the spleen, inflammation of the heart or tissues surrounding the heart, and severe bone marrow or central nervous system involvement are rare, life-threatening complications that are treated with steroid drugs. If the spleen should rupture, a doctor will immediately have to remove it surgically and start transfusions and other therapy for shock.

Although EBV remains in the body indefinitely following a bout of mononucleosis, the disease rarely recurs. Nearly all individuals who have repeated mono-like illnesses either have a seriously impaired immune system, such as transplant recipients, or are actually experiencing sequential infections with different viruses that can provoke similar symptoms. In addition, several scientific studies now have confirmed that EBV does not cause chronic fatigue syndrome.

Further Research

Scientists believe that increased knowledge of normal and abnormal immune responses will lead to an understanding of how EBV can cause a relatively benign illness, like mononucleosis, and also play a role in much more serious, sometimes fatal, diseases. Epstein and Barr, two British scientists after whom EBV is named, first found evidence of the virus in B lymphocytes of patients with a rare form of cancer of the lymph system. This cancer, known as Burkitt's lymphoma, occurs primarily in Africa.

Scientists have learned a lot about how EBV affects the body's cells in mononucleosis. EBV is known to increase the number of *B. lymphocytes*, which have receptors for the virus on their surfaces. The normal response of the body to this increase in B cells is a corresponding increase in *T. lymphocytes*, another component of the immune system, which change in appearance to become atypical cells. Some of these T cells apparently limit the spread of the virus from cell to cell; others suppress the production of the B cells. This suppression is what seems to eliminate the infection. Normally, the T cell response subsides as the patient recovers from mononucleosis.

Section 19.2

Mono: Tough for Teens and Twenty-Somethings

Food and Drug Administration (FDA), from *FDA Consumer*,
May-June 1998, Vol.32, No.3, Pg.32(4).

Missed parties. Postponed exams. Sitting out a season of team sports. And loneliness. These are a few of the ways that scourge of high school and college students known as "mono" can affect your life.

The disease whose medical name is infectious mononucleosis is most common in people 10 to 35 years old, with its peak incidence in those 15 to 17. Only 50 people out of 100,000 in the general population get mono, but it strikes as many as 2 out of 1,000 teens and twenty-somethings, especially those in high school, college, and the military. While mono is not usually considered a serious illness, it may have serious complications. Without a doubt your lifestyle will change for a few months.

You've probably heard people call mono the "kissing disease." But if your social life is in a slump, you may wonder. "How did I get this 'kissing disease' when I haven't kissed anyone romantically recently?"

Here's how. Mono is usually transmitted though saliva and mucus—which is where the "kissing disease" nickname comes from. But the kissing or close contact that transmits the disease doesn't happen right before you get sick. The virus that causes mono has a long incubation period: 30 to 50 days from the time you're exposed to it to the time you get sick. In addition, the virus can be transmitted in other ways, such as sipping from the same straw or glass as an infected person—or even being close when the person coughs or sneezes. Also, some people can have the virus in their systems without ever having symptoms and you can still catch it from them.

Two viruses can cause mono: Epstein-Barr virus (EBV) and cytomegalovirus (CMV). Both viruses are in the herpes family, whose other members include viruses responsible for cold sores and chickenpox.

EBV causes 85 percent of mono cases. About half of all children are infected with EBV before they're 5, but at that young age, it usually doesn't cause any symptoms. If you don't become infected with EBV until you're a teen or older, you're more likely to develop mono symptoms. After you're infected, the virus stays with you for life, but usually doesn't cause any additional symptoms. Still, every now and then you may produce viral particles in your saliva that can transmit the virus to other people, even though you feel perfectly fine. By age 40, 85 to 90 percent of Americans have EBV antibodies, indicating they have the virus in their systems and are immune to further EBV infection.

CMV is also a very common virus. About 85 percent of the U.S. population is infected with it by the time they reach adulthood. As with EBV, CMV is frequently symptomless, and mono most often results when infection occurs in the teens and 20s. Sore throat is less common in people who have CMV mono than in those infected with EBV.

As another one of its nicknames—glandular fever—implies, perhaps the most distinguishing mono symptom is enlarged glands or lymph nodes, especially in the neck, but also in the armpit and groin.

Another common mono symptom is fever. A temperature as high as 39.5 degrees Celsius (103 degrees Fahrenheit) is not uncommon. Other symptoms include a tired achy feeling, appetite loss, white patches on the back of the throat, and tonsillitis.

"My tonsils got so swollen they were touching each other in back," says Heidi Palombo of Annandale, Va., who had mono when she was a senior in college. She recalls her throat being "so hot and swollen that the only thing that felt good was ice water."

Cold drinks and frozen desserts are both ways to relieve sore throat symptoms. Doctors also recommend gargling with saltwater (about half a teaspoon salt to 8 ounces of warm water) and sucking on throat lozenges available over the counter in pharmacies and other stores. If throat or tonsils are infected, a throat culture should be taken so the doctor can prescribe an appropriate antibiotic. Ampicillin is usually not recommended because it sometimes causes a rash that can be confused with the pink, measleslike rash that 1 out of 5 mono patients develops.

For fever and achiness, you can take acetaminophen (marketed as Tylenol, Datril and others) or ibuprofen (marketed as Advil, Motrin,

Nuprin, and others). If you're under 20, don't take aspirin unless your doctor approves it. In children and teens, aspirin taken for viral illnesses has been associated with the potentially fatal disease Reye syndrome. Sometimes a person with mono may have trouble breathing because of swelling in the throat, and doctors have to use other medications and treatment. A person who has mono—or those caring for the person—should contact a doctor immediately if the person starts having breathing problems.

Some people with mono become overly sensitive to light and about half develop enlargement of the spleen, usually two to three weeks after they first become sick. Mild enlargement of the liver may also occur.

Whether or not the spleen is enlarged, people who have mono should not lift heavy objects or exercise vigorously—including participating in contact sports—for two months after they get sick, because these activities increase the risk of rupturing the spleen, which can be life-threatening. If you have mono and get a severe sharp, sudden pain on the left side of your upper abdomen, go to an emergency room or call 911 immediately.

Because its symptoms can be very similar to those of other illnesses, doctors often recommend tests to find out exactly what the problem is.

"I was misdiagnosed at first and told I was bit by a spider," writes John L. Gipson, of Kansas City, Mo., in a note he posted to a Website. "That's what I thought because I had killed a spider in my room. I figured I'd been bitten by a spider in my sleep. A few days after, I had no energy, a fever, and those peasized bumps on the back of my neck." Gipson returned to his doctor, who did blood tests and diagnosed mononucleosis.

Other diagnostic problems can result because enlarged lymphocytes, a type of white cell, are common with mono, but can also be a symptom of leukemia. Blood tests can distinguish between the type of white cell seen in leukemia and that with mono.

If your throat is sore, having a throat culture is usually a good idea for several reasons. First, the symptoms of mono and strep infection (including that caused by *Strep-A*, a particularly serious form of strep) are very similar. Second, strep throat or other throat infections can develop anytime during or shortly after in the disease. In any case, it's important that throat infections be diagnosed as soon as possible and treated with antibiotics that can kill the organism responsible for the infection.

The test most commonly used to tell whether you have mono or some other ailment is the mononucleosis spot test. This blood test detects the antibodies (proteins) that the body makes to fight EBV or CMV. Because it takes a while for antibodies to develop after infection, your doctor may need to order or repeat the test one to two weeks after you develop symptoms. At that time the test is about 85 percent accurate.

Other tests your doctor might order include a complete blood count (CBC) to see if your blood platelet count is lower than normal and if lymphocytes are abnormal, and a chemistry panel to see if liver enzymes are abnormal.

Bed rest is the most important treatment for uncomplicated mono. It's also important to drink plenty of fluids. Mono is not usually a reason to quarantine students. Many people are already immune to the viruses that cause it. But if you have mono you'll want to stay in bed and out of classes for several days, until the fever goes down and other symptoms abate. Even when you've started to get better, you can expect to have to curtail your activities for several weeks, and it can take two to three months or more until you feel your old self again.

The author of this article had mono herself when she was 16. Though she didn't mind getting out of all that homework (or at least putting it off), having to delay finals only added to her anxiety about college applications that many high school juniors experience. And then there was that guy who never called again.

When you add the time spent recuperating to the fact that most people are not exactly anxious to get close to a person with mono, you can understand why some students find themselves combating loneliness on top of their other troubles.

Getting through mono may be both challenging and depressing— and seem to take forever. But if you rest when your body tells you to, you can lessen the chances of complications and get back your life.

Chapter 20

Nongonococcal Urethritis (NGU)

Chapter Contents

Section 20.1

Diseases Characterized by Urethritis and Cervicitis

Centers for Disease Control and Prevention (CDC). 1998 Guidelines for Treatment of Sexually Transmitted Diseases. *MMWR* 1998;47(No. RR-1): Pg.1-118.

Management of Male Patients Who Have Urethritis

Urethritis, or inflammation of the urethra, is caused by an infection characterized by the discharge of mucopurulent or purulent material and by burning during urination. Asymptomatic infections are common. The only bacterial pathogens of proven clinical importance in men who have urethritis are *N. gonorrhoeae* and *C. trachomatis*. Testing to determine the specific disease is recommended because both of these infections are reportable to state health departments, and a specific diagnosis may improve compliance and partner notification. If diagnostic tools (e.g., a Gram stain and microscope) are unavailable, patients should be treated for both infections. The extra expense of treating a person who has nongonococcal urethritis (NGU) for both infections also should encourage the health-care provider to make a specific diagnosis. New nucleic acid amplification tests enable detection of *N. gonorrhoeae* and *C. trachomatis* on first-void urine; in some settings, these tests are more sensitive than traditional culture techniques.

Etiology

NGU is diagnosed if Gram-negative intracellular organisms cannot be identified on Gram stains. *C. trachomatis* is the most frequent cause (i.e., in 23%-55% of cases); however, the prevalence differs by age group, with lower prevalence among older men. The proportion of NGU cases caused by chlamydia has been declining gradually. Complications of NGU among men infected with *C. trachomatis* include epididymitis and Reiter's syndrome. Documentation of chlamydia infection is important because partner referral for evaluation and treatment would be indicated.

The etiology of most cases of nonchlamydial NGU is unknown. *Ureaplasma urealyticum* and possibly *Mycoplasma genitalium* are implicated in as many as one third of cases. Specific diagnostic tests for these organisms are not indicated.

Trichomonas vaginalis and HSV sometimes cause NGU. Diagnostic and treatment procedures for these organisms are reserved for situations in which NGU is nonresponsive to therapy.

Confirmed Urethritis

Clinicians should document that urethritis is present. Urethritis can be documented by the presence of any of the following signs:

- Mucopurulent or purulent discharge.

- Gram stain of urethral secretions demonstrating greater than or equal to 5 WBCs per oil immersion field. The Gram stain is the preferred rapid diagnostic test for evaluating urethritis. It is highly sensitive and specific for documenting both urethritis and the presence or absence of gonococcal infection. Gonococcal infection is established by documenting the presence of WBCs containing intracellular Gram-negative diplococci.

- Positive leukocyte esterase test on first-void urine, or microscopic examination of first-void urine demonstrating greater than or equal to 10 WBCs per high power field.

If none of these criteria is present, then treatment should be deferred, and the patient should be tested for *N. gonorrhoeae* and *C. trachomatis* and followed closely in the event of a positive test result. If the results demonstrate infection with either *N. gonorrhoeae* or *C. trachomatis*, the appropriate treatment should be given and sex partners referred for evaluation and treatment.

Empiric treatment of symptoms without documentation of urethritis is recommended only for patients at high risk for infection who are unlikely to return for a follow-up evaluation (e.g., adolescents who have multiple partners). Such patients should be treated for gonorrhea and chlamydia. Partners of patients treated empirically should be referred for evaluation and treatment.

Management of Patients Who Have Nongonococcal Urethritis

Diagnosis

All patients who have urethritis should be evaluated for the presence of gonococcal and chlamydial infection. Testing for chlamydia is strongly recommended because of the increased utility and availability of highly sensitive and specific testing methods and because a specific diagnosis might improve compliance and partner notification.

Treatment

Treatment should be initiated as soon as possible after diagnosis. Single-dose regimens have the important advantage of improved compliance and of directly observed therapy. If multiple-dose regimens are used, the medication should be provided in the clinic or health-care provider's office. Treatment with the recommended regimen can result in alleviation of symptoms and microbiologic cure of infection.

Recommended Regimens

Azithromycin 1 g orally in a single dose,

OR

Doxycycline 100 mg orally twice a day for 7 days.

Alternative Regimens

Erythromycin base 500 mg orally four times a day for 7 days,

OR

Erythromycin ethylsuccinate 800 mg orally four times a day for 7 days,

OR

Ofloxacin 300 mg twice a day for 7 days.

If only erythromycin can be used and a patient cannot tolerate high-dose erythromycin schedules, one of the following regimens can be used.

Erythromycin base 250 mg orally four times a day for 14 days,

OR

Erythromycin ethylsuccinate 400 mg orally four times a day for 14 days.

251:52

age.

Follow-Up for Patients Who Have Urethritis

Patients should be instructed to return for evaluation if symptoms persist or recur after completion of therapy. Symptoms alone, without documentation of signs or laboratory evidence of urethral inflammation, are not a sufficient basis for re-treatment. Patients should be instructed to abstain from sexual intercourse until therapy is completed.

Partner Referral

Patients should refer for evaluation and treatment all sex partners within the preceding 60 days. A specific diagnosis may facilitate partner referral; therefore, testing for gonorrhea and chlamydia is encouraged.

Recurrent and Persistent Urethritis

Objective signs of urethritis should be present before initiation of antimicrobial therapy. Effective regimens have not been identified for treating patients who have persistent symptoms or frequent recurrences after treatment. Patients who have persistent or recurrent urethritis should be re-treated with the initial regimen if they did not comply with the treatment regimen or if they were reexposed to an untreated sex partner. Otherwise, a wet mount examination and culture of an intraurethral swab specimen for *T. vaginalis* should be performed. Urologic examinations usually do not reveal a specific etiology. If the patient was compliant with the initial regimen and reexposure can be excluded, the following regimen is recommended.

Recommended Treatment for Recurrent/Persistent Urethritis

Metronidazole 2 g orally in a single dose,

PLUS

Erythromycin base 500 mg orally four times a day for 7 days,

OR

Erythromycin ethylsuccinate 800 mg orally four times a day for 7 days.

Special Considerations

HIV Infection

Gonococcal urethritis, chlamydial urethritis, and nongoncoccal, nonchlamydial urethritis may facilitate HIV transmission. Patients who have NGU and also are infected with HIV should receive the same treatment regimen as those who are HIV-negative.

Section 20.2

Single-Dose Treatment of Nongonococcal Urethritis

Used with permission from the Nov. 1, 1995 issue of
American Family Physician. © 1995 The American Academy of
Family Physicians. All rights reserved.

Most cases of nongonococcal urethritis, the most common sexually transmitted disease in men, are due to either *Chlamydia trachomatis* or *Ureaplasma urealyticum.* A seven-day course of doxycycline has been the usual empiric treatment for this condition. Stamm and colleagues compared the effectiveness of a single dose of azithromycin with that of the standard seven-day regimen of doxycycline in the treatment of nongonococcal urethritis.

Men 18 years of age or older were included in the study if they had a penile discharge consistent with urethritis that was shown on Gram's stain to be nongonococcal. Patients were excluded if they were allergic to the study drugs, if they were seropositive for the human immunodeficiency virus, if they had received antibiotics in the preceding two weeks or if they had a gastrointestinal problem that would prevent normal absorption of the study drug. Patients underwent evaluation with a history and physical examination and blood and urine testing. Patients were randomized to receive either 1,000 mg of azithromycin in a single dose or 100 mg of doxycycline twice daily for seven days; follow-up assessment was performed at two and five weeks after the start of treatment.

Of 452 patients initially enrolled, 248 men who received azithromycin and 123 who received doxycyline were available for evaluation. At the two-week follow-up, most of the men in both groups were cured. The cumulative cure rates were 81 percent for the azithromycin group and 77 percent for the doxycycline group. The two-week cure rate was 90 percent for patients in the azithromycin group and 89 percent for those in the doxycycline group; the five-week cure rates were 89 percent and 85 percent, respectively. The overall cure rate at both follow-up visits for men infected with *C. trachomatis* was 83 percent for the azithromycin group and 90 percent for the doxycycline group. For patients whose urethritis was due to *U. urealyticum*, the overall cure rates were 45 percent for the azithromycin group and 47 percent for the doxycycline group.

The authors conclude that a single dose of azithromycin is as effective as the traditional seven-day regimen of doxycycline in the treatment of nongonococcal urethritis. Although the authors acknowledge the higher cost of azithromycin ($10 to $30 versus approximately $5 for a course of doxycycline), they point out that compliance is much improved with use of a single-dose medication.

Chapter 21

Pelvic Inflammatory Disease (PID)

Chapter Contents

Section 21.1

Pelvic Inflammatory Disease Facts

Centers for Disease Control and Prevention (CDC). 1998 Guidelines for Treatment of Sexually Transmitted Diseases. *MMWR* 1998;47(No. RR-1).

PID comprises a spectrum of inflammatory disorders of the upper female genital tract, including any combination of endometritis, salpingitis, tubo-ovarian abscess, and pelvic peritonitis. Sexually transmitted organisms, especially *N. gonorrhoeae* and *C. trachomatis*, are implicated in most cases; however, microorganisms that can be part of the vaginal flora (e.g., anaerobes, *G. vaginalis*, *H. influenzae*, enteric Gram-negative rods, and *Streptococcus agalactiae*) also can cause PID. In addition, *M. hominis* and *U. urealyticum* might be etiologic agents of PID.

Diagnostic Considerations

Acute PID is difficult to diagnose because of the wide variation in the symptoms and signs. Many women with PID have subtle or mild symptoms that do not readily indicate PID. Consequently, delay in diagnosis and effective treatment probably contributes to inflammatory sequelae in the upper reproductive tract. Laparoscopy can be used to obtain a more accurate diagnosis of salpingitis and a more complete bacteriologic diagnosis. However, this diagnostic tool often is not readily available for acute cases, and its use is not easy to justify when symptoms are mild or vague. Moreover, laparoscopy will not detect endometritis and may not detect subtle inflammation of the fallopian tubes. Consequently, a diagnosis of PID usually is based on clinical findings. The clinical diagnosis of acute PID also is imprecise. Data indicate that a clinical diagnosis of symptomatic PID has a positive-predictive value (PPV) for salpingitis of 65%-90% in comparison with laparoscopy. The PPV of a clinical diagnosis of acute PID differs depending on epidemiologic characteristics and the clinical setting, with higher PPV among sexually active young (especially teenaged) women and among patients attending STD clinics or from settings in which rates of gonorrhea or chlamydia are high. In all settings, however, no single historical, physical, or laboratory finding is both sensitive and specific for the diagnosis of acute PID (i.e., can be used both to detect all cases of PID and to exclude all women without PID). Combinations of diagnostic findings that improve either sensitivity (i.e., detect more women who have PID) or specificity (i.e., exclude more women who do not have PID) do so only at the expense of the other. For example, requiring two or more findings excludes more women who do not have PID but also reduces the number of women with PID who are identified.

Many episodes of PID go unrecognized. Although some cases are asymptomatic, others are undiagnosed because the patient or the health-care provider fails to recognize the implications of mild or non-specific symptoms or signs (e.g., abnormal bleeding, dyspareunia, or vaginal discharge {atypical PID}). Because of the difficulty of diagnosis and the potential for damage to the reproductive health of women even by apparently mild or atypical PID, health-care providers should maintain a low threshold for the diagnosis of PID. Even so, the long-term outcome of early treatment of women with asymptomatic or atypical PID is unknown. The following recommendations for diagnosing PID are intended to help health-care providers recognize when PID should be suspected and when they need to obtain additional information to increase diagnostic certainty. These recommendations are based partially on the fact that diagnosis and management of other common causes of lower abdominal pain (e.g., ectopic pregnancy, acute appendicitis, and functional pain) are unlikely to be impaired by initiating empiric antimicrobial therapy for PID.

Empiric treatment of PID should be initiated in sexually active young women and others at risk for STDs if all the following minimum criteria are present and no other cause(s) for the illness can be identified:

- Lower abdominal tenderness,
- Adnexal tenderness, and
- Cervical motion tenderness.

More elaborate diagnostic evaluation often is needed, because incorrect diagnosis and management might cause unnecessary morbidity. These additional criteria may be used to enhance the specificity of the minimum criteria listed previously. Additional criteria that support a diagnosis of PID include the following:

- Oral temperature greater than 101 F (greater than 38.3 C),

255

- Abnormal cervical or vaginal discharge,

- Elevated erythrocyte sedimentation rate,

- Elevated C-reactive protein, and

- Laboratory documentation of cervical infection with *N. gonorrhoeae* or *C. trachomatis*.

The definitive criteria for diagnosing PID, which are warranted in selected cases, include the following:

- Histopathologic evidence of endometritis on endometrial biopsy,

- Transvaginal sonography or other imaging techniques showing thickened fluid-filled tubes with or without free pelvic fluid or tubo-ovarian complex, and

- Laparoscopic abnormalities consistent with PID.

Although treatment can be initiated before bacteriologic diagnosis of *C. trachomatis* or *N. gonorrhoeae* infection, such a diagnosis emphasizes the need to treat sex partners.

Treatment

PID treatment regimens must provide empiric, broad-spectrum coverage of likely pathogens. Antimicrobial coverage should include *N. gonorrhoeae*, *C. trachomatis*, anaerobes, Gram-negative facultative bacteria, and *streptococci*. Although several antimicrobial regimens have been effective in achieving a clinical and microbiologic cure in randomized clinical trials with short-term follow-up, few investigations have a) assessed and compared these regimens with regard to elimination of infection in the endometrium and fallopian tubes or b) determined the incidence of long-term complications (e.g., tubal infertility and ectopic pregnancy).

All regimens should be effective against *N. gonorrhoeae* and *C. trachomatis*, because negative endocervical screening does not preclude upper-reproductive tract infection. Although the need to eradicate anaerobes from women who have PID has not been determined definitively, the evidence suggests that this may be important. Anaerobic bacteria have been isolated from the upper-reproductive tract of women who have PID, and data from in vitro studies have revealed that anaerobes such as *Bacteroides fragilis* can cause tubal and epithelial destruction. In addition, bacterial vaginosis (BV) also is diagnosed in many women who have PID. Until treatment regimens that do not adequately cover these microbes have been shown to prevent sequelae as well as the regimens that are effective against these microbes, the recommended regimens should have anaerobic coverage.

Treatment should be initiated as soon as the presumptive diagnosis has been made, because prevention of long-term sequelae has been linked directly with immediate administration of appropriate antibiotics. When selecting a treatment regimen, health-care providers should consider availability, cost, patient acceptance, and antimicrobial susceptibility.

In the past, many experts recommended that all patients who had PID be hospitalized so that bed rest and supervised treatment with parenteral antibiotics could be initiated. However, hospitalization is no longer synonymous with parenteral therapy. No currently available data compare the efficacy of parenteral with oral therapy or inpatient with outpatient treatment settings. Until the results from ongoing trials comparing parenteral inpatient therapy with oral outpatient therapy for women who have mild PID are available, such decisions must be based on observational data and consensus opinion. The decision of whether hospitalization is necessary should be based on the discretion of the health-care provider.

The following criteria for hospitalization are based on observational data and theoretical concerns:

- Surgical emergencies such as appendicitis cannot be excluded;

- The patient is pregnant;

- The patient does not respond clinically to oral antimicrobial therapy;

- The patient is unable to follow or tolerate an outpatient oral regimen;

- The patient has severe illness, nausea and vomiting, or high fever;

- The patient has a tubo-ovarian abscess; or

- The patient is immunodeficient (i.e., has HIV infection with low CD4 counts, is taking immunosuppressive therapy, or has another disease).

Most clinicians favor at least 24 hours of direct inpatient observation for patients who have tubo-ovarian abscesses, after which time home parenteral therapy should be adequate.

There are no efficacy data comparing parenteral with oral regimens. Experts have extensive experience with both of the following regimens. Also, there are multiple randomized trials demonstrating the efficacy of each regimen. Although most trials have used parenteral treatment for at least 48 hours after the patient demonstrates substantial clinical improvement, this is an arbitrary designation. Clinical experience should guide decisions regarding transition to oral therapy, which may be accomplished within 24 hours of clinical improvement.

Parenteral Regimen A

Cefotetan 2 g IV every 12 hours,

OR

Cefoxitin 2 g IV every 6 hours,

PLUS

Doxycycline 100 mg IV or orally every 12 hours.

NOTE: Because of pain associated with infusion, doxycycline should be administered orally when possible, even when the patient is hospitalized. Both oral and IV administration of doxycycline provide similar bioavailability. In the event that IV administration is necessary, use of lidocaine or other short-acting local anesthetic, heparin, or steroids with a steel needle or extension of the infusion time may reduce infusion complications. Parenteral therapy may be discontinued 24 hours after a patient improves clinically, and oral therapy with doxycycline (100 mg twice a day) should continue for a total of 14 days. When tubo-ovarian abscess is present, many health-care providers use clindamycin or metronidazole with doxycycline for continued therapy rather than doxycycline alone, because it provides more effective anaerobic coverage.

Clinical data are limited regarding the use of other second- or third-generation cephalosporins (e.g., ceftizoxime, cefotaxime, and ceftriaxone), which also might be effective therapy for PID and might replace cefotetan or cefoxitin. However, they are less active than cefotetan or cefoxitin against anaerobic bacteria.

Parenteral Regimen B

Clindamycin 900 mg IV every 8 hours,

PLUS

Gentamicin loading dose IV or IM (2 mg/kg of body weight), followed by a maintenance dose (1.5 mg/kg) every 8 hours. Single daily dosing may be substituted.

NOTE: Although use of a single daily dose of gentamicin has not been evaluated for the treatment of PID, it is efficacious in other analogous situations. Parenteral therapy may be discontinued 24 hours after a patient improves clinically, and continuing oral therapy should consist of doxycycline 100 mg orally twice a day or clindamycin 450 mg orally four times a day to complete a total of 14 days of therapy. When tubo-ovarian abscess is present, many health-care providers use clindamycin for continued therapy rather than doxycycline, because clindamycin provides more effective anaerobic coverage.

Alternative Parenteral Regimens

Limited data support the use of other parenteral regimens, but the following three regimens have been investigated in at least one clinical trial, and they have broad spectrum coverage.

Ofloxacin 400 mg IV every 12 hours,

PLUS

Metronidazole 500 mg IV every 8 hours,

OR

Ampicillin/Sulbactam 3 g IV every 6 hours,

PLUS

Doxycycline 100 mg IV or orally every 12 hours,

OR

Ciprofloxacin 200 mg IV every 12 hours,

PLUS

Doxycycline 100 mg IV or orally every 12 hours,

PLUS

Metronidazole 500 mg IV every 8 hours.

Ampicillin/sulbactam plus doxycycline has good coverage against *C. trachomatis, N. gonorrhoeae,* and anaerobes and appears to be effective for patients who have tubo-ovarian abscess. Both IV ofloxacin and ciprofloxacin have been investigated as single agents. Because ciprofloxacin has poor coverage against *C. trachomatis,* it is recommended that doxycycline be added routinely. Because of concerns regarding the anaerobic coverage of both quinolones, metronidazole should be included with each regimen.

Oral Treatment

As with parenteral regimens, clinical trials of outpatient regimens have provided minimal information regarding intermediate and long-term outcomes. The following regimens provide coverage against the frequent etiologic agents of PID, but evidence from clinical trials supporting their use is limited. Patients who do not respond to oral therapy within 72 hours should be reevaluated to confirm the diagnosis and be administered parenteral therapy on either an outpatient or inpatient basis.

Regimen A

Ofloxacin 400 mg orally twice a day for 14 days,

PLUS

Metronidazole 500 mg orally twice a day for 14 days.

Oral ofloxacin has been investigated as a single agent in two well-designed clinical trials, and it is effective against both *N. gonorrhoeae* and *C. trachomatis.* Despite the results of these trials, ofloxacin's lack of anaerobic coverage is a concern; the addition of metronidazole provides this coverage.

Regimen B

Ceftriaxone 250 mg IM once,

OR

Cefoxitin 2 g IM plus Probenecid 1 g orally in a single dose concurrently once,

OR

Other parenteral third-generation cephalosporin (e.g., ceftizoxime or cefotaxime),

PLUS

Doxycycline 100 mg orally twice a day for 14 days. (Include this regimen with one of the above regimens.)

The optimal choice of a cephalosporin for Regimen B is unclear; although cefoxitin has better anaerobic coverage, ceftriaxone has better coverage against *N. gonorrhoeae*. Clinical trials have demonstrated that a single dose of cefoxitin is effective in obtaining short-term clinical response in women who have PID; however, the theoretical limitations in its coverage of anaerobes may require the addition of metronidazole. The metronidazole also will effectively treat BV, which also is frequently associated with PID. No data have been published regarding the use of oral cephalosporins for the treatment of PID.

Alternative Oral Regimens

Information regarding other outpatient regimens is limited, but one other regimen has undergone at least one clinical trial and has broad spectrum coverage. Amoxicillin/clavulanic acid plus doxycycline was effective in obtaining short-term clinical response in a single clinical trial; however, gastrointestinal symptoms might limit the overall success of this regimen. Several recent investigations have evaluated the use of azithromycin in the treatment of upper-reproductive tract infections; however, the data are insufficient to recommend this agent as a component of any of the treatment regimens for PID.

Follow-Up

Patients receiving oral or parenteral therapy should demonstrate substantial clinical improvement (e.g., defervescence; reduction in direct or rebound abdominal tenderness; and reduction in uterine, adnexal, and cervical motion tenderness) within 3 days after initiation of therapy. Patients who do not demonstrate improvement within this time period usually require additional diagnostic tests, surgical intervention, or both.

If the health-care provider prescribes outpatient oral or parenteral therapy, a follow-up examination should be performed within 72 hours, using the criteria for clinical improvement described previously. Some experts also recommend rescreening for *C. trachomatis* and *N.*

gonorrhoeae 4-6 weeks after therapy is completed. If PCR (polymerase chain reaction) or LCR (ligase chain reaction) is used to document a test of cure, rescreening should be delayed for 1 month after completion of therapy.

Management of Sex Partners

Sex partners of patients who have PID should be examined and treated if they had sexual contact with the patient during the 60 days preceding onset of symptoms in the patient. The evaluation and treatment are imperative because of the risk for reinfection and the strong likelihood of urethral gonococcal or chlamydial infection in the sex partner. Male partners of women who have PID caused by *C. trachomatis* and/or *N. gonorrhoeae* often are asymptomatic.

Sex partners should be treated empirically with regimens effective against both of these infections, regardless of the apparent etiology of PID or pathogens isolated from the infected woman.

Even in clinical settings in which only women are treated, special arrangements should be made to provide care for male sex partners of women who have PID. When this is not feasible, health-care providers should ensure that sex partners are referred for appropriate treatment.

Special Considerations

Pregnancy

Because of the high risk for maternal morbidity, fetal wastage, and preterm delivery, pregnant women who have suspected PID should be hospitalized and treated with parenteral antibiotics.

HIV Infection

Differences in the clinical manifestations of PID between HIV-infected women and HIV-negative women have not been well delineated. In early observational studies, HIV-infected women with PID were more likely to require surgical intervention. In a subsequent and more comprehensive observational study, HIV-infected women who had PID had more severe symptoms than HIV-negative women but responded equally well to standard parenteral antibiotic regimens. In another study, the microbiologic findings for HIV-infected and HIV-negative women were similar, except for higher rates of concomitant Candida and HPV infections and HPV-related cytologic abnormalities among HIV-infected women. Immunosuppressed HIV-infected women who have PID should be managed aggressively using one of the parenteral antimicrobial regimens recommended in this report.

Section 21.2

Adolescent Girls and Pelvic Inflammatory Disease

© 1998 American Medical Association, from *Archives of Pediatrics & Adolescent Medicine*, May 1998, Vol.152, No.5, Pg.449(6), by Jacques Benaim, Mary Pulaski, and Susan M. Coupey; reprinted with permission.

Sexually active adolescent girls aged 15 to 19 years are more likely to be hospitalized with pelvic inflammatory disease (PID) than are adult women aged 25 to 29 years. Although rates cited per 10,000 population are lower for adolescents (31.4) than for adults (56.9), only 50% of adolescent girls have had sexual intercourse and are thus at risk of infection compared with more than 90% of the older women.[1,2] In the adolescent age group, differences in both biology and sexual behavior are important contributors to the high sexually transmitted disease (STD) rate and the frequent extension of infection into the upper genital tract, resulting in PID. Immaturity of the epithelial lining of the cervix and lack of local immunity have been suggested as biological factors that put the adolescent at increased risk of infection with sexually transmitted pathogens.[3] In addition, behavioral factors common to adolescents, such as inconsistent use of either barrier or hormonal contraception, which reduce the risk of PID, lack of access to gynecologic health care to screen for asymptomatic infection, and fear of disclosure of sexual activity, contribute to the high PID rate in this age group.[4] Sequelae of PID are a major cause of reproductive morbidity in women, accounting for the majority of cases of acquired infertility and substantially increasing the risk of subsequent ectopic pregnancy.[5-7] Other serious health sequelae of PID include tubo-ovarian abscess and pelvic adhesions, often leading to dyspareunia and chronic pelvic pain.[8]

In 1991, the Centers for Disease Control and Prevention (CDC) issued guidelines for the prevention and management of PID in which they specifically singled out the adolescent age group for special consideration.[9] The CDC guidelines note that many women with PID have subtle, vague symptoms that are quite mild and, as a result, the condition is underdiagnosed and/or the seriousness of the infection is not appreciated. They recommend a "low threshold" for the diagnosis of PID. In addition, the guidelines indicate that the efficacy of outpatient management for preventing late sequelae is uncertain and could reduce the likelihood of successful eradication of upper genital tract pathogens because of both low serum levels of antibiotics given by the oral route and compliance issues. Adolescents are at the beginning of their reproductive lives, with a longer time frame in which to develop complications than adult women; they also have a greater likelihood of poor treatment adherence related to their living circumstances, psychosocial immaturity, and confidentiality issues. These concerns about the efficacy of outpatient management led the CDC experts to specifically recommend inpatient treatment with parenteral antibiotics for all adolescents diagnosed as having PID.[9] These recommendations were reiterated in the CDC's 1993 Sexually Transmitted Diseases Treatment Guidelines and in publications from other influential organizations.[10-12] For adult women, the CDC guidelines suggest consideration of inpatient treatment, but if outpatient treatment is undertaken, they recommend close follow-up within 72 hours of beginning antibiotic therapy. In addition, the guidelines recommend notification of sex partners and risk reduction counseling for all women diagnosed as having PID. Leading authorities in adolescent medicine and in pediatric emergency medicine echo these recommendations in major textbooks, as does the Institute of Medicine in its 1997 publication "The Hidden Epidemic: Confronting Sexually Transmitted Diseases."[13-15]

However, there are forces within the health care system, most notably the growth of managed care, that work against inpatient management of PID for economic rather than health-related reasons, and, indeed, overall hospitalization rates for PID declined during the 1980s by about 36% with no evidence of a decline in office visits for this diagnosis.[9] Although the decline in hospitalization rates occurred for all age groups, there was a relatively smaller decrease (10%) for 15 to 19-year-olds, suggesting that physicians still are more likely to treat this age group as inpatients. It is too soon to tell if the trend toward increased outpatient treatment will lead to higher rates of morbidity from sequelae of inadequately treated PID.

Many adolescents with PID will come for care to the emergency department with symptoms of abdominal pain, fever, dysuria, and/or vaginal discharge. One study examining emergency department use by rural adolescents aged 12 to 18 years found that females and older teens were more likely than males and younger teens to come to the emergency department for care and that, of the nearly 5000 adolescent emergency department visits examined, 9% of the females were given a discharge diagnosis of an obstetrics/gynecology problem (PID was included in this category).[16] The authors of the study noted that the highest hospital admission rates were among adolescents diagnosed with obstetrics/gynecology problems, but they also remarked that STDs were underrepresented as a diagnosis in their cohort and speculated that adolescent-specific risk factors may be difficult to address in the emergency department setting.

In many centers, the pediatric department cares for adolescents up to the age of 18 or even 21 years. Thus, pediatricians working in emergency departments are likely to see many adolescent girls with PID, and they are the ones who must make the decision regarding hospital admission vs. outpatient management. Pediatric emergency medicine is a newly board-certifiable subspecialty whose curriculum for fellowship training includes learning "age-appropriate pelvic examinations" as well as diagnosing and managing pelvic pain, salpingitis (PID), and vaginal discharge.[17] Most fellowship-trained emergency medicine pediatricians work in teaching hospitals affiliated with medical schools, and many are in leadership positions.[18] Such pediatric emergency medicine specialists are a critical component in the education of medical students and pediatric residents and thus have an impact on the practice of future pediatricians. In addition, when they make a diagnosis of PID in the emergency department, pediatric emergency medicine specialists often advise the referring primary care physician and health insurance carrier about appropriate treatment and follow-up for the patient. Thus, pediatric emergency medicine specialists' understanding of the diagnosis and management of PID in adolescents may be important in the control of this disease that extends far beyond their small numbers.

The purpose of this study was to describe the experience and practices of emergency department pediatricians in the United States related to the diagnosis and management of PID in adolescent girls. In addition, we wished to assess the physicians' attitudes toward STDs in adolescents and their perception of the adequacy of their training in adolescent STD management. Specifically, we were interested in the degree to which pediatric emergency medicine physicians complied with CDC guidelines related to hospital admission for PID, postdiagnosis counseling, and timing of follow-up care.

Results

Experience and Practices Related to PID

The large majority of pediatricians (51 [94%]) had made the diagnosis of PID in adolescent patients within the past 2 years. The diagnosis was made frequently (once a week or more often) by nearly half (24 [47%]) of the 51 pediatricians who had diagnosed PID. However, only 23 (45%) of the pediatricians diagnosing PID reported recommending routine hospital admission for adolescent girls with this diagnosis. There was no significant difference in patient admission recommendations between pediatricians who cared for adolescents only up to age 18 years and those who also cared for young adults up to age 21 years. Of the 37 pediatricians who ever treated adolescents with PID as outpatients, just over half (20 [54%]) reported recommending a follow-up visit within 72 hours as suggested in the CDC guidelines. The follow-up site most commonly recommended to patients with no primary care physician was an adolescent clinic (23 [62%]), with a minority of pediatricians recommending a gynecology clinic (9 [24%]). The majority of respondents (22/37 [59%]) reported that they arrange follow-up by giving the adolescent the telephone number of the referral site, whereas 9 (24%) reported providing date, time, and directions to the site.

Counseling after Diagnosis of an STD in Adolescent Girls

The large majority of the pediatricians surveyed (47 [87%]) reported routinely suggesting condom use after the diagnosis of an STD in a female adolescent. Similarly, 34 (63%) of respondents routinely suggested testing for human immunodeficiency virus on such occasions. Contraceptive counseling (other than condoms) after diagnosis of an STD was reported by less than half (23 [43%]) of the respondents. In addition, only 17 (31%) of the 54 pediatricians surveyed provided written notification for the patient to give to her sexual partner(s) informing him of the need for STD treatment.

Attitudes about STDs in Adolescent Girls

Almost two thirds of the respondents believed that the care of a female adolescent with an STD should be different from the care of a female adult with a similar condition. The majority (38 [70%]) of the pediatricians thought that adolescent girls were more prone than adult women to complications from STDs. In contrast, there was no agreement among the physicians when asked whether adolescent girls have increased biological susceptibility to acquiring an STD when compared with adult women, with 14 (26%) of respondents being unsure of the answer to this question and the others equally divided between yes and no answers.

Pediatricians' Perception of Their Training in Adolescent Health Care

Subjects were asked, "On a scale of 1 to 5, how do you feel your post-medical school training prepared you to care for adolescents with STDs?" where 1 indicated "didn't prepare me at all" and 5 indicated "prepared me extremely well." The mean ([+ of -] SD) response on this Likert-type scale for the total sample of pediatricians was 3.14 [+ of -] 1.27, indicating a moderate level of perceived adequacy of training in the area. When asked similarly about preparation for dealing with psychosocial problems of adolescent patients, the mean score was 2.6 [+ of -] 1.09, indicating that the pediatricians felt somewhat less well prepared in this area than in the area of STD care.

Comment

This survey of emergency department pediatricians confirms the important role of this group of physicians in the management of PID in adolescent girls. We found that PID is frequently diagnosed in pediatric emergency departments, with nearly one half of the pediatricians surveyed making this diagnosis once per week or more often. In addition, almost all the pediatricians surveyed reported that they have teaching responsibilities, confirming our hypothesis that they are in a position to influence trainees. The impact of these emergency department pediatricians on the management of PID in adolescent girls is therefore magnified by their importance to the training of future physicians in general and pediatricians in particular.

We found, however, that many emergency department pediatricians are not as aggressive in their management of PID in adolescents as the CDC guidelines and STD experts recommend. Our findings indicate that about half of the pediatric emergency physicians treated some adolescent girls with PID as outpatients. Although many pediatricians we surveyed indicated that they attempted to arrange close follow-up within 72 hours of beginning antibiotic therapy, many did not; 45% scheduled follow-up at longer intervals. This delay in follow-up is of some concern given the necessity to promptly evaluate response to therapy to minimize complications. Close follow-up of oral antibiotic therapy may be of particular importance in adolescents whose families may not help to reinforce medication compliance because they either do not appreciate the severity of the infection, or are unaware of the diagnosis, because of confidentiality issues related to the sexually transmitted nature of the disease.

We can only speculate about the reasons why many emergency department pediatricians are less aggressive in their management of PID in adolescents than STD experts recommend, since this issue was not directly assessed in the survey. On the basis of post-interview comments made by some physicians, several potential barriers can be considered. One such barrier may simply be that emergency department pediatricians are unaware of current recommendations for treatment of adolescents and how they differ from those of adults. Most of the pediatricians we surveyed believed that the care of adolescents with STDs ought to be different from the care of adult women and that adolescent girls are at higher risk of medical complications of STDs. These beliefs indicate that emergency department pediatricians understand the uniqueness of the adolescent developmental stage in relation to medical complications of sexual behavior. Despite these beliefs, however, many did not admit all adolescents with PID to the hospital for parenteral therapy or even arrange close outpatient follow-up. This may represent difficulty in handling the sensitive psychosocial issues related to adolescents and STDs. Many adolescents with PID are seen in community hospital emergency departments by physicians trained to treat adults. These clinicians may be less likely than the pediatric-trained physicians studied herein to acknowledge the uniqueness of the adolescent age group in relation to treatment of STDs and to follow guidelines for hospitalization. Thus, the problem of undertreatment may be much greater than suggested by this study alone.

We found in this survey that CDC recommendations pertaining to counseling after the diagnosis of STDs in adolescents were inconsistently followed. Most pediatricians surveyed would suggest HIV testing and condom use, but many do not provide optimal contraceptive counseling or partner notification. Effective partner notification procedures are especially important from a public health standpoint to prevent further spread of STDs. Despite increasing educational effort in adolescent medicine during pediatric training in recent years, some emergency department pediatricians may be uncomfortable with the care of adolescents, and this may influence their decision making related to PID management.[19] This discomfort may have been reflected in our finding in this study that the respondents had a relatively poor perception of the adequacy of their own training in dealing with psychosocial problems of adolescents. In addition, addressing such sociomedical issues as partner notification and pregnancy prevention may be perceived as too time consuming for the emergency department setting. However, with the use of effective medical communication skills, these patient education tasks can be accomplished efficiently in a short time, and it may be the only opportunity to reach some high-risk adolescents.

Many pediatricians we surveyed commented anecdotally that they would admit a girl with PID if she had a fever and looked sick but would suggest outpatient treatment if she had no systemic signs of illness other than pelvic pain and cervical motion tenderness. However, the most common organism causing PID in adolescents, *Chlamydia trachomatis*, often follows a subacute course without fever or elevation of the white blood cell count, despite serious underlying disease. The severity of the symptoms at initial examination should not be used as the main criterion for hospital admission in adolescents, and this is clearly addressed in the CDC guidelines. In addition, several interviewees commented that they had difficulty with reimbursement for inpatient treatment of PID, and this could represent an additional barrier to optimal treatment of adolescent girls with this illness. Managed care organizations and other insurers may require education to understand the medical necessity for parenteral treatment early in the course of this infection in adolescents even when clinical signs and symptoms are subacute. These are important issues to explore in further research, since they have potential solutions, such as using the CDC recommendations to support claims for reimbursement from third-party insurers. Similarly, increasing educational efforts in adolescent medicine during pediatric training could help to remove other potential barriers, such as discomfort in managing psychosocial issues.

This study has some limitations that are important to consider. Although the pediatricians surveyed were a random sample of the entire group, the response rate was only moderate, adding a potential source of bias. However, we found that respondents were demographically similar to nonrespondents in terms of sex and geographic location, suggesting that any systematic respondent bias is unlikely. This allows us to be confident that the descriptive data can be generalized to all members of the Section on Pediatric Emergency Medicine. The small sample size did not allow us to compare PID management practices by physicians' training, age, sex, and practice characteristics. Although such analysis may support or contradict some of our hypotheses on the reasons for physicians' management decisions, it could not have pointed to causality because of the cross-sectional design of the survey.

The findings of this study confirm the importance of pediatric emergency medicine physicians in the diagnosis of PID in adolescent girls and highlight some of the barriers to providing optimal management of this serious infection in this age group. Important avenues to explore in attempting to improve the treatment of PID in adolescents are the relative importance of barriers related to health care economics and third-party payers vs. those related to physicians' skills in psychosocial management of STD in adolescent girls and their awareness of current management guidelines.

References

1. Velebil, P.; Wingo, P.A.; Xia, Z., et al. Rate of hospitalization for gynecologic disorders among reproductive-age women in the United States. *Obstet Gynecol.* 1995; 86:764-769.

2. Bell, T.A.; Holmes, K.K. Age-specific risks of syphilis, gonorrhea, and hospitalized pelvic inflammatory disease in sexually experienced U.S. women. *Sex Transm Dis.* 1984;11:291-295.

3. Mosciki, A.B.; Winkler, B.; Irwin, C.E. Jr.; Schachter, J. Differences in biologic maturation, sexual behavior, and sexually transmitted disease between adolescents with and without cervical intraepithelial neoplasia. *J Pediatr.* 1989;115: 487-493.

4. Cates, W., Jr. The epidemiology and control of STD in adolescents. In: Schydlower, M.; Shafer, M.A., eds. AIDS and Other Sexually Transmitted Diseases. Vol 1. Philadelphia, Pa: Hanley & Belfus; 1990:409-427. *Adolescent Medicine State of the Art Reviews.*

5. Westrom, L.; Mardh, P.A. Acute pelvic inflammatory disease. In: Holmes, K.K.; Mardh, P.A.; Sparling, P.F.; Wiesner, P.J., eds. *Sexually Transmitted Diseases. 2nd ed.* New York, NY: McGraw-Hill Book Co; 1990:593-613.

6. Marchbanks, P.A.; Annegers, J.F.; Coulam, C.B.; Strathy, J.H.; Kurland, L.T. Risk factors for ectopic pregnancy: a population-based study. *JAMA.* 1988;259:1823-1827.

7. Coste, J.; Job-Spira, N.; Fernandez, H., et al. Risk factors for ectopic pregnancy: a case-control study in France, with special focus on infectious factors. *Am J Epidemiol.* 1991;133:839-849.

8. Sweet, R.L. Pelvic inflammatory disease. In: Sweet, R.L.; Gibbs, R.S., eds. *Infectious Diseases of the Female Genital Tract 2nd ed.* Baltimore, Md: Williams & Wilkins; 1990:241-266.

9. Centers for Disease Control and Prevention. Pelvic inflammatory disease: guidelines for prevention and management. *MMWR Morb Mortal Wkly Rep.* 1991; 40:1-25.

10. Centers for Disease Control and Prevention. 1993 Sexually transmitted diseases treatment guidelines. *MMWR Morb Mortal Wkly Rep.* 1993;42:78.

11. Biro, F. Adolescents and sexually transmitted diseases. *Maternal and Child Health Technical Information Bulletin.* August 1992:15.

12. Association of Reproductive Health Professionals. Pelvic inflammatory disease. *Clin Proc.* May 1994:8.

13. Rosenfeld, W.D.; Litman, N. Sexually transmitted diseases. In: Friedman, S.B,; Fisher, M.M.; Schonberg, S.K.; Alderman, E.M., eds. *Comprehensive Adolescent Health Care. 2nd ed.* St Louis, Mo: CV Mosby; 1998:1097-1118.

14. Paradise, J.E. Pediatric and adolescent gynecology. In: Fleischer, G.R.; Ludwig, S., eds. *Textbook of Pediatric Emergency Medicine.* Baltimore, Md: Williams &Wilkins; 1993:929-939.

15. Eng, T.R.; Butler, W.T., eds. *The Hidden Epidemic: Confronting Sexually Transmitted Diseases.* Washington, DC: Institute of Medicine, National Academy Press; 1997.

16. Lehmann, C.U.; Barr, J.; Kelly, P.J. Emergency department utilization by adolescents. *J Adolesc Health.* 1994;15:485-490.

17. Curriculum Subcommittee Section of Emergency Medicine, American Academy of Pediatrics. Pediatric emergency medicine (PEM) fellowship curriculum statement. *Pediatr Emerg Care.* 1991;7:48-53.

18. Nozick, C.A.; Singh, J. Training, attitudes, and income profiles of pediatric emergency physicians: the results of a 1993 survey of the American Academy of Pediatrics Section on Emergency Medicine. *Pediatr Emerg Care*. 1995;11: 20-24.

19. Cohen, M.I. Importance, implementation, and impact of the adolescent medicine components of the report of the task force on pediatric education. *J Adolesc Health*. 1980;1:1-8.

Chapter 22

Syphilis

Chapter Contents

Section 22.1

Syphilis Facts

Centers for Disease Control and Prevention (CDC). 1998 Guidelines for
Treatment of Sexually Transmitted Diseases. *MMWR* 1998;47(No. RR-1).
© 1999 Washington Post/Newsweek Interactive Co., from *The Washington
Post*, Oct 12, 1999, Pg.Z09, excerpted from "Health Officials Set Sights on
Syphilis; Citing Record Low U.S. Incidence," by Susan Okie;
reprinted with permission.

Background

Syphilis is a sexually transmitted infection caused by a bacterium,
Treponema pallidum, that can damage tissues in many organs of the
body. The initial symptoms—a painless sore, followed by a rash—often go unnoticed and disappear without treatment. However, the bacteria remain in the body, producing a "latent" infection that may injure
the brain, spinal cord, major blood vessels, bones or other tissues.

Infections may be detected by serologic testing during the latent
stage. Latent syphilis acquired within the preceding year is referred
to as early latent syphilis; all other cases of latent syphilis are either
late latent syphilis or syphilis of unknown duration. Treatment for
late latent syphilis, as well as tertiary syphilis, theoretically may require a longer duration of therapy because organisms are dividing
more slowly; however, the validity and importance of this concept have
not been determined.

Diagnostic Considerations and Use of Serologic Tests

Darkfield examinations and direct fluorescent antibody tests of lesion
exudate or tissue are the definitive methods for diagnosing early syphilis. A presumptive diagnosis is possible with the use of two types of serologic tests for syphilis: a) nontreponemal (e.g., Venereal Disease Research
Laboratory {VDRL} and RPR [rapid plasma reagin]) and b) treponemal
(e.g., fluorescent treponemal antibody absorbed {FTA-ABS} and microhemagglutination assay for antibody to *T. pallidum* {MHA-TP}). The
use of only one type of test is insufficient for diagnosis because false-
positive nontreponemal test results occasionally occur secondary to

various medical conditions. Nontreponemal test antibody titers usually correlate with disease activity, and results should be reported quantitatively. A fourfold change in titer, equivalent to a change of two dilutions (e.g., from 1:16 to 1:4 or from 1:8 to 1:32), usually is considered necessary to demonstrate a clinically significant difference between two nontreponemal test results that were obtained by using the same serologic test. It is expected that the nontreponemal test will eventually become nonreactive after treatment; however, in some patients, nontreponemal antibodies can persist at a low titer for a long period, sometimes for the remainder of their lives. This response is referred to as the serofast reaction. Most patients who have reactive treponemal tests will have reactive tests for the remainder of their lives, regardless of treatment or disease activity. However, 15%-25% of patients treated during the primary stage might revert to being serologically nonreactive after 2-3 years. Treponemal test antibody titers correlate poorly with disease activity and should not be used to assess treatment response.

Sequential serologic tests should be performed by using the same testing method (e.g., VDRL or RPR), preferably by the same laboratory. The VDRL and RPR are equally valid, but quantitative results from the two tests cannot be compared directly because RPR titers often are slightly higher than VDRL titers.

HIV-infected patients can have abnormal serologic test results (i.e., unusually high, unusually low, and fluctuating titers). For such patients with clinical syndromes suggestive of early syphilis, use of other tests (e.g., biopsy and direct microscopy) should be considered. However, for most HIV-infected patients, serologic tests appear to be accurate and reliable for the diagnosis of syphilis and for evaluation of treatment response.

No single test can be used to diagnose all cases of neurosyphilis. The diagnosis of neurosyphilis can be made based on various combinations of reactive serologic test results, abnormalities of cerebrospinal fluid (CSF) cell count or protein, or a reactive VDRL-CSF with or without clinical manifestations. The CSF leukocyte count usually is elevated (greater than 5 WBCs/mm3) when neurosyphilis is present, and it also is a sensitive measure of the effectiveness of therapy. The VDRL-CSF is the standard serologic test for CSF; when reactive in the absence of substantial contamination of CSF with blood, it is considered diagnostic of neurosyphilis. However, the VDRL-CSF may be nonreactive when neurosyphilis is present. Some experts recommend performing an FTA-ABS test on CSF. The CSF FTA-ABS is less specific (i.e., yields more false-positive results) for neurosyphilis than the

VDRL-CSF. However, the test is believed to be highly sensitive, and some experts believe that a negative CSF FTA-ABS test excludes neurosyphilis.

Treatment

Parenteral penicillin G is the preferred drug for treatment of all stages of syphilis. The preparation(s) used (i.e., benzathine, aqueous procaine, or aqueous crystalline), the dosage, and the length of treatment depend on the stage and clinical manifestations of disease.

The efficacy of penicillin for the treatment of syphilis was well established through clinical experience before the value of randomized controlled clinical trials was recognized. Therefore, almost all the recommendations for the treatment of syphilis are based on expert opinion reinforced by case series, clinical trials, and 50 years of clinical experience.

Parenteral penicillin G is the only therapy with documented efficacy for neurosyphilis or for syphilis during pregnancy. Patients, who report a penicillin allergy, including pregnant women with syphilis in any stage and patients with neurosyphilis, should be desensitized and treated with penicillin. Skin testing for penicillin allergy may be useful in some settings, because the minor determinants needed for penicillin skin testing are unavailable commercially.

The Jarisch-Herxheimer reaction is an acute febrile reaction—often accompanied by headache, myalgia, and other symptoms—that might occur within the first 24 hours after any therapy for syphilis; patients should be advised of this possible adverse reaction. The Jarisch-Herxheimer reaction often occurs among patients who have early syphilis. Antipyretics may be recommended, but no proven methods prevent this reaction. The Jarisch-Herxheimer reaction may induce early labor or cause fetal distress among pregnant women. This concern should not prevent or delay therapy.

Management of Sex Partners

Sexual transmission of *T. pallidum* occurs only when mucocutaneous syphilitic lesions are present; such manifestations are uncommon after the first year of infection. However, persons exposed sexually to a patient who has syphilis in any stage should be evaluated clinically and serologically according to the following recommendations:

- Persons who were exposed within the 90 days preceding the diagnosis of primary, secondary, or early latent syphilis in a sex partner might be infected even if seronegative; therefore, such persons should be treated presumptively.

- Persons who were exposed greater than 90 days before the diagnosis of primary, secondary, or early latent syphilis in a sex partner should be treated presumptively if serologic test results are not available immediately and the opportunity for follow-up is uncertain.

- For purposes of partner notification and presumptive treatment of exposed sex partners, patients with syphilis of unknown duration who have high nontreponemal serologic test titers (i.e., greater than or equal to 1:32) may be considered as having early syphilis. However, serologic titers should not be used to differentiate early from late latent syphilis for the purpose of determining treatment.

- Long-term sex partners of patients who have late syphilis should be evaluated clinically and serologically for syphilis and treated on the basis of the findings of the evaluation.

The time periods before treatment used for identifying at-risk sex partners are a) 3 months plus duration of symptoms for primary syphilis, b) 6 months plus duration of symptoms for secondary syphilis, and c) 1 year for early latent syphilis.

Primary and Secondary Syphilis

Treatment

Parenteral penicillin G has been used effectively for four decades to achieve a local cure (i.e., healing of lesions and prevention of sexual transmission) and to prevent late sequelae. However, no adequately conducted comparative trials have been performed to guide the selection of an optimal penicillin regimen (i.e., the dose, duration, and preparation). Substantially fewer data are available concerning nonpenicillin regimens.

Recommended Regimen for Adults

Patients who have primary or secondary syphilis should be treated with the following regimen.

Benzathine penicillin G 2.4 million units IM in a single dose.

NOTE: Recommendations for treating pregnant women and HIV-infected patients for syphilis are discussed in separate sections.

Recommended Regimen for Children

After the newborn period, children in whom syphilis is diagnosed should have a CSF examination to detect asymptomatic neurosyphilis, and birth and maternal medical records should be reviewed to assess whether the child has congenital or acquired syphilis. Children with acquired primary or secondary syphilis should be evaluated (including consultation with child-protection services) and treated by using the following pediatric regimen.

Benzathine penicillin G 50,000 units/kg IM, up to the adult dose of 2.4 million units in a single dose.

Other Management Considerations

All patients who have syphilis should be tested for HIV infection. In geographic areas in which the prevalence of HIV is high, patients who have primary syphilis should be retested for HIV after 3 months if the first HIV test result was negative. This recommendation will become particularly important if it can be demonstrated that intensive antiviral therapy administered soon after HIV seroconversion is beneficial.

Patients who have syphilis and who also have symptoms or signs suggesting neurologic disease (e.g., meningitis) or ophthalmic disease (e.g., uveitis) should be evaluated fully for neurosyphilis and syphilitic eye disease; this evaluation should include CSF analysis and ocular slit-lamp examination. Such patients should be treated appropriately according to the results of this evaluation.

Invasion of CSF by *T. pallidum* accompanied by CSF abnormalities is common among adults who have primary or secondary syphilis. However, neurosyphilis develops in only a few patients after treatment with the regimens described in this report. Therefore, unless clinical signs or symptoms of neurologic or ophthalmic involvement are present, lumbar puncture is not recommended for routine evaluation of patients who have primary or secondary syphilis.

Follow-Up

Treatment failures can occur with any regimen. However, assessing response to treatment often is difficult, and no definitive criteria for cure or failure have been established. Serologic test titers may decline more slowly for patients who previously had syphilis. Patients should be reexamined clinically and serologically at both 6 months and 12 months; more frequent evaluation may be prudent if follow-up is uncertain.

Patients who have signs or symptoms that persist or recur or who have a sustained fourfold increase in nontreponemal test titer (i.e., in comparison with either the baseline titer or a subsequent result) probably failed treatment or were reinfected. These patients should be re-treated after reevaluation for HIV infection. Unless reinfection with *T. pallidum* is certain, a lumbar puncture also should be performed.

Failure of nontreponemal test titers to decline fourfold within 6 months after therapy for primary or secondary syphilis identifies persons at risk for treatment failure. Such persons should be reevaluated for HIV infection. Optimal management of such patients is unclear. At a minimum, these patients should have additional clinical and serologic follow-up. HIV-infected patients should be evaluated more frequently (i.e., at 3-month intervals instead of 6-month intervals). If additional follow-up cannot be ensured, re-treatment is recommended. Some experts recommend CSF examination in such situations.

When patients are re-treated, most experts recommend re-treatment with three weekly injections of benzathine penicillin G 2.4 million units IM, unless CSF examination indicates that neurosyphilis is present.

Special Considerations

Penicillin Allergy

Nonpregnant penicillin-allergic patients who have primary or secondary syphilis should be treated with one of the following regimens. Close follow-up of such patients is essential.

Recommended Regimens

Doxycycline 100 mg orally twice a day for 2 weeks,

OR

Tetracycline 500 mg orally four times a day for 2 weeks.

There is less clinical experience with doxycycline than with tetracycline, but compliance is likely to be better with doxycycline. Therapy for a patient who cannot tolerate either doxycycline or tetracycline should depend on whether the patient's compliance with the therapy regimen and with follow-up examinations can be ensured.

Pharmacologic and bacteriologic considerations suggest that ceftriaxone should be effective, but data concerning ceftriaxone are limited and clinical experience is insufficient to enable identification of late failures. The optimal dose and duration have not been established for ceftriaxone, but a suggested daily regimen of 1 g may be considered if treponemacidal levels in the blood can be maintained for 8-10 days. Single-dose ceftriaxone therapy is not effective for treating syphilis.

For nonpregnant patients whose compliance with therapy and follow-up can be ensured, an alternative regimen is erythromycin 500 mg orally four times a day for 2 weeks. However, erythromycin is less effective than the other recommended regimens.

Patients whose compliance with therapy or follow-up cannot be ensured should be desensitized and treated with penicillin. Skin testing for penicillin allergy may be useful in some circumstances in which the reagents and expertise to perform the test adequately are available.

Pregnancy

Pregnant patients who are allergic to penicillin should be desensitized, if necessary, and treated with penicillin.

Latent Syphilis

Latent syphilis is defined as those periods after infection with *T. pallidum* when patients are seroreactive, but demonstrate no other evidence of disease. Patients who have latent syphilis and who acquired syphilis within the preceding year are classified as having early latent syphilis. Patients can be demonstrated as having early latent syphilis if, within the year preceding the evaluation, they had a) a documented seroconversion, b) unequivocal symptoms of primary or secondary syphilis, or c) a sex partner who had primary, secondary, or early latent syphilis. Almost all other patients have latent syphilis of unknown duration and should be managed as if they had late latent syphilis. Nontreponemal serologic titers usually are higher during early latent syphilis than late latent syphilis. However, early latent syphilis cannot be reliably distinguished from late latent syphilis solely on the basis of nontreponemal titers. Regardless of the level of the nontreponemal titers, patients in whom the illness does not meet the definition of early syphilis should be treated as if they have late latent infection. All sexually active women with reactive nontreponemal serologic tests should have a pelvic examination before syphilis staging is completed to evaluate for internal mucosal lesions. All patients who have syphilis should be tested for HIV infection.

Treatment of latent syphilis is intended to prevent occurrence or progression of late complications. Although clinical experience supports the effectiveness of penicillin in achieving these goals, limited evidence is available for guidance in choosing specific regimens. There is minimal evidence to support the use of nonpenicillin regimens.

Recommended Regimens for Adults

The following regimens are recommended for nonallergic patients who have normal CSF examinations (if performed):

Early Latent Syphilis:

Benzathine penicillin G 2.4 million units IM in a single dose.

Late Latent Syphilis or Latent Syphilis of Unknown Duration:

Benzathine penicillin G 7.2 million units total, administered as three doses of 2.4 million units IM each at 1-week intervals.

Recommended Regimens for Children

After the newborn period, children in whom syphilis is diagnosed should have a CSF examination to exclude neurosyphilis, and birth and maternal medical records should be reviewed to assess whether the child has congenital or acquired syphilis. Older children with acquired latent syphilis should be evaluated as described for adults and treated using the following pediatric regimens. These regimens are for non-allergic children who have acquired syphilis and whose results of the CSF examination were normal.

Early Latent Syphilis:

Benzathine penicillin G 50,000 units/kg IM, up to the adult dose of 2.4 million units in a single dose.

Late Latent Syphilis or Latent Syphilis of Unknown Duration:

Benzathine penicillin G 50,000 units/kg IM, up to the adult dose of 2.4 million units, administered as three doses at 1-week intervals (total 150,000 units/kg up to the adult total dose of 7.2 million units).

Other Management Considerations

All patients who have latent syphilis should be evaluated clinically for evidence of tertiary disease (e.g., aortitis, neurosyphilis, gumma, and iritis). Patients who have syphilis and who demonstrate any of the following criteria should have a prompt CSF examination:

- Neurologic or ophthalmic signs or symptoms;

- Evidence of active tertiary syphilis (e.g., aortitis, gumma, and iritis);

- Treatment failure; and

- HIV infection with late latent syphilis or syphilis of unknown duration.

If dictated by circumstances and patient preferences, a CSF examination may be performed for patients who do not meet these criteria. If a CSF examination is performed and the results indicate abnormalities consistent with neurosyphilis, the patient should be treated for neurosyphilis.

Follow-Up

Quantitative nontreponemal serologic tests should be repeated at 6, 12, and 24 months. Limited data are available to guide evaluation of the treatment response for patients who have latent syphilis. Patients should be evaluated for neurosyphilis and re-treated appropriately if a) titers increase fourfold, b) an initially high titer (greater than or equal to 1:32) fails to decline at least fourfold (i.e., two dilutions) within 12-24 months, or c) signs or symptoms attributable to syphilis develop in the patient.

Special Considerations

Penicillin Allergy

Nonpregnant patients who have latent syphilis and who are allergic to penicillin should be treated with one of the following regimens.

Recommended Regimens

Doxycycline 100 mg orally twice a day,

OR

Tetracycline 500 mg orally four times a day.

Both drugs should be administered for 2 weeks if the duration of infection is known to have been less than 1 year; otherwise, they should be administered for 4 weeks.

Pregnancy

Pregnant patients who are allergic to penicillin should be desensitized and treated with penicillin.

Tertiary Syphilis

Tertiary syphilis refers to gumma and cardiovascular syphilis, but not to neurosyphilis. Nonallergic patients without evidence of neurosyphilis should be treated with the following regimen.

Recommended Regimens

Benzathine penicillin G 7.2 million units total, administered as three doses of 2.4 million units IM at 1-week intervals.

Other Management Considerations

Patients who have symptomatic late syphilis should have a CSF examination before therapy is initiated. Some experts treat all patients who have cardiovascular syphilis with a neurosyphilis regimen. The complete management of patients who have cardiovascular or gummatous syphilis is beyond the scope of these guidelines. These patients should be managed in consultation with an expert.

Follow-Up

Information is lacking with regard to follow-up of patients who have late syphilis. The clinical response depends partially on the nature of the lesions.

Special Considerations

Penicillin Allergy

Patients allergic to penicillin should be treated according to the recommended regimens for late latent syphilis.

Pregnancy

Pregnant patients who are allergic to penicillin should be desensitized, if necessary, and treated with penicillin.

Neurosyphilis

Treatment

Central nervous system disease can occur during any stage of syphilis. A patient who has clinical evidence of neurologic involvement with syphilis (e.g., ophthalmic or auditory symptoms, cranial nerve palsies, and symptoms or signs of meningitis) should have a CSF examination. Syphilitic uveitis or other ocular manifestations frequently are associated with neurosyphilis; patients with these symptoms should be treated according to the recommendations for neurosyphilis. A CSF examination should be performed for all such patients to identify those with abnormalities who should have follow-up CSF examinations to assess treatment response. Patients who have neurosyphilis or syphilitic eye disease (e.g., uveitis, neuroretinitis, or optic neuritis) and who are not allergic to penicillin should be treated with the following regimen:

Recommended Regimens

Aqueous crystalline penicillin G 18-24 million units a day, administered as 3-4 million units IV every 4 hours for 10-14 days.

If compliance with therapy can be ensured, patients may be treated with the following alternative regimen:

Alternative Regimen

Procaine penicillin 2.4 million units IM a day, PLUS Probenecid 500 mg orally four times a day, both for 10-14 days.

The durations of the recommended and alternative regimens for neurosyphilis are shorter than that of the regimen used for late syphilis in the absence of neurosyphilis. Therefore, some experts administer benzathine penicillin, 2.4 million units IM, after completion of these neurosyphilis treatment regimens to provide a comparable total duration of therapy.

Other Management Considerations

Other considerations in the management of patients who have neurosyphilis are as follows:

- All patients who have syphilis should be tested for HIV.

- Many experts recommend treating patients who have evidence of auditory disease caused by syphilis in the same manner as for neurosyphilis, regardless of the findings on CSF examination. Although systemic steroids are used frequently as adjunctive therapy for otologic syphilis, such drugs have not been proven beneficial.

Follow-Up

If CSF pleocytosis was present initially, a CSF examination should be repeated every 6 months until the cell count is normal. Follow-up CSF examinations also can be used to evaluate changes in the VDRL-CSF or CSF protein after therapy; however, changes in these two parameters are slower, and persistent abnormalities are of less importance. If the cell count has not decreased after 6 months, or if the CSF is not entirely normal after 2 years, re-treatment should be considered.

Special Considerations

Penicillin Allergy

Data have not been collected systematically for evaluation of therapeutic alternatives to penicillin for treatment of neurosyphilis. Patients who report being allergic to penicillin should either be desensitized to penicillin or be managed in consultation with an expert. In some situations, skin testing to confirm penicillin allergy may be useful.

Pregnancy

Pregnant patients who are allergic to penicillin should be desensitized, if necessary, and treated with penicillin.

Syphilis in HIV-Infected Persons

Diagnostic Considerations

Unusual serologic responses have been observed among HIV-infected persons who have syphilis. Most reports involved serologic titers that were higher than expected, but false-negative serologic test results or delayed appearance of seroreactivity also have been reported. Nevertheless, both treponemal and nontreponemal serologic tests for syphilis can be interpreted in the usual manner for most patients who are coinfected with *T. pallidum* and HIV.

When clinical findings suggest that syphilis is present, but serologic tests are nonreactive or unclear, alternative tests (e.g., biopsy of a lesion, darkfield examination, or direct fluorescent antibody staining of lesion material) may be useful.

Neurosyphilis should be considered in the differential diagnosis of neurologic disease in HIV-infected persons.

Treatment

In comparison with HIV-negative patients, HIV-infected patients who have early syphilis may be at increased risk for neurologic complications and may have higher rates of treatment failure with currently recommended regimens. The magnitude of these risks, although not defined precisely, is probably minimal. No treatment regimens for syphilis are demonstrably more effective in preventing neurosyphilis in HIV-infected patients than the syphilis regimens recommended for HIV-negative patients. Careful follow-up after therapy is essential.

Primary and Secondary Syphilis in HIV-Infected Persons

Treatment

Treatment with benzathine penicillin G, 2.4 million units IM, as for HIV-negative patients, is recommended. Some experts recommend additional treatments (e.g., three weekly doses of benzathine penicillin G as suggested for late syphilis) or other supplemental antibiotics in addition to benzathine penicillin G 2.4 million units IM.

Other Management Considerations

CSF abnormalities often occur among both asymptomatic HIV-infected patients in the absence of syphilis and HIV-negative patients who have primary or secondary syphilis. Such abnormalities in HIV-infected patients who have primary or secondary syphilis are of unknown prognostic significance. Most HIV-infected patients respond appropriately to the currently recommended penicillin therapy;

however, some experts recommend CSF examination before therapy and modification of treatment accordingly.

Follow-Up

It is important that HIV-infected patients be evaluated clinically and serologically for treatment failure at 3, 6, 9, 12, and 24 months after therapy. Although of unproven benefit, some experts recommend a CSF examination after therapy (i.e., at 6 months).

HIV-infected patients who meet the criteria for treatment failure should be managed the same as HIV-negative patients (i.e., a CSF examination and re-treatment). CSF examination and re-treatment also should be strongly considered for patients whose nontreponemal test titer does not decrease fourfold within 6-12 months. Most experts would re-treat patients with 7.2 million units of benzathine penicillin G (administered as three weekly doses of 2.4 million units each) if CSF examinations are normal.

Special Considerations

Penicillin Allergy

Penicillin-allergic patients who have primary or secondary syphilis and HIV infection should be managed according to the recommendations for penicillin-allergic HIV-negative patients.

Latent Syphilis in HIV-Infected Persons

Diagnostic Considerations

HIV-infected patients who have early latent syphilis should be managed and treated according to the recommendations for HIV-negative patients who have primary and secondary syphilis. HIV-infected patients who have either late latent syphilis or syphilis of unknown duration should have a CSF examination before treatment.

Treatment

A patient with late latent syphilis or syphilis of unknown duration and a normal CSF examination can be treated with 7.2 million units of benzathine penicillin G (as three weekly doses of 2.4 million units each). Patients who have CSF consistent with neurosyphilis should be treated and managed as described for neurosyphilis.

Follow-Up

Patients should be evaluated clinically and serologically at 6, 12, 18, and 24 months after therapy. If, at any time, clinical symptoms develop or nontreponemal titers rise fourfold, a repeat CSF examination should be performed and treatment administered accordingly. If between 12 and 24 months the nontreponemal titer fails to decline fourfold, the CSF examination should be repeated, and treatment administered accordingly.

Special Considerations

Penicillin Allergy

Penicillin regimens should be used to treat all stages of syphilis in HIV-infected patients. Skin testing to confirm penicillin allergy may be used. Patients may be desensitized, then treated with penicillin.

Section 22.2

Syphilis during Pregnancy

Centers for Disease Control and Prevention (CDC).
1998 Guidelines for Treatment of Sexually Transmitted Diseases.
MMWR 1998;47(No. RR-1).

All women should be screened serologically for syphilis during the early stages of pregnancy. In populations in which utilization of prenatal care is not optimal, RPR-card test screening and treatment (i.e., if the RPR-card test is reactive) should be performed at the time a pregnancy is diagnosed. For communities and populations in which the prevalence of syphilis is high or for patients at high risk, serologic testing should be performed twice during the third trimester, at 28 weeks of gestation and at delivery. (Some states mandate screening at delivery for all women.) Any woman who delivers a stillborn infant after 20 weeks of gestation should be tested for syphilis. No infant should leave the hospital without the maternal serologic status having been determined at least once during pregnancy.

Diagnostic Considerations

Seropositive pregnant women should be considered infected unless an adequate treatment history is documented clearly in the medical records and sequential serologic antibody titers have declined.

Treatment

Penicillin is effective for preventing maternal transmission to the fetus and for treating fetal-established infection. Evidence is insufficient to determine whether the specific, recommended penicillin regimens are optimal.

Recommended Regimens

Treatment during pregnancy should be the penicillin regimen appropriate for the stage of syphilis.

Other Management Considerations

Some experts recommend additional therapy in some settings. A second dose of benzathine penicillin 2.4 million units IM may be administered 1 week after the initial dose for women who have primary, secondary, or early latent syphilis. Ultrasonographic signs of fetal syphilis (i.e., hepatomegaly and hydrops) indicate a greater risk for fetal treatment failure; such cases should be managed in consultation with obstetric specialists.

Women treated for syphilis during the second half of pregnancy are at risk for premature labor and/or fetal distress if the treatment precipitates the Jarisch-Herxheimer reaction. These women should be advised to seek obstetric attention after treatment if they notice any contractions or decrease in fetal movements. Stillbirth is a rare complication of treatment, but concern for this complication should not delay necessary treatment. All patients who have syphilis should be offered testing for HIV infection.

Follow-Up

Coordinated prenatal care and treatment follow-up are important, and syphilis case management may help facilitate prenatal enrollment. Serologic titers should be repeated in the third trimester and at delivery. Serologic titers may be checked monthly in women at high risk for reinfection or in geographic areas in which the prevalence of syphilis is high. The clinical and antibody response should be appropriate for the stage of disease. Most women will deliver before their serologic response to treatment can be assessed definitively.

Special Considerations

Penicillin Allergy

There are no proven alternatives to penicillin for treatment of syphilis during pregnancy. Pregnant women who have a history of penicillin allergy should be desensitized and treated with penicillin. Skin testing may be helpful.

Tetracycline and doxycycline usually are not used during pregnancy. Erythromycin should not be used, because it does not reliably cure an infected fetus. Data are insufficient to recommend azithromycin or ceftriaxone.

Section 22.3

Record Low U.S. Incidence of Syphilis

Syphilis, an infection that has plagued kings and paupers around the globe for centuries, may soon be eliminated from the United States.

Reported new cases, already at a historic low, declined further in 1998, and in 1999 health officials announced the kickoff of a campaign to eliminate syphilis in this country.

"We have an unprecedented opportunity to eliminate syphilis . . . because disease rates are at an all-time low and because the disease is so concentrated geographically," said Judith Wasserheit, director of the division of sexually transmitted disease prevention at the U.S. Centers for Disease Control and Prevention (CDC).

Syphilis is a sexually transmitted infection that, if untreated, can damage the brain and other organs and can be passed from a mother to her unborn infant, causing stillbirth or birth defects. It can also produce a genital sore called a chancre that increases an infected person's susceptibility to the human immunodeficiency virus (HIV), which causes AIDS. Transmission of syphilis has been controlled in most other industrialized countries, but in the United States the disease has continued to rise and fall in approximately 10-year cycles.

In recent years, new U.S. cases have been increasingly concentrated in a few counties and urban areas, especially in the South. Twenty-eight counties or independent cities, representing less than 1 percent of all U.S. counties, accounted for half of last year's 6,993 reported cases of primary and secondary syphilis, according to data released by the CDC. Such cases represent recently acquired infections.

Baltimore City reported the largest number of cases of any jurisdiction—456—but that figure represented a 31 percent decrease from the 1997 total of 665. The District ranked 16th with 81 reported cases, which also was 31 percent below the D.C.'s 1997 total of 117 cases.

Health officials emphasize that cases reported to health departments represent a fraction of all new cases, but provide an indication of the frequency of syphilis in a community. Reported cases also reflect the quality of local health services, so a city's or county's total may be deceptively low if there are barriers to treatment or if public health workers are not doing an adequate job of interviewing people with new infections and contacting their sexual partners for testing.

"Syphilis is really sort of a barometer of community health," Wasserheit said. Nationally, the number of new syphilis cases reported last year was 19 percent lower than in 1997 and 86 percent lower than the number reported in 1990. In that year, the peak of the most recent syphilis epidemic, there were 50,578 new cases of the disease.

Syphilis is a sexually transmitted infection caused by a bacterium, *Treponema pallidum*, that can damage tissues in many organs of the body. The initial symptoms—a painless sore, followed by a rash—often go unnoticed and disappear without treatment. However, the bacteria remain in the body, producing a "latent" infection that may injure the brain, spinal cord, major blood vessels, bones or other tissues.

Syphilis rates within the population vary among ethnic groups. The rate has historically been highest among African Americans, and in 1998 it was still much higher (17.1 cases per 100,000 population) than the national average (2.6 cases per 100,000) or the rates among other racial or ethnic groups. The data indicated that African Americans were 34 times more likely to be reported with syphilis than whites.

"Syphilis is a completely preventable disease that can be cured with one dose of penicillin, yet it takes a staggering toll on the African

American community," said Helene Gayle, director of the CDC's National Center for HIV, STD and TB Prevention, in a statement. "Syphilis remains one of the most glaring examples of racial inequities in health status facing this nation."

U.S. Surgeon General David Satcher and CDC director Jeffrey P. Koplan joined state and local health officials in Nashville last Thursday to launch a national campaign to eliminate syphilis. Wasserheit said the campaign will focus on reducing transmission of the infection, with the goal of having fewer than 1,000 new cases reported annually and at least 90 percent of U.S. counties syphilis-free by 2005. Last year, about 80 percent of U.S. counties reported no new cases of syphilis.

As part of the elimination plan, the CDC is providing additional funds for syphilis control to 33 states and cities with a heavy burden of disease or a high potential for an outbreak. Baltimore and Washington, as well as Maryland and Virginia, are among the recipients.

The plan calls for expanded surveillance for syphilis, rapid testing in clinics and other settings, expanded laboratory services, improved partnerships with social service organizations, schools, churches and other agencies, and efforts to enhance community awareness of the disease. Federal health officials estimate that fully implementing the plan would cost $37 million. So far, Congress has appropriated $10 million for syphilis elimination, Wasserheit said.

Peter Moore, acting chief of the bureau of STD (sexually transmitted disease) control in the D.C. Health Department, said the District received $175,000 from the CDC in September for syphilis elimination activities and is applying to receive $210,000 next year. He said some of the money will probably be used for syphilis education and testing by community outreach workers, and that part of it may also be used to open one of the neighborhood health centers in Northwest Washington on some evenings and weekends, specifically to treat patients with sexually transmitted diseases.

The health department closed an STD clinic in Northwest Washington in 1995. Currently the only public STD clinic in the District is in Southeast Washington at D.C. General Hospital. Moore said despite the need for better STD treatment services in Northwest Washington, he is encouraged by the 31 percent drop in new cases reported from the District during 1998. "I think it's a real decline," he said.

Wasserheit said if the national elimination campaign succeeds, sporadic cases of syphilis may still occur, but "syphilis would no longer spread within the United States. It would no longer be a health threat, just as . . . people living in the United States don't need to worry about cholera [or] malaria."

Chapter 23

Trichomoniasis

Chapter Contents

Section 23.1

Trichomoniasis Facts

Centers for Disease Control and Prevention (CDC).
1998 Guidelines for Treatment of Sexually Transmitted Diseases.
MMWR 1998;47(No. RR-1).

Trichomoniasis is caused by the protozoan *T. vaginalis*. Most men who are infected with *T. vaginalis* do not have symptoms of infection, although a minority of men have NGU. Many women do have symptoms of infection. Of these women, *T. vaginalis* characteristically causes a diffuse, malodorous, yellow-green discharge with vulvar irritation; many women have fewer symptoms. Vaginal trichomoniasis might be associated with adverse pregnancy outcomes, particularly premature rupture of the membranes and preterm delivery.

Treatment

Recommended Regimen

Metronidazole 2 g orally in a single dose.

Alternative Regimen

Metronidazole 500 mg twice a day for 7 days.

Metronidazole is the only oral medication available in the United States for the treatment of trichomoniasis. In randomized clinical trials, the recommended metronidazole regimens have resulted in cure rates of approximately 90%-95%; ensuring treatment of sex partners might increase the cure rate. Treatment of patients and sex partners results in relief of symptoms, microbiologic cure, and reduction of transmission. Metronidazole gel is approved for treatment of BV, but, like other topically applied antimicrobials that are unlikely to achieve therapeutic levels in the urethra or perivaginal glands, it is considerably less efficacious for treatment of trichomoniasis than oral preparations of metronidazole and is not recommended for use. Several other topically applied antimicrobials have been used for treatment of trichomoniasis, but it is unlikely that these preparations will have greater efficacy than metronidazole gel.

Follow-Up

Follow-up is unnecessary for men and women who become asymptomatic after treatment or who are initially asymptomatic. Infections with strains of *T. vaginalis* that have diminished susceptibility to metronidazole can occur; however, most of these organisms respond to higher doses of metronidazole. If treatment failure occurs with either regimen, the patient should be re-treated with metronidazole 500 mg twice a day for 7 days. If treatment failure occurs repeatedly, the patient should be treated with a single 2g dose of metronidazole once a day for 3-5 days. Patients with culture-documented infection who do not respond to the regimens described in this section and in whom reinfection has been excluded should be managed in consultation with an expert; consultation is available from CDC. Evaluation of such cases should include determination of the susceptibility of *T. vaginalis* to metronidazole.

Management of Sex Partners

Sex partners should be treated. Patients should be instructed to avoid sex until they and their sex partners are cured. In the absence of a microbiologic test of cure, this means when therapy has been completed and patient and partner(s) are asymptomatic.

Special Considerations

Allergy, Intolerance, or Adverse Reactions

Effective alternatives to therapy with metronidazole are not available. Patients who are allergic to metronidazole can be managed by desensitization.

Pregnancy

Patients can be treated with 2 g of metronidazole in a single dose.

HIV Infection

Patients who have trichomoniasis and also are infected with HIV should receive the same treatment regimen as those who are HIV-negative.

Section 23.2

Genital Tract Infections:
How Best to Treat Trichomoniasis

© 1996 Cliggott Publishing Company, from *Consultant*, August 1996,
Vol.36, No.8, Pg.1769(6), excerpted from "Genital Tract Infections: How Best
to Treat Trichomoniasis, Bacterial vaginosis, and Candida Infection,"
by Michael S. Policar; reprinted with permission.

As the CDC has outlined, several significant changes have occurred
in the treatment of genital tract infections. For example, new, more convenient medications have been approved; organisms have become resistant to previously reliable agents; and, in this era of cost-containment,
the pressure on physicians to make a correct diagnosis and institute
effective therapy on the first visit has escalated.

Clinical Considerations

Infection by *Trichomonas vaginalis* virtually always is sexually
transmitted, although not necessarily by intercourse (it can be transmitted by fingers or the sharing of sex toys). *T. vaginalis* tends to have
wider local invasion than other vaginal pathogens; it can involve the
Skene's glands, the endocervix, and even the urethra and the trigone
of the bladder. Because of these hard to reach reservoirs, this infection can be cured only with systemic therapy. Sexual partners of patients with trichomoniasis also must be treated to prevent reinfection.

Trichomoniasis can be asymptomatic for many years; between
5% and 10% of nonsymptomatic women of reproductive age are colonized by *T. vaginalis*. Transmission can be by the current sexual partner or any sexual partner the patient has had during her entire life.
Symptoms signal that colonization has converted to overt or frank disease.

Diagnosis

Women with trichomoniasis usually complain of vaginal itching and
irritation as well as a profuse, watery foul-smelling vaginal discharge.

On examination, the vaginal and cervical epithelium can appear inflamed or normal. The discharge is characteristically frothy or bubbly and sometimes is yellow or green. The appearance of a bubbly discharge is a clue that either trichomoniasis or BV is the cause.

A saline wet mount procedure is required to detect motile trichomonads. *T. vaginalis* is extremely sensitive to light, heat, air, and the osmolality of the suspension solution; thus, a fresh normal saline solution is essential to avoid killing the protozoa. Laboratories should change their solution monthly or every 2 months, since old, hypertonic solutions kill these organisms on contact and are a major cause of trichomoniasis underdiagnosis.

The vaginal pH in patients with trichomoniasis is between 6 and 7.5. However, pH testing is not required in uncomplicated cases. Other tests do not contribute to the diagnosis.

What if trichomonads are found in a Pap smear? Assume that the patient has trichomoniasis; a saline wet mount is redundant. Notify and treat such patients to prevent spread of the infection and to avert eventual symptoms. Treatment is worthwhile, especially if the patient is of reproductive age.

Therapy

The agent of choice is metronidazole, 2 g by mouth as a single dose. Four 500-mg tablets at once or over a 5- to 10-minute period.

During the first trimester of pregnancy, oral metronidazole is contraindicated but clotrimazole cream or metronidazole gel can be applied for symptomatic relief. During the second and third trimesters, oral metronidazole is administered.

Topical gels should not be used as first-line therapy for trichomoniasis, since the cure rate with these preparations is less than 50%. The usual reason for treatment failure is reinfection by an untreated or new sexual partner, although reports of metronidazole-resistant strains are increasing. If trichomoniasis persists despite therapy, prescribe oral metronidazole, twice daily for a total daily dose of 500 mg for 7 days. If this regimen fails, use high-dose metronidazole (2 g by mouth every day for 3 to 5 days) plus topical metronidazole gel.

Sexual partners should be encouraged to come to the office so that seizure disorder or anemia (metronidazole is known to lower the seizure threshold and cause reversible neutropenia) can be ruled out. An examination generally is not necessary, however, unless other genital tract infections, such as gonorrhea, Chlamydia infection, or syphilis are suspected.

Chapter 24

Vaginal Infections

Vaginitis Due to Vaginal Infections

Vaginitis is an inflammation of the vagina characterized by discharge, odor, irritation, and/or itching. The cause of vaginitis may not always be determined adequately solely on the basis of symptoms or a physical examination. For a correct diagnosis, a doctor should perform laboratory tests including microscopic evaluation of vaginal fluid. A variety of effective drugs are available for treating vaginitis.

Vaginitis often is caused by infections, which cause distress and discomfort. Some infections are associated with more serious diseases. The most common vaginal infections are bacterial vaginosis, trichomoniasis, and vaginal yeast infection or candidiasis. Some vaginal infections are transmitted through sexual contact, but others such as yeast infections probably are not, depending on the cause.

Bacterial Vaginosis

Bacterial vaginosis (BV) is the most common cause of vaginitis symptoms among women of childbearing age. Previously called non-specific vaginitis or Gardnerella-associated vaginitis, BV is associated with sexual activity. BV reflects a change in the vaginal ecosystem. This imbalance, including pH changes, occurs when different types of bacteria outnumber the normal ones. Instead of *Lactobacillus bacteria* being the most numerous, increased numbers of organisms such

---

1998 National Institute of Allergy and Infectious Diseases (NIAID).

as *Gardnerella vaginalis*, Bacteroides, Mobiluncus, and *Mycoplasma hominis* are found in the vaginas of women with BV. Investigators are studying the role that each of these microbes may play in causing BV, but they do not yet understand the role of sexual activity in developing BV. A change in sexual partners and douching may increase the risk of acquiring bacterial vaginosis.

Symptoms

The primary symptom of BV is an abnormal, odorous vaginal discharge. The fish-like odor is noticeable especially after intercourse. Nearly half of the women with clinical signs of BV, however, report no symptoms. A physician may observe these signs during a physical examination and may confirm the diagnosis by doing tests of vaginal fluid.

Diagnosis

A healthcare worker can examine a sample of vaginal fluid under a microscope, either stained or in special lighting, to detect the presence of the organisms associated with BV. They can make a diagnosis based on the absence of *lactobacilli*, the presence of numerous "clue cells" (cells from the vaginal lining that are coated with BV organisms), a fishy odor, and decreased acidity or change in pH of vaginal fluid.

Treatment

All women with BV should be informed of their diagnoses, including the possibility of sexual transmission, and offered treatment. They can be treated with antibiotics such as metronidazole or clindamycin. Generally, male sex partners are not treated. Many women with symptoms of BV do not seek medical treatment, and many asymptomatic women decline treatment.

Complications

Researchers have shown an association between BV and pelvic inflammatory disease (PID), which can cause infertility and tubal (ectopic) pregnancy. BV also can cause adverse outcomes of pregnancy such as premature delivery and low-birth-weight infants. Therefore, the U.S. Centers for Disease Control and Prevention (CDC) recommends that doctors check all pregnant women for BV who previously have delivered a premature baby, whether or not the women have symptoms. If these women have BV, they should be treated with oral metronidazole or oral clindamycin. A pregnant woman who has not delivered a premature baby should be treated if she has symptoms and laboratory evidence of BV. BV is also associated with increased risk of gonorrhea and HIV infection (HIV, human immunodeficiency virus, causes AIDS).

Vaginal Yeast Infection

Vaginal yeast infection or vulvovaginal candidiasis is a common cause of vaginal irritation. Doctors estimate that approximately 75 percent of all women will experience at least one symptomatic yeast infection during their lifetimes. Yeast are always present in the vagina in small numbers, and symptoms only appear with overgrowth. Several factors are associated with increased symptomatic infection in women, including pregnancy, uncontrolled diabetes mellitus, and the use of oral contraceptives or antibiotics. Other factors that may increase the incidence of yeast infection include using douches, perfumed feminine hygiene sprays, and topical antimicrobial agents, and wearing tight, poorly ventilated clothing and underwear. Whether or not yeast can be transmitted sexually is unknown. Because almost all women have the organism in the vagina, it has been difficult for researchers to study this aspect of the natural history.

Symptoms

The most frequent symptoms of yeast infection in women are itching, burning, and irritation of the vagina. Painful urination and/or intercourse are common. Vaginal discharge is not always present and may be minimal. The thick, whitish-gray discharge is typically described as cottage-cheese-like in nature, although it can vary from watery to thick in consistency. Most male partners of women with yeast infection do not experience any symptoms of the infection. A transient rash and burning sensation of the penis, however, have been reported after intercourse if condoms were not used. These symptoms are usually self-limiting.

Diagnosis

Because few specific signs and symptoms are usually present, this condition cannot be diagnosed by the patient's history and physical examination. The doctor usually diagnoses yeast infection through microscopic examination of vaginal secretions for evidence of yeast forms. Scientists funded by the National Institute of Allergy and Infectious Diseases (NIAID) have developed a rapid simple test for yeast infection, which will soon be available for use in doctors' offices. If such a test were available for home screening, it would help them to appropriately use yeast medication.

Treatment

Various antifungal vaginal medications are available to treat yeast infection. Women can buy some antifungal creams, tablets, or suppositories (butoconazole, miconazole, clotrimazole, and tioconazole) over the counter for use in the vagina. But because BV, trichomoniasis, and yeast infection are difficult to distinguish on the basis of symptoms alone, a woman with vaginal symptoms should see her physician for an accurate diagnosis before using these products. Other products available over the counter contain antihistamines or topical anesthetics that only mask the symptoms and do not treat the underlying problem. Women who have chronic or recurring yeast infections may need to be treated with vaginal creams for extended periods of time.

Recently, effective oral medications have become available. Women should work with their physicians to determine possible underlying causes of their chronic yeast infections. HIV-infected women may have severe yeast infections that are often unresponsive to treatment.

Other Causes of Vaginitis

Although most vaginal infections in women are due to bacterial vaginosis, trichomoniasis, or yeast, there may be other causes as well. These causes may include allergic and irritative factors or other STDs. Noninfectious allergic symptoms can be caused by spermicides, vaginal hygiene products, detergents, and fabric softeners. Cervical inflammation from these products often is associated with abnormal vaginal discharge, but can be distinguished from true vaginal infections by appropriate diagnostic tests.

In an effort to control vaginitis, research is under way to determine the factors that promote the growth and disease-causing potential of vaginal microbes. No longer considered merely a benign annoyance, vaginitis is the object of serious investigation as scientists attempt to clarify its role in such conditions as pelvic inflammatory disease and pregnancy-related complications.

Part Three

Risk and Prevention Issues

Chapter 25

Stds: Clinical Prevention Guidelines

The prevention and control of STDs is based on five major concepts: first, education of those at risk on ways to reduce the risk for STDs; second, detection of asymptomatically infected persons and of symptomatic persons unlikely to seek diagnostic and treatment services; third, effective diagnosis and treatment of infected persons; fourth, evaluation, treatment, and counseling of sex partners of persons who are infected with an STD; and fifth, preexposure vaccination of persons at risk for vaccine-preventable STDs. Although this focuses primarily on the clinical aspects of STD control, prevention of STDs is based on changing the sexual behaviors that place persons at risk for infection. Moreover, because STD control activities reduce the likelihood of transmission to sex partners, prevention for individuals constitutes prevention for the community.

Clinicians have the opportunity to provide client education and counseling and to participate in identifying and treating infected sex partners in addition to interrupting transmission by treating persons who have the curable bacterial and parasitic STDs. The ability of the health-care provider to obtain an accurate sexual history is crucial in prevention and control efforts. The accurate diagnosis and timely reporting of STDs by the clinician is the basis for effective public health surveillance.

Centers for Disease Control and Prevention (CDC). 1998 Guidelines for Treatment of Sexually Transmitted Diseases. *MMWR* 1998;47(No. RR-1).

Prevention Messages

Preventing the spread of STDs requires that persons at risk for transmitting or acquiring infections change their behaviors. The essential first step is for the health-care provider to proactively include questions regarding the patient's sexual history as part of the clinical interview. When risk factors have been identified, the provider has an opportunity to deliver prevention messages. Counseling skills (i.e., respect, compassion, and a nonjudgmental attitude) are essential to the effective delivery of prevention messages. Techniques that can be effective in facilitating a rapport with the patient include using open-ended questions, using understandable language, and reassuring the patient that treatment will be provided regardless of considerations such as ability to pay, citizenship or immigration status, language spoken, or lifestyle.

Prevention messages should be tailored to the patient, with consideration given to the patient's specific risk factors for STDs. Messages should include a description of specific actions that the patient can take to avoid acquiring or transmitting STDs (e.g., abstinence from sexual activity if STD-related symptoms develop).

Sexual Transmission

The most effective way to prevent sexual transmission of HIV infection and other STDs is to avoid sexual intercourse with an infected partner. Counseling that provides information concerning abstinence from penetrative sexual intercourse is crucial for a) persons who are being treated for an STD or whose partners are undergoing treatment and b) persons who wish to avoid the possible consequences of sexual intercourse (e.g., STD/HIV and pregnancy).

- Both partners should get tested for STDs, including HIV, before initiating sexual intercourse.

- If a person chooses to have sexual intercourse with a partner whose infection status is unknown or who is infected with HIV or another STD, a new condom should be used for each act of intercourse.

Injecting-Drug Users

The following prevention messages are appropriate for injecting-drug users:

- Enroll or continue in a drug-treatment program.

- Do not, under any circumstances, use injection equipment (e.g., needles and syringes) that has been used by another person.

- If needles can be obtained legally in the community, obtain clean needles.

- Persons who continue to use injection equipment that has been used by other persons should first clean the equipment with bleach and water. (Disinfecting with bleach does not sterilize the equipment and does not guarantee that HIV is inactivated. However, for injecting-drug users, thoroughly and consistently cleaning injection equipment with bleach should reduce the rate of HIV transmission when equipment is shared.)

Preexposure Vaccination

Preexposure vaccination is one of the most effective methods used to prevent transmission of certain STDs. HBV infection frequently is sexually transmitted, and hepatitis B vaccination is recommended for all unvaccinated patients being evaluated for an STD. In the United States, hepatitis A vaccines from two manufacturers were licensed recently. Hepatitis A vaccination is recommended for several groups of patients who might seek treatment in STD clinics; such patients include homosexual or bisexual men and persons who use illegal drugs. Vaccine trials for other STDs are being conducted, and vaccines for these STDs may become available within the next several years.

Prevention Methods

Male Condoms

When used consistently and correctly, condoms are effective in preventing many STDs, including HIV infection. Multiple cohort studies, including those of serodiscordant sex partners, have demonstrated a strong protective effect of condom use against HIV infection. Because condoms do not cover all exposed areas, they may be more effective in preventing infections transmitted between mucosal surfaces than those transmitted by skin-to-skin contact. Condoms are regulated as medical devices and are subject to random sampling and testing by the Food and Drug Administration (FDA). Each latex condom manufactured in the United States is tested electronically for holes before packaging. Rates of condom breakage during sexual intercourse and withdrawal are low in the United States (i.e., usually two broken condoms per 100 condoms used). Condom failure usually results from inconsistent or incorrect use rather than condom breakage. Patients should be advised that condoms must be used consistently and correctly to be highly effective in preventing STDs. Patients also should be instructed in the correct use of condoms. The following recommendations ensure the proper use of male condoms:

- Use a new condom with each act of sexual intercourse.
- Carefully handle the condom to avoid damaging it with fingernails, teeth, or other sharp objects.
- Put the condom on after the penis is erect and before genital contact with the partner.
- Ensure that no air is trapped in the tip of the condom.
- Ensure that adequate lubrication exists during intercourse, possibly requiring the use of exogenous lubricants.
- Use only water-based lubricants with latex condoms. Oil-based lubricants (e.g., petroleum jelly, shortening, mineral oil, massage oils, body lotions, and cooking oil) can weaken latex.
- Hold the condom firmly against the base of the penis during withdrawal, and withdraw while the penis is still erect to prevent slippage.

Female Condoms

Laboratory studies indicate that the female condom—a lubricated polyurethane sheath with a ring on each end that is inserted into the vagina—is an effective mechanical barrier to viruses, including HIV. Other than one investigation of recurrent trichomoniasis, no clinical studies have been completed to evaluate the efficacy of female condoms in providing protection from STDs, including HIV. If used consistently and correctly, the female condom should substantially reduce the risk for STDs. When a male condom cannot be used appropriately, sex partners should consider using a female condom.

Condoms and Spermicides

Whether condoms lubricated with spermicides are more effective than other lubricated condoms in protecting against the transmission of HIV and other STDs has not been determined. Furthermore, spermicide-coated condoms have been associated with *Escherichia coli* urinary tract infection in young women. Whether condoms used with vaginal application of spermicide are more effective than condoms used without vaginal spermicides also has not been determined. Therefore, the consistent use of condoms, with or without spermicidal lubricant or vaginal application of spermicide, is recommended.

Vaginal Spermicides, Sponges, and Diaphragms

As demonstrated in several randomized controlled trials, vaginal spermicides used alone without condoms reduce the risk for cervical gonorrhea and chlamydia. However, vaginal spermicides offer no protection against HIV infection, and spermicides are not recommended for HIV prevention. The vaginal contraceptive sponge, which is not available in the United States, protects against cervical gonorrhea and chlamydia, but its use increases the risk for candidiasis. In case-control and cross-sectional studies, diaphragm use has been demonstrated to protect against cervical gonorrhea, chlamydia, and trichomoniasis; however, no cohort studies have been conducted. Vaginal sponges or diaphragms should not be assumed to protect women against HIV infection. The role of spermicides, sponges, and diaphragms for preventing STDs in men has not been evaluated.

Nonbarrier Contraception, Surgical Sterilization, and Hysterectomy

Women who are not at risk for pregnancy might incorrectly perceive themselves to be at no risk for STDs, including HIV infection. Nonbarrier contraceptive methods offer no protection against HIV or other STDs. Hormonal contraception has been associated in some cohort studies with cervical STDs and increased acquisition of HIV; however, data concerning this latter finding are inconsistent. Women who use hormonal contraception, have been surgically sterilized, or have had hysterectomies should be counseled regarding the use of condoms and the risk for STDs, including HIV infection.

HIV Prevention Counseling

Knowledge of HIV status and appropriate counseling are important components in initiating behavior change. Therefore, HIV counseling is an important HIV prevention strategy, although its efficacy in reducing risk behaviors is still being evaluated. By ensuring that counseling is empathic and client-centered, clinicians can develop a realistic appraisal of the patient's risk and help the patient develop a specific and realistic HIV prevention plan.

Counseling associated with HIV testing has two main components: pretest and posttest counseling. During pretest counseling, the clinician should conduct a personalized risk assessment, explain the meaning of positive and negative test results, ask for informed consent for the HIV test, and help the patient develop a realistic, personalized risk-reduction plan. During posttest counseling, the clinician should inform the patient of the results, review the meaning of the results, and reinforce prevention messages. If the patient has a confirmed positive HIV test result, posttest counseling should include referral for follow-up medical services and, if needed, social and psychological services. HIV-negative patients at continuing risk for HIV infection also may benefit from referral for additional counseling and prevention services.

Partner Notification

For most STDs, partners of patients should be examined. When exposure to a treatable STD is considered likely, appropriate antimicrobials should be administered even though no clinical signs of infection are evident and laboratory test results are not yet available. In many states, the local or state health department can assist in notifying the partners of patients who have selected STDs (e.g., HIV infection, syphilis, gonorrhea, hepatitis B, and chlamydia).

Health-care providers should advise patients who have an STD to notify sex partners, including those without symptoms, of their exposure and encourage these partners to seek clinical evaluation. This type of partner notification is known as patient referral. In situations in which patient referral may not be effective or possible, health departments should be prepared to assist the patient either through contract referral or provider referral. Contract referral is the process by which patients agree to self-refer their partners within a defined time period. If the partners do not obtain medical evaluation and treatment within that period, then provider referral is implemented. Provider referral is the process by which partners named by infected patients are notified and counseled by health department staff.

Interrupting the transmission of infection is crucial to STD control. For treatable and vaccine-preventable STDs, further transmission and reinfection can be prevented by referral of sex partners for diagnosis, treatment, vaccination (if applicable), and counseling. When health-care providers refer infected patients to local or state health departments for provider-referral partner notification, the patients may be interviewed by trained professionals to obtain the names of their sex partners and information regarding the location of these partners for notification purposes. Every health department protects the privacy of patients in partner-notification activities. Because of the advantage of confidentiality, many patients prefer that public health officials notify partners. However, the ability of public health officials to provide appropriate prophylaxis to contacts of all patients who have STDs may be limited. In situations where the number of anonymous partners is substantial (e.g., situations among persons who exchange sex for drugs), targeted screening of persons at risk may be more effective at stopping the transmission of disease than provider-referral partner notification. Guidelines for management of sex partners and recommendations for partner notification for specific STDs are included for each STD addressed in this report.

Reporting and Confidentiality

The accurate identification and timely reporting of STDs are integral components of successful disease control efforts. Timely reporting is important for assessing morbidity trends, targeting limited resources, and assisting local health authorities in identifying sex partners who may be infected. STD/HIV and acquired immunodeficiency syndrome (AIDS) cases should be reported in accordance with local statutory requirements.

Syphilis, gonorrhea, and AIDS are reportable diseases in every state. Chlamydial infection is reportable in most states. The requirements for reporting other STDs differ by state, and clinicians should be familiar with local STD reporting requirements. Reporting may be provider and/or laboratory-based. Clinicians who are unsure of local reporting requirements should seek advice from local health departments or state STD programs.

STD and HIV reports are maintained in strictest confidence; in most jurisdictions, such reports are protected by statute from subpoena. Before public health representatives conduct follow-up of a positive STD-test result, these persons should consult the patient's health-care provider to verify the diagnosis and treatment.

Chapter 26

A Contemporary Approach to Curbing STDs

If the AIDS epidemic had generated alarm and common sense in equal proportions, other sexually transmitted diseases (STDs) might not be nearly as prevalent as they are today. The World Health Organization estimates a global STD incidence of 250 million new cases per year.[1] HIV infections, accounting for some 7 million of these, are far outpaced by chlamydia, genital herpes, gonorrhea, human papillomavirus (HPV) infection, and trichomoniasis. Even the prospect of a universally fatal disease has had a limited influence on human behavior. One quip spawned in the last two decades aptly sums up a lingering attitude toward STDs: "I'm looking for an old-fashioned lover—somebody with gonorrhea."

Dangerous Liaisons

In truth, every STD should be considered serious business. Hepatitis B and syphilis have always had the capacity to kill a percentage of those infected. Chlamydia trachomatis infection and gonorrhea have been identified as the most common causes of pelvic inflammatory disease (PID). In turn, PID-associated scarring of the fallopian tubes is an important cause of chronic pelvic pain, potentially fatal ectopic pregnancy, and infertility. Infection with HPV, some strains of which cause genital warts, is the major risk factor for squamous intraepithelial lesions of the cervix and invasive cervical carcinoma.[2]

When acquired during pregnancy, syphilis can be transmitted across the placenta to the developing fetus, while prenatal gonorrhea can induce premature delivery and sight—threatening eye infections. Chlamydia can also cause ocular infection in the newborn, as well as neonatal pneumonia and, probably, prematurity. Neonatal herpes infection poses a risk of permanent CNS deficits.

Bacterial vaginosis, once considered little more than a nuisance, has also proved to be a substantial public health problem. Although bacterial vaginosis is not specifically categorized as an STD, it has been linked to having multiple sex partners. The condition occurs when normal components of vaginal flora, including anaerobic bacteria and *Gardnerella vaginalis*, crowd out the ordinarily predominant *Lactobacillus* species.

In one recent study, a diagnosis of bacterial vaginosis during the second trimester of pregnancy increased the risk of delivering a premature, low-birth-weight infant by 40%.[3] Data from another trial indicated that treatment with erythromycin base and oral metronidazole at about the 24th week of gestation reduced the rate of premature delivery in women who had both bacterial vaginosis and a preexisting risk for preterm delivery.[4] Other potential consequences of bacterial vaginosis include intra-amniotic infection and PID.

In the United States, reducing the prevalence of STDs is likely to help curb the spread of AIDS. Obviously, the sexual behaviors that increase the risk of HIV infection are the same as those that can expose people to other STDs. Also, lesions or inflammation in the genital tract are thought to allow HIV to be transmitted more efficiently. People with STDs who are exposed to HIV are estimated to have at least twice—and perhaps as much as 50 times—the risk of acquiring HIV infection as those without an STD who've had similar HIV exposure.

That risk should be a point of concern for a large segment of the U.S. population. In this country, an estimated 1 in 4 people between the ages of 15 and 55 will get at least one STD in the course of a lifetime.[5] At any one time, genital herpes, which afflicts some 30 million people in the United States, and HPV infection, harbored by an estimated 24-40 million people, are the most prevalent STDs. Because viral infections are currently incurable, the numbers only climb higher. While surveillance for trichomoniasis isn't routine, the parasitic infection is presumed to occur in as many as 3 million people in the nation each year.[5]

Reported cases of bacterial STDs wax and wane. Of these STDs, chlamydia is astonishingly widespread, with more than 4 million U.S.

cases estimated to occur each year.[6] Particularly common among sexually active adolescents and young adults, chlamydia has infiltrated every segment of the population, regardless of location or socioeconomic status. Annually, direct and indirect costs of associated illness exact a toll that surpasses $2.4 billion. The incidence of chlamydia appears to be rising, but that phenomenon is partly attributed to increased testing, detection of asymptomatic infections, and reporting.

Annual gonorrhea incidence rates have fallen consistently over the last 20 years—149.5 per 100,000 population in 1995. Yet they remain high when compared to those reported in Europe 5-40 per 100,000.[7] What's more, as overall prevalence has declined, the number of cases occurring among the urban poor, particularly adolescents and blacks, has not been reduced by a similar magnitude. Gonorrhea rates are many-fold higher among blacks than whites, primarily due to more limited contact with the health care system.

Similarly, syphilis and chancroid tend to occur in specific pockets of the nation, mainly among marginalized populations living in poverty. Factors thought to fuel disease dissemination include the sex-for-drugs barter that has become common among drug dealers and their clients. In 1990, the annual incidence of primary and secondary syphilis was higher in this country than it had been since the 1940s 20 cases per 100,000 people.[7]

Incidence rates among blacks were 62 times those reported in whites. Cases were clustered in big cities and the South. Although nationally 1995 rates had fallen to 6.3 per 100,000 population, dramatic racial and ethnic differentials persist, and the United States continues to have the highest syphilis rates of all industrialized nations.

Chancroid, a relatively uncommon infection, is endemic to particular regions, but distinct outbreaks also occur. Fewer than 4,300 cases were reported to the Centers for Disease Control and Prevention (CDC) in 1990; 88% of the cases occurred in five states.[8] In contrast, the CDC received fewer than 1,000 reports in 1981. But chancroid is also thought to be more common than figures suggest, mainly because it is difficult to distinguish from other genital ulcers. Additional STDs that occur more sporadically include *lymphogranuloma venereum* and *granuloma inguinale*.

The Invisible Infection

The most urgent message to remember is that a significant proportion of persons with STDs have no apparent signs or symptoms.

Most new infections are acquired from people who are unaware that they have a transmissible disease. Chlamydia is notoriously hard to detect without using laboratory diagnostic tools—a culture, DNA amplification techniques, or immunodiagnostic methods. Studies suggest that 50-80% of affected women are asymptomatic. In addition, any urogenital signs, such as cervical friability or increased discharge, are not specific for chlamydia. Males are more likely to notice a telltale urethritis, but infections can also be asymptomatic.

It's also vital to recognize that even STDs generally believed to have obvious symptoms offer no hint of their presence in most cases. For example, only a small fraction of participants in serologic studies who demonstrated antibodies to herpes simplex virus type 2 (HSV-2) ever experienced symptoms of infection. The observation is ascribed to asymptomatic shedding of virus, a fairly common event. Keep in mind as well that most of those who do experience an episode are not likely to have frequent symptomatic recurrences. To further complicate matters, so-called atypical presentations are not truly unusual. Genital herpes infection cannot be ruled out in a patient who does not have the characteristic painful vesicular lesions. Minor bumps, lumps, scratches, or sores are worthy of suspicion.

Nonetheless, people who harbor the virus but have never had overt symptoms of HSV infection are fully capable of transmitting the disease to partners. In fact, experts believe this group is primarily responsible for the spread of HSV. Asymptomatic women can also infect their newborn infants—an observation sparked by the appearance of HSV disease in babies whose mothers had no detectable lesions.

In the same way, HPV infection is usually imperceptible on the basis of signs and symptoms. The majority of those who've been infected don't have abnormal Pap smears, cervical cancer, or genital warts. Of the more than 70 identified types of HPV, 23 infect the uterine cervix.[2] While half of these are associated with squamous intraepithelial lesions or invasive cervical cancer, only four strains account for more than 80% of invasive cervical cancers. So, while most such cervical cancers are connected to HPV, cervical cancer isn't an absolute consequence of HPV infection. Then again, it's possible to be infected with multiple strains of HPV over time.

Even infections that are usually symptomatic, such as gonorrhea or trichomoniasis, can be present for extended periods without development of symptoms or signs. The crucial point, then, is that every STD can be asymptomatic. It's a mistake for patients to assume that they can easily identify possibly infected sexual partners—or for physicians to expect all patients with STDs to have visible signs of infection.

Risk Assessment

STDs don't always manifest with distinct clinical features—an inability to conceive may be the first clue to a previous chlamydial or gonococcal infection. Determining which of your patients are at highest risk of infection means taking a thorough sexual history, a difficult but imperative task. Questions about sexual practices are as important as questions about alcohol, cigarettes, other substance abuse, diet, and exercise. Without this information, you can't be sure you're addressing all of a patient's potential health problems.

Don't make assumptions that prevent you from introducing delicate subjects. For example, married patients aren't always monogamous. Remember that all sexually active people are candidates for STDs. Further, patients who have multiple sexual partners at the same time aren't necessarily at greater hazard than those who practice serial monogamy. Some degree of risk is introduced any time patients change sexual partners, no matter how faithful or enduring the previous affiliation. Adolescents are especially inclined to engage in a string of short-term but otherwise committed sexual relationships. You probably should presume, however, that all adults, married or not, are sexually active unless you have good reason to believe otherwise.

Ask patients if they are sexually active, whether they've recently changed partners, and how many partners they've had in the past several months. Record any history of STDs. Find out about sexual orientation. One straightforward approach is to ask patients whether they have sex with men, women, or both, and whether contact has been vaginal, anal, or oral. Ask the patient about condom use and whether other contraceptive methods are employed. Here are other basic screening questions:

- Do you have any pain or discomfort during intercourse?
- Do you have any pain or discomfort when you urinate?
- Do you have a discharge from your vagina or a discharge from your penis?
- Do you have bleeding after sex?
- Do you have lower abdominal pain?
- Do you have any genital bumps or sores?
- Does your sexual partner have partners other than you?
- Does your sexual partner have any of these symptoms?

Make these inquiries when you evaluate a patient for the first time and at regular intervals thereafter. It's not unreasonable to do a sexual risk assessment of adolescents and young adults every time you see them in your office. Be sure to offer long-time patients who've been in mutually monogamous relationships an opportunity to talk. You might begin by asking how the patient's partner is. Follow up with a question such as, is there anything we should discuss with respect to your sexual life?

Your discussions should take place privately, without the patient's partner (or parents) present. Assure patients that the information they give you is confidential. Frame questions in a way that's most likely to make patients comfortable about answering. For example, make it clear that this is an important health matter, not a moral issue. Let patients know that they can and should discuss these issues with another health care professional—whether affiliated with your office or not—if they aren't willing to speak to you.

With practice, you'll become as adept at taking a sexual history as you are at exploring other aspects of a patient's life. You'll also know how you can modify questions on the basis of what you've learned from previous efforts. If the prospect is daunting, consider enrolling in a special training course.

Screening and Diagnosis

Because the consequences of untreated chlamydia can be devastating, experts recommend routine screening at least once a year for all sexually active females younger than 20. The CDC also recommends screening of women aged 20-24 who use barrier contraceptives inconsistently or who have had a new sex partner or more than one sex partner in the last three months, women older than 24 who meet both of these criteria, and any woman with mucopurulent cervicitis. One recent study determined that the incidence of PID was reduced by more than half when women at high risk of infection were identified, tested, and, when necessary, treated.[9]

Although chlamydia is extremely common among adolescents and young adults, its incidence decreases with increasing age. Once patients are out of their 20s, you don't need to screen all of them. Consider screening, however, for patients—symptomatic or not—who have entered into a new relationship, have multiple partners, or are afraid their partners may have given them an infection. Explain that testing for chlamydia is as much a part of good medical practice as breast examinations or Pap smears.

Routine screening for other STDs is not usually worthwhile, but that may vary with the population you treat. For example, possible exceptions include gonorrhea screening in areas with a high incidence of the disease and bacterial vaginosis screening among pregnant women. Symptomatic patients should always be tested and, when appropriate, treated.

Both chlamydia and gonorrhea are more accurately and easily diagnosed than ever, thanks to the recent widespread availability of DNA amplification tests. Previously, the most reliable test capable of finding chlamydia was cell culture, which has a sensitivity of 80-90% at best? Gonorrhea has traditionally been detected with bacterial culture. While cultures have served as the so-called gold standard, they are technically complicated and time-consuming. Transportation of laboratory samples requires special transport media and specific storage temperatures. Organisms that die en route will not be detected. Polymerase chain reaction (PCR), used to detect the presence of *C. trachomatis*, and ligase chain reaction (LCR), used to diagnose chlamydia or gonorrhea, are more precise, with sensitivities of 90% or better. These technologies allow identification of DNA sequences present in the organisms. The tests are complicated and more expensive than other methods currently in use but produce results in hours rather than days. They're also quite specific, producing few false-positive results.

Perhaps most impressive, though, LCR and PCR tests can find traces of the organisms in urine samples. For the first time, specimens can be collected without inserting a swab or brush into the endocervical canal or urethra. That offers the potential to screen for both STDs in facilities that don't have the capability to perform pelvic examinations. Infections can be diagnosed during a routine physical examination. Or, LCR and PCR can be used to screen high-risk asymptomatic patients who generally avoid the health care system. For instance, routine screening could take place in community centers, juvenile detention centers, or school-based clinics.

Immunodiagnostic studies, such as enzyme immunoassay or immunofluorescent antibody tests, have proved useful in detecting *C. trachomatis* as well. These are less sensitive than cell cultures, but they are also faster, less expensive, and technically less demanding. Antigen-detection methods are used to diagnose other STDs as well, as is microscopy.

Treatment and Prevention

The treatment recommendations issued by the CDC in 1993 continue to serve as the most appropriate guide to STD therapy.[11] The drug that has provided a most valuable addition to the STD armamentarium is single-dose azithromycin therapy for chlamydia. Its availability allows physicians to circumvent compliance problems by administering the complete course of treatment on the spot. Patients with infections caused by *C. trachomatis* cannot always be counted on to take the full seven-day course of doxycycline hyclate, though it remains a widely used treatment.

Experts predict that other STD-related applications for azithromycin will be more thoroughly explored. Already the drug is used to treat nongonococcal urethritis in men, and its value in PID and syphilis is also under scrutiny. Topical vaginal preparations of clindamycin phosphate and metronidazole for treatment of bacterial vaginosis have provided feasible alternatives for women who can't or won't take oral drugs. Two new drugs indicated for the treatment of recurrent genital herpes have been approved since the 1993 CDC guidelines were published. Famciclovir, 125 mg bid for five days, and valacyclovir HC1, 500 mg bid for five days, generally offer patients a more convenient dosage schedule than oral acyclovir. Whether all three drugs are equally effective is still unclear. Recently, valacyclovir has been approved for treatment of initial episodes of genital herpes. The dosage is 1 g bid for 10 days. Therapy is most effective when administered within 48 hours of the onset of signs and symptoms.

When treating patients for STDs, remember that different infections may have similar symptoms. In many cases, you'll want to initiate therapy before a laboratory confirms your suspicions. Base the treatment on what you believe the causative agent to be, and then change if necessary. Patients undergoing treatment for gonorrhea should always receive concurrent therapy for chlamydia. The sexual partners of patients should be examined and treated too, unless the infection being treated is bacterial vaginosis or HPV. In these cases, little evidence suggests that treatment of partners provides any benefit.

Patients with concurrent HIV infection may require modifications of their drug regimens since they are prone to more serious episodes of infection. For example, HIV-infected patients undergoing treatment for chancroid warrant close monitoring and, possibly, longer courses of therapy. Some physicians tend to choose erythromycin base over azithromycin or ceftriaxone sodium because there is relatively little information on the efficacy of the latter two in patients with HIV infection.

Immunocompromised patients, including those with HIV infection, often require more aggressive therapy to clear genital herpes lesions—

400 mg of acyclovir 3-5 times per day until the lesions resolve, for example—and suppressive therapy may be appropriate. In addition, patients with both HIV infection and syphilis may require supplemental antibiotic therapy; many experts believe these patients are also more susceptible to neurologic complications. Consider neurosyphilis in the differential diagnosis when evaluating neurologic signs and symptoms in this group.

Therapy adjustments must often be made for pregnant patients with STDs. Certain drugs, including the fluoroquinolone class of antibiotics and tetracycline, should not be used during pregnancy.

Don't be dismissive of nongonococcal, non-chlamydial causes of vaginal discharge, and advise your patients to take these seriously as well. Delayed or inappropriate treatment allows infection to flourish, increasing the chance of complications and further transmission. Improper therapy also wastes money. Differentiation of bacterial vaginosis, trichomoniasis, and vaginal yeast infections is easy to accomplish and takes very little time.

Educate your patients so that they're more inclined to avoid subsequent STD risks. Remind patients that they didn't expect or intend to get an STD and that a change in behavior could prevent another. Ask patients if they've considered changing risky behaviors or attempted to do so. Help them devise strategies that might work for them. Avoid lectures on the evils of STDs and unsafe sexual practices—you might well lose your listener. On repeat visits, ask about their progress. Ask if they've encountered any problems, and assist them in resolving those problems.

Patients tend to have similar questions when they hear that they have an STD. One is whether it's treatable, and for bacterial infections the answer is Yes. You may also be asked if it's absolutely necessary to inform partners. When patients are reluctant, explain that not doing so puts them at risk of reinfection in the event of additional sexual contact with these partners and also puts others in the community at risk. In certain cases, you may be required by law to report the infection. Other common concerns include how long the infection has been there and where it came from. While a patient's history might sometimes allow you to roughly deduce when, your patient is better equipped to tell you who.

References

1. Quinn, T.C., Recent advances in diagnosis of sexually transmitted diseases. *Sex Transm Dis* 1994;21 (suppl 2):S19-S27.

2. *National Institutes of Health Consensus Development Conference Statement: Cervical Cancer.* April 1-3, 1996, Bethesda, Md, National Cancer Institute, National Institutes of Health, 1996.

3. Hiller, S.L.; Nugent, R.P.; Eschenbach, D.A,, et al, Association between bacterial vaginosis and preterm delivery of a low-birth-weight infant. *N Engl J Med* 1995; 333:1737-1742.

4. Hauth, J.C.; Goldenberg, R.L.; Andrews, W.W., et al, Reduced incidence of preterm delivery with metronidazole and erythromycin in women with bacterial vaginosis. *N Engl J Med* 1995;333:1732-1736.

5. Knowles, J., *Sexually Transmitted Infections: The Facts.* New York, Planned Parenthood Federation of America, Inc., 1995.

6. Recommendations for the prevention and management of Chlamydia trachomatis infections, 1993. *MMWR* 1993;42:1-v.

7. Pict, P.; Islam, M.Q., Sexually transmitted diseases in the 1990s: Global epidemiology and challenges for control. *Sex Transm Dis* 1994;21 (suppl 2):S7-S13.

8. Schulte, J.M.; Martich, F.A.; Schmid, G.P., Chancroid in the United States, 19811990: Evidence for underreporting of cases. *MMWR* 1992;41:57-61.

9. Scholes, D.; Stergachis, A.; Heidrich, F.E., et al, Prevention of pelvic inflammatory disease by screening for cervical chlamydial infection. *N Engl J Med* 1996;334:1362-1366.

10. Quinn, T.C.; Zenilman, J.; Rompalo, A., Sexually transmitted diseases: Advances in diagnosis and treatment. *Adv Intern Med* 1994;39:149-196.

11. Centers for Disease Control and Prevention: 1993 Sexually Transmitted Diseases Treatment Guidelines. *MMWR* 1993;42(RR-14):i-102.

Chapter 27

Sex Turns Dangerous

When physicians and patients fail to talk frankly about sexually transmitted diseases, the "hidden epidemic" that continues to thwart public health intervention.

There isn't anything even remotely sexy about sexually transmitted diseases. And therein lies the problem: In this society, "sexy" topics get plenty of attention, while serious matters pertaining to sex are more apt to be swept under the rug.

Experts say that's especially true with STDs, which now represent about 85% of the infectious diseases reported to the federal Centers for Disease Control and Prevention. Yet, secrecy and discomfort about sexual issues prevent many people, including health care providers, from talking openly about them.

"It requires more intimacy to talk about sex than to actually have it," Beth Meyerson, chief of the bureau of STD/HIV in the Missouri Dept. of Health, told participants at the National STD Prevention Conference here in December 1996.

A major topic at the three-day conference, sponsored by the CDC and the American Social Health Assn., was the recently released report by the Institute of Medicine, "The Hidden Epidemic: Confronting Sexually Transmitted Diseases (*AMNews*, Dec. 9, 1996). The report describes STDs as a hidden problem not only because of people's reluctance to discuss them, but also because many are asymptomatic and thus difficult to diagnose. For example, fully two-thirds of STD infections cannot be detected without a screening test, said Kathleen E. Toomey, MD, state epidemiologist and director, epidemiology and prevention branch, Division of Public Health, Georgia Dept. of Human Resources. Thus, more training is needed so primary care physicians can better identify and treat STDs.

Many Infections, Little Awareness

Of the estimated 12 million Americans infected with an STD, most are unaware they even have a disease. The United States also has the world's highest rates of STDs, often 10 to 15 times higher than other Western industrialized nations. About a quarter of the cases occur among adolescents.

Yet awareness and knowledge about STDs lag, and there is no national strategy to address the problem, the IOM says.

Prevention efforts have been hampered on many levels by the "biological characteristics of STDs, societal problems, unbalanced media messages, lack of awareness, fragmentation of STD-related services, inadequate training of health care professionals, inadequate health insurance coverage and access to services, and insufficient investment in STD prevention," the report said.

HIV was not included in the report because it is now the most-recognized STD, and HIV-prevention efforts are relatively well untried, the IOM panel said. Such is not the case with other STDs, however.

According to a recent Kaiser Family Foundation survey:

- More than 10% of American adults can't name a single STD.

- One in five think all STDs are incurable.

- More than 50% are unaware that having an STD increases the risk of becoming infected with HIV.

STDs associated with increased HIV risk include chancroid, syphilis and genital herpes and inflammatory STDs, such as gonorrhea, Chlamydia infection and trichomoniasis.

One explanation for the increased HIV risk is that STDs may damage or weaken the mucosal and cutaneous surfaces of the genital tract that normally act as a barrier against HIV. According to the Institute of Medicine, many, if not most, heterosexually transmitted HIV infections could be prevented by reducing other STDs. HIV infection also puts individuals at higher risk of contracting another STD, meaning that someone exposed to an HIV-infected individual would also be at higher risk for other STDs. Some STD screening tests are so new that physicians may be unaware of them. An ongoing challenge is getting information about scientific advances to physicians quickly, said Judith Wasserheit, MD, MPH, director of the Division of STD Prevention in the CDCs National Center for HIV, STD and TB.

Reporting Gap Clouds Picture

States require providers to report syphilis, gonorrhea, Chlamydia, chancroid, hepatitis B and AIDS. But private physicians still need to do a much better job of reporting, said CDC Director David Satcher, MD, PhD. "Private providers are not adequately reporting the data on sexually transmitted diseases.... We don't know as much as we could know if we had adequate reporting at every level." There also are formidable scientific challenges, including the ongoing development and recognition of new STD pathogens, the shift to viral STDs, and an increase in antibiotic-resistant strains, Dr. Wasserheit said.

Health officials are trying to move beyond the traditional, clinical approach to STD control by calling for more behavioral and community-based interventions, said Helene D. Gayle, MD, MPH, director of the National Center for HIV, STD and TB. "Our focus has shifted to thinking beyond what are the different microbes involved in causing sexually transmitted infection, to the consequences and impact of these infections on the health of people and on their lives," Dr. Gayle said.

"We're also strengthening our partnerships at all levels of the public sector and developing greater collaboration with academia, community-based organizations and other members of the private sector," she said. "No single agency can take on STD prevention and control alone; partnerships are essential."

Another reason STDs are of growing concern is their role in reproductive disease. For anatomical reasons, women and female adolescents are at higher risk for STDs that can lead to fertility problems and lowered life expectancy. For example, human papillomavirus, or genital warts, has been associated with a number of reproductive cancers, most notably cervical cancer. Of the more than 25 infectious organisms transmitted through sexual contact, the most underrecognized are those that are viral: HPV, herpes simplex virus and sexually transmitted hepatitis B. Only hepatitis B, the STD with the second-highest mortality rate (the first is AIDS), has a preventive vaccine. None of the viral STDs is curable.

"These diseases are causing a tremendous amount of morbidity, and yet these are diseases that are in their infancy in terms of what we can do control-wise," said John Douglas, MD, associate director of the Denver Disease Control Service. Unless the emphasis is shifted to prevention—vaccines and microbicides—"we are going to watch this epidemic continue to move," said Nancy J. Alexander, PhD, chief of the contraceptive development branch in the Center for Population Research at the National Institute of Child Health and Human Development.

Searching for Ideal Contraceptive

Complications due to STDs also are more severe and occur more frequently in women. They are also more likely to remain undiagnosed. With the exception of abstinence, consistent and correct use of a latex condom is the most effective prevention method against both bacterial and viral STDs. But condom use requires male consent and cooperation, which doesn't always occur. Consequently there's a great need for female-controlled prevention methods, especially those that offer dual protection against unwanted pregnancy and STDs, including HIV.

Due to the lack of well-designed randomized clinical trials, there's little information on the ability of spermicides to prevent STDs and HIV, said Penelope J. Hitchcock, chief of the STD branch of Division of Microbiology and Infectious Disease in the National Institute of Allergy and Infectious Diseases. "That's a bad enough situation in itself given that these products have been on the market almost 30 years. But the specter of risk has been raised [because] these products, depending on the concentration of spermicides and the frequency of use, can actually change the surface of the vaginal and cervical epithelium, causing irritation and inflammation, increasing the risk of HIV infection." To date, only one small study, involving about 50 women, has looked at the efficacy of the female condom, and found it to be virtually ineffective against STD infection, Hitchcock said. Furthermore, its effectiveness as a contraceptive was "not impressive," resulting in a pregnancy risk of 12% to 24%.

"If you can still get pregnant three days a month, and you can get an infection 30 days a month, we may not be looking at a great device," Hitchcock said. Abstinence—a foolproof protection against both pregnancy and disease—also has a downside: It offers no option for wanted pregnancy.

"Currently we have no methods to prevent infections that [also] permit pregnancy," Hitchcock said. "I would maintain that, as a species, that's an untenable position for us to be in." "For people in very high-risk environments we're talking about making a life-threatening choice to decide to have a child."

Better Integration, More Training

One of the recommendations of the IOM report centered on improving current STD-related services, including better integration into primary care. But the institute was tepid in its recommendations on physician training and education, said Meyerson of the Missouri Dept. of Health. "I expected to see a call for rigorous change in medical school curricula. I expected to see specific articulation of what must change... that clinical standards for education in medical school be developed now." "Not only must we improve clinical STD knowledge among medical students, we are going to have to teach and provide adequate STD risk assessment to clinicians who are already in practice."

A review of 102 medical schools by H. Trent MacKay, MD, MPH, and colleagues looking at STD and HIV training, found that typically about 23 hours of training were spread among several departments, said Dr. MacKay, medical epidemiologist in the Division of STD Prevention in the National Center for HIV, STD and TB Prevention. "It's competing with a whole host of other areas of interest, and if there isn't someone on the faculty who champions that particular subject the chance is that there isn't going to be much of a focus on it," he said.

The CDC funds two programs to improve STD education in medical schools: STD/HIV Prevention Training Centers, which are based at local health departments but operate jointly with medical schools; and the Faculty Expansion Program, which supports five housestaff positions for two years at schools unaffiliated with a prevention training center. The CDC also funds a two-year STD prevention fellowship that's aimed at individuals who are postdoctorate, typically MDs or PhDs.

"The hope is that these individuals will go on to become faculty members and bridge the gap between schools of medicine, universities and health departments," Dr. MacKay said. People think STDs are treated solely or primarily in public health clinics, but probably the majority of treatment for STDs, particularly for women, occurs in other settings, he said.

"One of our real concerns is that with the advent of managed care a lot of STD care will be shifted into managed care settings, where physicians who may not have much training in STDs will be treating what can be very complicated problems," Dr. MacKay said. "We see a need to train housestaff... so they are prepared to treat STDs in whatever setting they practice."

To help patients achieve and maintain long-term sexual health, a physician needs well-honed communication and negotiation skills, which are difficult to teach in a busy STD or family practice clinic, Meyerson said. "The first step is one of promoting free and open discussion about healthy sexuality," said IOM committee member Edward W. Hook III, MD, professor of medicine and epidemiology at the University of Alabama at Birmingham and director of the STD control program for the Jefferson County Dept. of Health.

Chapter 28

Condoms and Sexually Transmitted Diseases

This chapter is to help you understand why it's important to use condoms (rubbers, prophylactics) to help reduce the spread of sexually transmitted diseases. These diseases include AIDS, chlamydia, genital herpes, genital warts, gonorrhea, hepatitis B, and syphilis. You can get them through having sex—vaginal, anal, or oral.

The surest way to avoid these diseases is to not have sex altogether (abstinence). Another way is to limit sex to one partner who also limits his or her sex in the same way (monogamy). Condoms are not 100% safe, but if used properly, will reduce the risk of sexually transmitted diseases, including AIDS. Protecting yourself against the AIDS virus is of special concern because this disease is fatal and has no cure.

About two-thirds of the people with AIDS in the United States got the disease during sexual intercourse with an infected partner. Experts believe that many of these people could have avoided the disease by using condoms.

Condoms are used for both birth control and reducing the risk of disease. That's why some people think that other forms of birth control—such as the IUD, diaphragm, cervical cap or pill—will protect them against diseases, too. But that's not true. So if you use any other form of birth control, you still need a condom in addition to reduce the risk of getting sexually transmitted diseases.

A condom is especially important when an uninfected pregnant woman has sex, because it can also help protect her and her unborn

---

1996 U.S. Food and Drug Administration (FDA).

child from a sexually transmitted disease. Note well: Condoms are not 100% safe, but if used properly, will reduce the risk of sexually transmitted diseases, including AIDS.

Facts about Sexually Transmitted Diseases

- Sexually transmitted diseases (STDs) affect 12 million men and women in the United States each year.

- Anyone can become infected through sexual intercourse with an infected person.

- Many of those infected are teenagers or young adults.

- Changing sexual partners adds to the risk of becoming infected.

- Sometimes, early in the infection, there may be no symptoms, or symptoms may be easily confused with other illnesses.

Sexually transmitted diseases can cause:

- Tubal pregnancies, sometimes fatal to the mother and always fatal to the unborn child

- Death or severe damage to a baby born to an infected woman

- Sterility (loss of ability to get pregnant)

- Cancer of the cervix in women

- Damage to other parts of the body, including the heart, kidneys, and brain

- Death to infected individuals

See a doctor if you have any of these symptoms of STDs:

- Discharge from the vagina, penis, and/or rectum

- Pain or burning during urination and/or intercourse

- Pain in the abdomen (women), testicles (men), and buttocks and legs (both)

- Blisters, open sores, warts, rash, and/or swelling in the genital area, sex organs, and/or mouth

330

- Flu-like symptoms, including fever, headache, aching muscles, and/or swollen glands

You can get more information about preventing sexually transmitted diseases by calling the National AIDS Hotline, the National Sexually Transmitted Diseases Hotline, or your state or local hotlines.

Who Should Use a Condom?

A person who takes part in risky sexual behavior should always use a condom. The highest risk comes from having intercourse—vaginal, anal, or oral—with a person who has a sexually transmitted disease. If you have sex with an infected person, you're taking a big chance. If you know your partner is infected, the best rule is to avoid intercourse (including oral sex). If you do decide to have sex with an infected partner, you should always be sure a condom is used from start to finish, every time.

And it's risky to have sex with someone who has shared needles with an infected person. It's also risky to have sex with someone who had sex with an infected person in the past. If your partner had intercourse with a person infected with HIV (the AIDS virus), he or she could pass it on to you. That can happen even if the intercourse was a long time ago and even if you partner seems perfectly healthy.

With sexually transmitted diseases, you often can't tell whether your partner has been infected. If you're not sure about yourself or your partner, you should choose to not have sex at all. But if you do have sex, be sure to use a condom that covers the entire penis to reduce your risk of being infected. This includes oral sex where the penis is in contact with the mouth. If you think you and your partner should be using condoms but your partner refuses, then you should say NO to sex with that person.

Will a Condom Guarantee I Won't Get a Sexually Transmitted Disease?

No. There's no absolute guarantee even when you use a condom. But most experts believe that the risk of getting AIDS and other sexually transmitted diseases can be greatly reduced if a condom is used properly. In other words, sex with condoms isn't totally "safe sex," but it is "less risky" sex.

How Can I Get the Most Protection from Condoms?

- Choose the right kind of condoms to prevent disease.
- Store them properly.
- Remember to use a new condom every time you have sex.
- Use the condom the right way, from start to finish.

How Does a Condom Protect Against Sexually Transmitted Diseases?

A condom acts as a barrier or wall to keep blood, or semen, or vaginal fluids from passing from one person to the other during intercourse. These fluids can harbor germs such as HIV (the AIDS virus). If no condom is used, the germs can pass from the infected partner to the uninfected partner.

How Do I Choose the Right Kind of Condoms to Prevent Disease?

Always read the label. Look for two things:

- The condoms should be made of latex (rubber). Tests have shown that latex condoms can prevent the passage of the AIDS, hepatitis and herpes viruses. But natural (lambskin) condoms may not do this. In the future, manufacturers may offer condoms of other materials and designs for disease prevention. As with all new products that make medical claims, such as "prevention of sexually transmitted disease," these new condoms would have to be reviewed by the Food and Drug Administration (FDA) before they are allowed to be sold.

- The package should say that the condoms are to prevent disease. If the package doesn't say anything about preventing disease, the condoms may not provide the protection you want, even though they may be the most expensive ones you can buy. Novelty condoms will not say anything about either disease prevention or pregnancy prevention on the package. They are intended only for sexual stimulation, not protection. Condoms which do not cover the entire penis are not labeled for disease prevention and should not be used for this purpose. For proper protection, a condom must unroll to cover the entire penis. This is another good reason to read the label carefully.

What Is the Government Doing about Condom Quality?

The FDA is working with condom manufacturers to help ensure that the latex condoms you buy are not damaged. Manufacturers "spot check" their condoms using a "water-leak" test. FDA inspectors do a similar test on sample condoms they take from warehouses. The condoms are filled with water and checked for leaks. An average of 996 of 1000 condoms must pass this test. (Don't try the water-leak test on condoms you plan to use, because this kind of testing weakens condoms.) Government testing can not guarantee that condoms will always prevent the spread of sexually transmitted diseases. How well you are protected will also depend a great deal on which condoms you choose and how you store, handle and use them.

Are Condoms Strong Enough for Anal Intercourse?

The Surgeon General has said, "Condoms provide some protection, but anal intercouse is simply too dangerous to practice." Condoms may be more likely to break during anal intercourse than during other types of sex because of the greater amount of friction and other stresses involved. Even if the condom doesn't break, anal intercourse is very risky because it can cause tissue in the rectum to tear and bleed. These tears allow disease germs to pass more easily from one partner to the other.

Should Spermicides Be Used with Condoms?

In test tubes, a spermicide called nonoxynol-9 (a chemical used to kill the man's sperm for birth control) has been shown to kill the germs that cause sexually transmitted diseases. Some experts believe nonoxynol-9 may kill the AIDS virus during intercourse, too. So you might want to use a spermicide along with a latex condom as an added precaution in case the condom breaks during intercourse.

Condoms with spermicides have an expiration date. Pay attention to that date.

How Do I Buy Spermicides and How Should They Be Used?

Spermicides generally come in the form of jellies, creams or foams. You can buy them in pharmacies and some grocery stores. You can also buy condoms with a small amount of spermicide already applied.

333

But some experts believe it's a good idea to add more spermicide to the amount that comes on the condom.

If you do add spermicide, place a small amount inside the condom at its tip. After the condom is on the penis, put more on the outside. Spermicides can also be put inside the woman's vagina. Follow the directions for use.

If you have oral sex, use a condom without a spermicide. Although swallowing small amounts of spermicide has not proven harmful in animal test, we don't know if this is always true for people. Spermicide products and condoms with spermicides have expiration dates. Don't buy or use a package that is outdated.

Should I Use a Lubricant with a Condom?

Some condoms are already lubricated with dry silicone, jellies, or creams. If you buy condoms not already lubricated, it's a good idea to apply some yourself. Lubricants may help prevent condoms from breaking during use and may prevent irritation, which might increase the chance of infection.

If you use a separate lubricant, be sure to use one that's water-based and made for this purpose. If you're not sure which to choose, ask your pharmacist. Never use a lubricant that contains oils, fats, or greases such as petroleum-based jelly, baby oil or lotion, hand or body lotions, cooking shortenings, or oily cosmetics like cold cream. They can seriously weaken latex, causing a condom to tear easily.

Does it Matter Which Styles of Condoms I Use?

It's most important to choose latex condoms that say "disease prevention" on the package. Other features are a matter of personal choice.

What Do the Dates Mean on the Package?

Some packages show "DATE MFG." This tells you when the condoms were made. It is not an expiration date. Other packages may show an expiration date. The condoms should not be purchased or used after that date.

Are Condoms from Vending Machines Any Good?

It depends. Vending machine condoms may be OK:

- If you know you are getting a latex condom,

- If they are labeled for disease prevention,

- If you know the spermicide (if any) is not outdated, and

- If the machine is not exposed to extreme temperature and direct sunlight.

How Should Condoms Be Stored?

You should store condoms in a cool, dry place out of direct sunlight, perhaps in a drawer or closet. If you want to keep one with you, put it in a loose pocket, wallet, or purse for no more than a few hours at a time.

Extreme temperature—especially heat—can make latex brittle or gummy (like an old balloon). So don't keep these latex products in a hot place like a glove compartment.

How Should Condoms Be Handled?

Gently! When opening the packet, don't use your teeth, scissors or sharp nails. Make sure you can see what you're doing.

What Defects Should I Look for?

If the condom material sticks to itself or is gummy, the condom is no good. Also check the condom tip for other damage that is obvious (brittleness, tears, and holes). Don't unroll the condom to check it because this could cause damage.

Never use a damaged condom.

How Should I Use a Condom?

Follow these guidelines

- Use a new condom for every act of intercourse.

- If the penis is uncircumcised, pull the foreskin back before putting the condom on.

- Put the condom on after the penis is erect (hard) and before any contact is made between the penis and any part of the partner's body.

- If using a spermicide, put some inside the condom tip.

- If the condom does not have a reservoir tip, pinch the tip enough to leave a half-inch space for semen to collect.

- While pinching the half-inch tip, place the condom against the penis and unroll it all the way to the base. Put more spermicide or lubricant on the outside.

- If you feel a condom break while you are having sex, stop immediately and pull out. Do not continue until you have put on a new condom and used more spermicide.

- After ejaculation and before the penis gets soft, grip the rim of the condom and carefully withdraw from your partner.

- To remove the condom from the penis, pull it off gently, being careful semen doesn't spill out.

- Wrap the used condom in a tissue and throw it in the trash where others won't handle it. Because condoms may cause problems in sewers, don't flush them down the toilet. Afterwards, wash your hands with soap and water.

- Finally, beware of drugs and alcohol! They can affect your judgment, so you may forget to use a condom. They may even affect your ability to use a condom properly.

Sexually Transmitted Diseases, Including AIDS, Can Be Prevented!

Learn the facts so that you can protect yourself and others from getting infected. Condoms are not 100% safe, but if used properly, will reduce the risk of sexually transmitted diseases, including AIDS. If you have unprotected sex now, you can contract sexually transmitted diseases. Later, if you decide to have children, you might pass the disease on to them.

If you would like more information about condoms and how to prevent sexually transmitted diseases, talk with your doctor or call the National AIDS Hotline. It's open 24 hours a day. Trained operators will answer your questions and can send you more information.

Condom Shopping Guide

Use this handy shopping guide as a reminder of what to look for when buying condoms, lubricants and spermicides.

Be sure to choose:

- Latex
- Disease prevention claim on package label

Also consider:

- With spermicide
- Separate spermicide (gel, cream, foam)
- With lubricant
- Separate lubricant (Select only water-based lubricants made for this purpose.)

Chapter 29

Condom Use Sends Positive Message to Partner

While as many as 85 percent of college students may be sexually active, only 40 percent have ever used a condom, according to one study.

Numerous theories have been cited for this failure, but an overwhelming factor is the embarrassment of bringing the subject up at all. A study by a professor of speech communication and two graduate students at the University of Georgia (UGA) in Athens, Georgia USA, however, has shown for the first time that the use of condoms, especially in first-time sex, may lead to closer, more intimate, and longer-lasting relationships. And it sends the message that the male is less likely to have a sexually transmitted disease.

"The folklore of this issue is that insisting on condom use sends a negative message to a partners," said John Hocking, a professor at UGA. "But we found that for both males and females, insisting on condom use sends a positive message to the partner. It may well be that both males and females would prefer that condoms be used but that they don't bring the subject up because they're afraid of the partner's perception. This information could have a major impact on public health, we believe."

The study by Hocking and graduate students Don Turk and Alex Ellinger, was published in the August 19, 1999, issue of the *Journal of Adolescence*. The research involved some 268 University of Georgia students, who took part in what Hocking calls an "extremely effective and realistic" role-playing survey. Male and female participants imagined that they were about to engage in first-time sex with his or her new partner, and participants were randomly assigned to a condom or no condom condition in which the partner either insisted on using one or made it clear that one would not be used. The participants then responded in writing to measures designed to assess their post-sex attitudes toward the partner, the relationship, and the sexual experience.

The issue of condom use has long perplexed researchers in a number of studies. One research group found in 1992 that only 6 percent of 588 randomly selected undergraduates talked about condom use prior to intercourse. Another study discovered that although some 44 percent of their sample used a condom during their most recent sexual encounter, only 6 percent recalled talking about the use of condoms prior to sex.

One serious problem in understanding the dilemma, obviously, is that it can be conducted only through surveys. Hocking believes the design of his study, with its controls and scientific rigor, give for the first time a serious look at how men and women communicate on issues like condoms prior to sexual encounters. "The conclusion we found was startling," said doctoral student Don Turk. "If you insist on the use of condoms, your partner will like you better."

Scientists have been divided for years on the validity of research conducted through role-playing. But growing evidence, Hocking said, shows that role-playing can be a powerful predictor of behavior if it is designed well. Participants in the study at the University of Georgia took part in one-hour sessions in which those involved were given either a male or female version of a 13-page packet that contained role-playing materials.

A pilot study with some 20 participants was successful enough to move forward with a full study. "The pilot study helped us craft our research so that the participants could decide for themselves how long they had been dating their imaginary partner before their first sexual encounter," said Hocking. The stage was set by having participants read to themselves a scenario in which a male and female student meet, date, and decide to have sex. At the point at which sex looks likely, some role-playing booklets made it clear that their partner insisted on using a condoms (for male) or that one be used (for females) and others made it clear the partner proceeded with sex without use of a condom.

Those in the study were then asked to rate how they felt after the encounter. Each participant was asked if he or she felt confident-insecure, responsible-irresponsible, desirable-undesirable, physically attractive-physically unattractive, in control-out of control, scared-calm, moral-immoral, at risk-risk free, and at ease or worried. They were also asked to evaluate their imaginary partners on the basis of being responsible-irresponsible, promiscuous-chaste, heterosexual-bisexual, attractive-unattractive, care about me-does not care about me, physically attractive-physically unattractive, moral-immoral, someone I respect-someone I do not respect, likely to have a sexually transmitted disease-not likely to have an STD.

The results of the study were consistent and surprising to the researchers. "Those participants whose partners insisted on condom use evaluated those partners as more deserving of respect," said Hocking. "Insistence on condom use also led to feelings of greater safety and less regret following the sexual encounter. And the use of a condom had no apparent effect on beliefs about the partner's perception that the participant had an STD."

Thus it may well be that both males and females would prefer condoms be used but that the issue is just never discussed. Males may fear their partner's negative perception of them if the subject is brought up. "The response of the partners clearly showed that people feel much better in many ways if a condom is used," said Turk.

While the authors admit that the "role-play nature of the present research cannot be generalized with complete confidence to an actual sexual encounter," they suggested that the study gives powerful clues about why condoms are too infrequently used. They noted that further studies on the issue should be done, especially in regard to the relationship between condom use and socioeconomic status and the length of the relationship.

"In addition, the scenario we used described one particular kind of sex a first-time heterosexual encounter with a boyfriend or girlfriend," said Hocking. "We don't know if the results would apply to other kinds of sex, such as repeat sex with the same girlfriend or boyfriend, casual sex such as one-night stands, or same-sex encounters."

Still, the study indicates that condom use can be positive for both partners in ways that have not been widely recognized. Hocking and Turk believe that the results could be incorporated immediately into sex education classes. Students, they said, could be truthfully told, "If you use a condom, or insist that your partner does, your partner will like you more, respect you more, be more likely to want a long-term relationship with you, feel that the sexual encounter was more intimate and meaningful, and be no less likely to think that you have a sexually transmitted disease, or that you think that he or she has one either."

"The best available empirical evidence indicates that use of a condom sends a positive message to your partner about you, about the relationship and the experience and about what you think of them," Hocking added.

Chapter 30

Vaccine-Preventable STDs

One of the most effective means of preventing the transmission of STDs is preexposure immunization. Currently licensed vaccines for the prevention of STDs include those for hepatitis A and hepatitis B. Clinical development and trials are underway for vaccines against a number of other STDs, including HIV and HSV. As more vaccines become available, immunization possibly will become one of the most widespread methods used to prevent STDs.

Five different viruses (i.e., hepatitis A-E) account for almost all cases of viral hepatitis in humans. Serologic testing is necessary to confirm the diagnosis. For example, a health-care provider might assume that an injecting-drug user with jaundice has hepatitis B when, in fact, outbreaks of hepatitis A among injecting-drug users often occur. The correct diagnosis is essential for the delivery of appropriate preventive services. To ensure accurate reporting of viral hepatitis and appropriate prophylaxis of household contacts and sex partners, all case reports of viral hepatitis should be investigated and the etiology established through serologic testing.

Hepatitis A

Hepatitis A is caused by infection with the hepatitis A virus (HAV). HAV replicates in the liver and is shed in the feces. Virus in the stool

---

Centers for Disease Control and Prevention (CDC). 1998 Guidelines for Treatment of Sexually Transmitted Diseases. *MMWR* 1998;47(No. RR-1).

is found in the highest concentrations from 2 weeks before to 1 week after the onset of clinical illness. Virus also is present in serum and saliva during this period, although in much lower concentrations than in feces. The most common mode of HAV transmission is fecal-oral, either by person-to-person transmission between household contacts or sex partners or by contaminated food or water. Because viremia occurs in acute infection, bloodborne HAV transmission can occur; however, such cases have been reported infrequently. Although HAV is present in low concentrations in the saliva of infected persons, no evidence indicates that saliva is involved in transmission.

Of patients who have acute hepatitis A, less than or equal to 20% require hospitalization; fulminant liver failure develops in 0.1% of patients. The overall mortality rate for acute hepatitis A is 0.3%, but it is higher (1.8%) for adults aged greater than 49 years. HAV infection is not associated with chronic liver disease.

In the United States during 1995, 31,582 cases of hepatitis A were reported. The most frequently reported source of infection was household or sexual contact with a person who had hepatitis A, followed by attendance or employment at a day care center; recent international travel; homosexual activity; injecting-drug use; and a suspected food or waterborne outbreak. Many persons who have hepatitis A do not identify risk factors; their source of infection may be other infected persons who are asymptomatic. The prevalence of previous HAV infection among the U.S. population is 33% (CDC, unpublished data).

Outbreaks of hepatitis A among homosexual men have been reported in urban areas, both in the United States and in foreign countries. In one investigation, the prevalence of HAV infection among homosexual men was significantly higher (30%) than that among heterosexual men (12%). In New York City, a case-control study of homosexual men who had acute hepatitis A determined that case-patients were more likely to have had more anonymous sex partners and to have engaged in group sex than were the control subjects; oral-anal intercourse (i.e., the oral role) and digital-rectal intercourse (i.e., the digital role) also were associated with illness.

Treatment

Because HAV infection is self-limited and does not result in chronic infection or chronic liver disease, treatment is usually supportive. Hospitalization may be necessary for patients who are dehydrated because of nausea and vomiting or who have fulminant hepatitis A. Medications that might cause liver damage or that are metabolized by the liver should be used with caution. No specific diet or activity restrictions are necessary.

Prevention

General measures for hepatitis A prevention (e.g., maintenance of good personal hygiene) have not been successful in interrupting outbreaks of hepatitis A when the mode of transmission is from person to person, including sexual contact. To help control hepatitis A outbreaks among homosexual and bisexual men, health education messages should stress the modes of HAV transmission and the measures that can be taken to reduce the risk for transmission of any STD, including enterically transmitted agents such as HAV. However, vaccination is the most effective means of preventing HAV infection.

Two types of products are available for the prevention of hepatitis A: immune globulin (IG) and hepatitis A vaccine. IG is a solution of antibodies prepared from human plasma that is made with a serial ethanol precipitation procedure that inactivates HBV and HIV. When administered intramuscularly before exposure to HAV, or within 2 weeks after exposure, IG is greater than 85% effective in preventing hepatitis A. IG administration is recommended for a variety of exposure situations (e.g., for persons who have sexual or household contact with patients who have hepatitis A). The duration of protection is relatively short (i.e., 3-6 months) and dose dependent.

Inactivated hepatitis A vaccines have been available in the United States since 1995. These vaccines, administered as a two-dose series, are safe, highly immunogenic, and efficacious. Immunogenicity studies indicate that 99%-100% of persons respond to one dose of hepatitis A vaccine; the second dose provides long-term protection. Efficacy studies indicate that inactivated hepatitis A vaccines are 94%-100% effective in preventing HAV infection[2].

Preexposure Prophylaxis

Vaccination with hepatitis A vaccine for preexposure protection against HAV infection is indicated for persons who have the following risk factors and who are likely to seek treatment in settings where STDs are being treated.

- Men who have sex with men. Sexually active men who have sex with men (both adolescents and adults) should be vaccinated.

- Illegal drug users. Vaccination is recommended for users of illegal injecting and noninjecting drugs if local epidemiologic evidence indicates previous or current outbreaks among persons with such risk behaviors.

Postexposure Prophylaxis

Persons who were exposed recently to HAV (i.e., household or sexual contact with a person who has hepatitis A) and who had not been vaccinated before the exposure should be administered a single IM dose of IG (0.02 mL/kg) as soon as possible, but not greater than 2 weeks after exposure. Persons who received at least one dose of hepatitis A vaccine greater than or equal to 1 month before exposure to HAV do not need IG.

Hepatitis B

Hepatitis B is a common STD. During the past 10 years, sexual transmission accounted for approximately 30%-60% of the estimated 240,000 new HBV infections that occurred annually in the United States. Chronic HBV infection develops in 1%-6% of persons infected as adults. These persons are capable of transmitting HBV to others, and they are at risk for chronic liver disease. In the United States, HBV infection leads to an estimated 6,000 deaths annually; these deaths result from cirrhosis of the liver and primary hepatocellular carcinoma.

The risk for perinatal HBV infection among infants born to HBV-infected mothers is 10%-85%, depending on the mother's hepatitis B antigen (HbeAg) status. Chronic HBV infection develops in approximately 90% of infected newborns; these children are at high risk for chronic liver disease. Even when not infected during the perinatal period, children of HBV-infected mothers are at high risk for acquiring chronic HBV infection by person-to-person transmission during the first 5 years of life.

Treatment

No specific treatment is available for persons who have acute HBV infection. Supportive and symptomatic care usually are the mainstays of therapy. During the past decade, numerous antiviral agents have been investigated for treatment of chronic HBV infection. Alpha-2b interferon has been 40% effective in eliminating chronic HBV infection; persons who became infected during adulthood were most likely to respond to this treatment. Antiretroviral agents (e.g., lamivudine) have been effective in eliminating HBV infection, and a number of other compounds are being evaluated. The goal of antiviral treatment is to stop HBV replication. Response to treatment can be demonstrated by normalization of liver function tests, improvement in liver histology, and seroreversion from HBeAg-positive to HBeAg-negative. Long-term follow-up of treated patients suggests that the remission of chronic hepatitis induced by alpha interferon is of long duration. Patient characteristics associated with positive response to interferon therapy include low pretherapy HBV DNA levels, high pretherapy alanine aminotransferase levels, short duration of infection, acquisition of disease in adulthood, active histology, and female sex.

Prevention

Although methods used to prevent other STDs should prevent HBV infection, hepatitis B vaccination is the most effective means of preventing infection. The epidemiology of HBV infection in the United States indicates that multiple age groups must be targeted to provide widespread immunity and effectively prevent HBV transmission and HBV-related chronic liver disease[1]. Vaccination of persons who have a history of STDs is part of a comprehensive strategy to eliminate HBV transmission in the United States. This comprehensive strategy also includes prevention of perinatal HBV infection by a) routine screening of all pregnant women, b) routine vaccination of all newborns, c) vaccination of older children at high risk for HBV infection (e.g., Alaskan Natives, Pacific Islanders, and residents in households of first-generation immigrants from countries in which HBV is of high or intermediate endemicity), d) vaccination of children aged 11-12 years who have not previously received hepatitis B vaccine, and e) vaccination of adolescents and adults at high risk for infection.

Preexposure Prophylaxis

With the implementation of routine infant hepatitis B vaccination and the wide-scale implementation of vaccination programs for adolescents, vaccination of adults at high risk for HBV has become a priority in the strategy to eliminate HBV transmission in the United States. All persons attending STD clinics and persons known to be at high risk for HBV infection (e.g., persons with multiple sex partners, sex partners of persons with chronic HBV infection, and injecting-drug users) should be offered hepatitis B vaccine and advised of their risk for HBV infection (as well as their risk for HIV infection) and the means to reduce their risk (i.e., exclusivity in sexual relationships, use of condoms, and avoidance of nonsterile drug-injection equipment).

Persons who should receive hepatitis B vaccine include the following:

- Sexually active homosexual and bisexual men;

- Sexually active heterosexual men and women, including those a) in whom another STD was recently diagnosed, b) who had more than one sex partner in the preceding 6 months, c) who received treatment in an STD clinic, and d) who are prostitutes;

- Illegal drug users, including injecting-drug users and users of illegal noninjecting drugs;

- Health-care workers;

- Recipients of certain blood products;

- Household and sexual contacts of persons who have chronic HBV infection;

- Adoptees from countries in which HBV infection is endemic;

- Certain international travelers;

- Clients and employees of facilities for the developmentally disabled;

- Infants and children; and

- Hemodialysis patients.

Screening for Antibody Versus Vaccination Without Screening

The prevalence of previous HBV infection among sexually active homosexual men and among injecting-drug users is high. Serologic screening for evidence of previous infection before vaccinating adult members of these groups may be cost-effective, depending on the costs of laboratory testing and vaccine. At the current cost of vaccine, prevaccination testing on adolescents is not cost-effective. For adults attending STD clinics, the prevalence of HBV infection and the vaccine cost may justify prevaccination testing. However, because prevaccination testing may lower compliance with vaccination, the first dose of vaccine should be administered at the time of testing. The additional doses of hepatitis vaccine should be administered on the basis of the prevaccination test results. The preferred serologic test for prevaccination testing is the total antibody to hepatitis B core antigen (anti-HBc), because it will detect persons who have either resolved or chronic infection. Because anti-HBc testing will not identify persons immune to HBV infection as a result of vaccination, a history of hepatitis B vaccination should be obtained, and fully vaccinated persons should not be revaccinated.

Vaccination Schedules

Hepatitis B vaccine is highly immunogenic. Protective levels of antibody are present in approximately 50% of young adults after one dose of vaccine; in 85%, after two doses; and greater than 90%, after three doses. The third dose is required to provide long-term immunity. The most often used schedule is vaccination at 0, 1-2, and 4-6 months. The first and second doses of vaccine must be administered at least 1 month apart, and the first and third doses at least 4 months apart. If the vaccination series is interrupted after the first or second dose of vaccine, the missing dose should be administered as soon as possible. The series should not be restarted if a dose has been missed. The vaccine should be administered IM in the deltoid, not in the buttock.

Postexposure Prophylaxis

Exposure to Persons Who Have Acute Hepatitis B

Sexual Contacts

Patients who have acute HBV infection are potentially infectious to persons with whom they have sexual contact. Passive immunization with hepatitis B immune globulin (HBIG) prevents 75% of these infections. Hepatitis B vaccination alone is less effective in preventing infection than HBIG and vaccination. Sexual contacts of patients who have acute hepatitis B should receive HBIG and begin the hepatitis B vaccine series within 14 days after the most recent sexual contact. Testing of sex partners for susceptibility to HBV infection (anti-HBc) can be considered if it does not delay treatment greater than 14 days.

Nonsexual Household Contacts

Nonsexual household contacts of patients who have acute hepatitis B are not at high risk for infection unless they are exposed to the patient's blood (e.g., by sharing a toothbrush or razor blade). However, vaccination of household contacts is encouraged, especially for children and adolescents. If the patient remains HBsAg-positive after 6 months (i.e., becomes chronically infected), all household contacts should be vaccinated.

Exposure to Persons Who Have Chronic HBV Infection

Hepatitis B vaccination without the use of HBIG is highly effective in preventing HBV infection in household and sexual contacts of persons who have chronic HBV infection, and all such contacts should be vaccinated. Postvaccination serologic testing is indicated for sex partners of persons who have chronic hepatitis B infections and for infants born to HBsAg-positive women.

Special Considerations

Pregnancy

Pregnancy is not a contraindication to hepatitis B vaccine or HBIG vaccine administration.

HIV Infection

HBV infection in HIV-infected persons is more likely to lead to chronic HBV infection. HIV infection also can impair the response to hepatitis B vaccine. Therefore, HIV-infected persons who are vaccinated should be tested for hepatitis B surface antibody 1-2 months after the third vaccine dose. Revaccination with three more doses should be considered for those who do not respond initially to vaccination. Those who do not respond to additional doses should be advised that they might remain susceptible to HBV infection.

Chapter 31

Non-Sexual Transmission of STDs: Tattoos, Body Pierces, and Medical Safety

More and more young people are decorating their bodies with tattoos and pierces. Understanding the fad can help you ensure your patients' safety. David Rothman, PhD, a professor of social medicine at Columbia University's College of Physicians and Surgeons in New York City, says he doesn't know a single person who has a tattoo. Rothman's 23-year-old daughter Micol, a second-year medical student at Columbia, knew a couple of women in her undergraduate days at Brown University in Providence, R.I., who had discreet tattoos in places where they might not be commonly observed. In contrast, Kris Sperry, MD, deputy chief medical examiner of Fulton Co., Ga., has no trouble believing an estimate he has heard that one-quarter of all the 15 to 25-year-olds in the United States have tattoos. It all depends on whom you know, and how much of them you see.

Many physicians see a cross-section of people, and there is no question that they are encountering more examples of "body modification" now than ever before. Men and women in all walks of life are getting tattooed, and are piercing their faces, navels, nipples and genitals. In Chicago, for example, there was one tattoo parlor in 1974, according to David Kottker, a local sculptor-turned-tattooist. Ten years later there were about 10; now there are more than 20, some of which also do piercing. There is no federal regulation of tattooing or piercing, and

© 1995 American Medical Association, from *American Medical News*, Dec. 18, 1995, Vol.38, No.47, Pg.17(4), "Risky Fashions," by Delia O'Hara; reprinted with permission.

local regulation is spotty. New York City outlawed the practice in 1961 after 13 tattoo-related cases of hepatitis B were reported despite a two-year experiment with regulating the city's tattoo parlors. As a spokesman for New York City's public health department noted, however, the fact that it's illegal doesn't mean nobody gets tattooed there.

Still, tattooing has come a long way since the days when boards of health—if they checked in with tattooists at all—typically required tattoo parlors to keep "a bucket of Lysol under the sink, and asked that it be changed once a week," says Mick Beasley, a Glen Burnie, Md., tattooist.

What Are the Risks?

Beasley and other advocates of body modification say the risks are few when the procedures are done properly. Some people have allergic reactions to the ink, but Beasley says that in her experience such reactions are minor and transitory; Dr. Sperry puts the risk from a bee sting well above that from a tattoo. "People who form keloids should avoid tattoos," Dr. Sperry says.

Beasley and Dr. Sperry also say there is little to no risk of contracting HIV from body-modification procedures. "The volume of blood extant during a tattoo is not enough to cause AIDS. And you need an intermuscular stick, not just a dermal scratch," says Dr. Sperry, who is heavily inked. But the Centers for Disease Control and Prevention take a different view. Although "there have been no cases reported of HIV transmission that have been ascribed to tattooing, we do think the potential exists," says Peter Drotman, MD, assistant director for public health in the division of HIV and AIDS prevention. No one knows the minimum amount of inoculum that must be present to allow for HIV transmission, he says.

The biggest established threat is hepatitis. Some experts are concerned that tattooing and piercing will expose an entirely new population to infection as the fad gains popularity among otherwise low-risk, middle and upper-class young people. "A lot of this is done on impulse. One young person has something like this done, and then all the friends want one, too. It's a herd instinct," says gastroenterologist-internist Willis C. Maddrey, MD, vice chair of the Hepatitis Education Campaign of the American Gastroenterological Society and the American Society for Gastrointestinal Endoscopy. This tendency toward impetuousness means young people may not take the time to shop around for a commercial piercing or tattooing business with adequate safeguards to minimize the risk of hepatitis exposure.

"Our recommendation is that anyone considering undergoing a tattooing or piercing operation should ask for evidence of proper sterilization," says Dr. Maddrey. He is also adviser to "Get Hip to Hep," a public awareness campaign launched by the American Liver Foundation and the Blues Heaven Foundation with funding from Schering Laboratories.

According to "Get Hip," 27 states have no minimum hygiene standards for tattoo parlors. For that reason, the campaign suggests tattooing and piercing may be factors in the approximately 40% of all hepatitis B and C cases with no known source of infection. "Tattooing and body piercing may provide additional routes for blood-to-blood transmission of hepatitis," the campaign's literature warns. "Although transmission of blood-borne hepatitis via tattooing may be rare in comparison with the most common modes of transmission, this may change as tattooing and other nonmedical invasive procedures become more widespread."

Dr. Maddrey says the risk could be greatly reduced if more young people received vaccinations against hepatitis B. Most public health and prevention authorities currently recommend vaccinations for certain health care workers, homosexual men, intravenous drug users, children born to infected mothers and others considered at high risk for hepatitis exposure.

Effort to Self-Police

Practitioners of tattooing and body piercing attribute infection problems to "amateurs" who use improper equipment and techniques. According to Beasley, reputable tattooists use stainless-steel solid-core needles, which are attached to a stainless-steel bar that fits into a tube. The tube is inserted into a hand-held electrical machine, which punctures the skin about 2,300 times per minute. Working with one color at a time, the tattooist pushes the pigment—a food-grade dry powder suspended in a solution of distilled water—up under the skin.

When administered properly, the machine does not come in contact with blood, Beasley says. In reputable tattoo parlors, she adds, the needle and tube are removed after use, the needle is broken off and disposed of in a sharps container, and the tube is cleaned in an ultrasonic tank, then autoclaved and sterilized.

Michaela Grey, director of training seminars at the Gauntlet, a chain of body piercing shops, says that reputable piercers use hollow-core needles, which at the Gauntlet are autoclaved before use, used on one person and then thrown away. Grey is among those who have organized to improve safety conditions. In 1994, she founded the Assn. of Professional Piercers to advocate for standardized practices. "Reputable piercers do want to talk to doctors and legislators," she says.

Beasley is executive director of the Alliance of Professional Tattooists, which has conducted nine-hour seminars on preventing disease transmission for more than 700 professional tattooists nationwide, she says. Dr. Sperry is the group's medical adviser. Despite these efforts at self-policing, Eugene Schoenfeld, MD, who hosts a popular San Francisco radio call-in program targeted to young adults, says he tries to discourage callers from body modification.

"I tell them that colleagues at San Francisco's county hospital have seen some ugly infections, especially of genital piercings," says the psychiatrist, who once wrote a syndicated newspaper column under the pseudonym Dr. Hippocrates. He says he typically gets one or two calls per program about genital or nipple piercing. "I generally try not to take an authoritarian tone, but it seems to me to be a strange fad," Dr. Schoenfeld says.

Grey contends that many physicians are simply "phobic about piercing." The Gauntlet keeps of list of "piercing-friendly" physicians. San Francisco internist Flash Gordon, MD, is one of those on the store's list. He says he often sees patients who don't want to bring piercing-related problems to their usual physicians. Dr. Gordon concedes that people with hyperactive skin reactions, diabetes or immune system problems should avoid any body modifications. But he notes that most candidates tend to be "young and fairly healthy, so they'll probably do well."

"I'd like to emphasize that a non-judgmental attitude is important," says Dr. Gordon, who adds that he is not pierced or tattooed himself. "The physician should let the patient know what the risks are and then let him decide. Most doctors don't have a problem taking care of somebody who gets hurt skiing or Roller Blading, which are thrill-seeking behaviors that carry a certain risk. If a physician feels and acts disgusted, he can't practice good medicine."

Dr. Maddrey agrees that physicians should convey the health risks in an objective manner. "From a medical standpoint, we might think this is a reasonable thing for patients to avoid. But if someone wants to do it, we shouldn't impose our social values."

Outsider Fashion Trend

Tattooists and piercers like to talk about the increasingly common-place nature of the practices, about the grandmothers and CEOs and bureaucrats who are swelling the ranks of their customers. But Dr. Rothman, the social medicine professor, who studies the ideas that various cultures hold about the integrity of the body, says that these practices have a long way to go before they lose the "outsider" implications they carry here and elsewhere. Piercing and tattooing "come up against some deep beliefs about what you can and cannot do with the body, Where writing on the body is forbidden"—as it is in the Judeo-Christian tradition, among others—these practices "have the potential to be subversive," Dr. Rothman says.

Dr. Schoenfeld describes a colleague, the chief of staff at a northern California hospital, who has expressed interest in getting a tattoo. If she does so, Dr. Rothman argues that she will be placing herself outside the mainstream, at least in her own mind. Dr. Gordon agrees. "I think these practices are a way of saying, I might not be able to make much difference in what the world does to me, but at least I can do what I want, with my body."

Chapter 32

Syringe Exchange Programs

As of December 1997, more than one third (36%) of the 641,086 cases of acquired immunodeficiency syndrome (AIDS) reported to CDC were directly or indirectly associated with injecting-drug use[1]. Syringe exchange programs (SEPs) are one of the strategies employed to prevent infection with human immunodeficiency virus (HIV) among injecting-drug users (IDUs). The goal of SEPs is to reduce the transmission of HIV and other bloodborne infections associated with reuse of blood-contaminated syringes for drug injection by providing sterile syringes in exchange for used, potentially contaminated syringes. This chapter summarizes a survey of U.S. SEP activities during January-December 1997 and compares the findings with those of two previous surveys during 1994-1995 and 1996[2,3]. The findings indicate continued expansion in the number, geographic coverage, and activity of SEPs in the United States.

In November 1997, the Beth Israel Medical Center (BIMC) in New York City, in collaboration with the North American Syringe Exchange Network (NASEN), mailed questionnaires to the directors of 113 SEPs in the United States that were members of NASEN. From December 1997 through March 1998, BIMC contacted SEP directors to conduct structured telephone interviews based on the mailed questionnaires. SEP directors were asked about their program's legal status, number of syringes exchanged during 1997, program operations, services provided, budgets, and community and law enforcement relations.

Centers for Disease Control (CDC), from *MMWR*, August 14, 1998/ 47(31);652-655.

Of the 113 SEPs, 100 (89%) participated in the survey. Of these, 54 began operating before 1995; 20, in 1995; 18, in 1996; and 8, in 1997. One SEP closed in 1997. These 100 SEPs reported operating in 80 cities in 30 states, the District of Columbia, and Puerto Rico; 52 (52%) of the SEPs were located in four states (California {19}, New York {14}, Washington {11}, and Connecticut {8}). Nine cities had at least two SEPs (31 SEPs in the nine cities). In the 1996 survey, 87 SEPs reported operating in 71 cities in 26 states, the District of Columbia, and Puerto Rico and during 1994-1995, a total of 60 SEPs reported operating in 46 cities and in 21 states[2,3].

In 1997, a total of 96 of the 100 SEPs provided information about the number of syringes and reported exchanging approximately 17.5 million syringes (median: 57,343 syringes per SEP). The 10 largest volume SEPs (i.e., those that exchanged greater than or equal to 500,000 syringes) exchanged approximately 10.3 million (59%) of all syringes exchanged. The SEP in San Francisco reported exchanging the largest number of syringes (1.9 million) in 1997. During 1996, a total of 84 SEPs reported exchanging approximately 14 million syringes (median: 36,017) and in 1994, a total of 55 SEPs exchanged 8 million syringes (median: 39,014).

Most of the 100 SEPs provided other public health and social services: 99% offered instruction in the use of condoms and dental dams to prevent sexual transmission of HIV and other sexually transmitted diseases (STDs); 96% provided IDUs with information about safer injection techniques and/or use of bleach to disinfect injection equipment; and 94% referred clients for substance abuse treatment programs. Health-care services offered on site included HIV counseling and testing (64%), tuberculosis skin testing (20%), STD screening (20%), and primary health care (19%).

In this survey, SEPs were defined as legal if they operated in a state that had no law requiring a prescription to purchase a hypodermic syringe (i.e., a prescription law) or had an exemption to the state prescription law allowing the SEP to operate; illegal-tolerated if they operated in a state with a prescription law but had received a formal vote of support or approval from a local elected body (e.g., city council); and illegal-underground if the SEP operated in a state with a prescription law but had not received formal support from local elected officials. In 1997, a total of 52 SEPs were legal, 16 were illegal-tolerated, and 32 were illegal-underground.

SEPs reported receiving financial support from various sources including foundations, individuals, and state and local governments. Current federal law prohibits the use of federal funds to carry out any program of distributing sterile needles or syringes for the hypodermic injection of any illegal drug.

The 100 SEPs operated in various settings, including home visits (37%) (syringe pick-up/drop-off sites), storefront locations (35%), vans (35%), sidewalk tables (23%), on-foot outreach (23%), cars (19%), locations where IDUs gather to inject drugs (i.e., shooting galleries) (17%), and health clinics (11%). Sixty-nine (69%) SEPs operated in multiple settings. Ninety-five SEPs reported data on the hours of program operation each week; they reported providing 2078.5 hours (median: 18 hours; range: 1-112 hours) of SEP services each week.

Reported by: D Paone, EdD, DC Des Jarlais, PhD, MP Singh, MPH, D Grove, Q Shi, PhD, Beth Israel Medical Center, New York; M Krim, PhD, American Foundation for AIDS Research, New York, New York; D Purchase, North American Syringe Exchange Network, Tacoma, Washington; RH Needle, PhD, P Hartsock, PhD, Community Research Br, Div of Epidemiology and Prevention, National Institute on Drug Abuse, National Institutes of Health; Div of HIV/AIDS Prevention-Intervention, Research, and Support, National Center for HIV, STD, and TB Prevention, CDC.

Editorial Note

The findings in this survey indicate continued growth in the number, geographic coverage, and activity of SEPs in the United States. From 1994-1995 to 1997, there were increases in the number of SEPs participating in these surveys (67% {from 60 to 100}), the number of cities with SEPs (74% {from 46 to 80}), and the number of syringes exchanged (119% {from 8 million to 17.5 million}). However, the scope of SEP activity may be underestimated because some of the known SEPs in the United States did not participate in this survey and some may not be members of NASEN.

The 10 largest volume SEPs are responsible for approximately half of all syringes exchanged in 1997, and the 24 smallest volume SEPs (i.e., those that exchanged less than 10,000 syringes) reported exchanging only less than 1% of total syringes (mean: 3431.5 syringes per program). An IDU makes approximately 1000 illicit drug injections per year[4]. Larger volume SEPs could have greater community impact in allowing IDUs to use a sterile syringe for every injection.

Many IDUs who participate in SEPs are high-risk drug users, suggesting that SEPs can reach persons at risk for bloodborne infections (including HIV and hepatitis C) and other public health problems[5,6]. IDUs who participate in SEPs increase the proportion of drug injections in which a syringe is used only once, thereby reducing the reuse of potentially contaminated syringes[7]. In addition, IDUs using syringes obtained from SEPs have lower rates of HIV incidence (compared to IDUs using syringes obtained from the illicit market)[8]. Compared with clients referred to substance abuse treatment programs from other sources, IDUs referred by SEPs have comparably good short-term treatment outcomes [9].

SEPs are one component of a community's comprehensive approach currently used to prevent HIV infection among IDUs, their sexual partners, and their children. Access to sterile syringes for drug users who continue to inject also can be provided through the sale of syringes in pharmacies. In addition to SEPs, comprehensive programs for reducing the spread of HIV and other bloodborne infections should include community outreach programs, substance abuse treatment programs, HIV-prevention programs in jails and prisons, prevention of initiation of drug injection, health care for HIV-infected IDUs, and HIV risk-reduction counseling and testing for IDUs and their sexual partners[10].

References

1. CDC. HIV/AIDS surveillance report, 1997. Atlanta, Georgia. US Department of Health and Human Services, Public Health Service, 1997. Vol 9, no. 2).

2. CDC. Syringe exchange programs—United States, 1994-1995. *MMWR* 1995;44:684-5,691.

3. CDC. Update: Syringe exchange programs—United States, 1996. *MMWR* 1997;46:565-8.

4. Lurie, P.; Jones, T.S.; Foley, J., A sterile syringe for every drug user injection: how many injections take place annually and how might pharmacists contribute to syringe distribution? *J Acquir Immune Defic Syndr Hum Retrovirol*, 1998;18(suppl 1):S126-S132.

5. Bruneau, J.; Lamothe, F.; Lachance, N., et al, Injection behaviors in HIV seroconversion among IV drug users in Montreal. Geneva, Switzerland: Presented at the XII International Conference on AIDS, June 28-July 3, 1998. (Abstract 23221).

6. Schechter, M.; Strathdee, S.L.; Currie, D.M., et al, Harm reduction, not harm production: needle exchange does not promote

HIV transmission among injection drug users in Vancouver, Canada. Geneva, Switzerland: Presented at the XII International Conference on AIDS, June 28-July 3, 1998. (Abstract 33379).

7. Heimer, R.; Khoshnood, K.; Bigg, D.; Guydish, J., Syringe use and re-use: effects of needle exchange programs in three cities. *J Acquir Immune Defic Syndr Hum Retrovirol* 1998;18(suppl 1):S37-S44.

8. Des Jarlais, D.C.; Marmor, M.; Paone, D., et al, HIV incidence among injecting drug users in New York City syringe-exchange programs. *Lancet* 1996;348:987-91.

9. Brooner, R.; Kidorf, M.; King, V.; Beilenson, P.; Svikis, D.; Vlahov, D., Drug abuse treatment success among needle exchange participants. *Public Health Rep* 1998;113(suppl 1):129-39.

10. Jones, T.S.; Vlahov, D.. Use of sterile syringes and aseptic drug preparation are important components of HIV prevention among injection drug users. *J Acquir Immune Defic Syndr Hum Retrovirol* 1998;18(suppl 1):S1-S5.

Part Four

Diagnosis and Treatment of Sexually Transmitted Diseases

Chapter 33

Guidelines for the Treatment of Sexually Transmitted Diseases

The Centers for Disease Control and Prevention (CDC) has released the "1998 Guidelines for the Treatment of Sexually Transmitted Diseases." The guidelines were developed by the CDC after consultation with a group of experts who met in Atlanta in 1997. Chair of the expert panel was David Atkins, M.D., M.P.H., of the Agency for Health Care Policy and Research.

The 116-page guidelines include prevention, diagnosis and treatment information for all common sexually transmitted diseases and are organized by syndrome. Included are new recommendations for the treatment of primary and recurrent genital herpes and management of pelvic inflammatory disease, a new patient-applied medication for the treatment of human papillomavirus infection and a revised approach to the management of victims of sexual assault. Revised sections describe the evaluation of urethritis and the diagnostic evaluation of congenital syphilis. The guidelines also include expanded sections concerning sexually transmitted diseases in infants, children and pregnant women, and the management of patients who have asymptomatic human immunodeficiency virus (HIV) infection, genital warts and genital herpes.

Recommendations are also provided for diseases characterized by genital ulcers; management of patients who have a history of penicillin allergy; diseases characterized by vaginal discharge; pelvic inflammatory disease; epididymitis; human papillomavirus infection; proctitis, proctocolitis and enteritis; and vaccine-preventable sexually transmitted diseases, including recommendations for the use of hepatitis A and hepatitis B vaccines.

The 1998 guidelines update CDC recommendations from 1993 for screening, diagnosis and treatment. Some of the advances in treatment made since the last guidelines were published include the following:

- Highly effective single-dose oral therapies have been developed for almost all common curable sexually transmitted diseases.

- Improved treatments are now available for herpes simplex virus type 2 and human papillomavirus infection.

- A simple urine test has been introduced for the diagnosis of chlamydia in clinical and nonclinical settings.

- Recommendations for hepatitis A and hepatitis B include vaccination of all sexually active youth.

- Improved treatments for sexually transmitted diseases in pregnant women may produce fewer side effects and reduce the number of infants born prematurely.

Special Populations

The following information has been excerpted from the section of the guidelines that covers special populations:

Pregnant Women

Intrauterine or perinatally transmitted sexually transmitted diseases can have fatal or severely debilitating effects on a fetus. Pregnant women and their sex partners should be questioned about sexually transmitted diseases and should be counseled about the possibility of perinatal infections. The recommended screening tests include the following:

- A serologic test for syphilis should be performed in all pregnant women at the first prenatal visit. In populations in which prenatal care is not optimally used, rapid plasma reagin (RPR)-card test screening, with treatment if that test is reactive, should be performed at the time a pregnancy is confirmed. For patients at high risk, screening should be repeated in the third trimester and again at delivery. Some states also mandate screening of all women at delivery. No infant should be discharged from the hospital without the syphilis serologic status of its mother having been determined at least one time during pregnancy and, preferably, again, at delivery. Any woman who delivers a stillborn infant should be tested for syphilis.

- A serologic test for hepatitis B surface antigen (HBsAg) should be performed for all pregnant women at the first renatal visit. HBsAg testing should be repeated late in the pregnancy for women who are HBsAg negative but who are at high risk for hepatitis B virus infection (e.g., injecting drug users and women who have concomitant sexually transmitted diseases).

- A test for *Neisseria gonorrhoeae* should be performed at the first prenatal visit for women at risk of gonorrhea or for women living in an area where the prevalence of *N. gonorrhoeae* is high. A repeat test should be performed during the third trimester for those at continued risk.

- A test for *Chlamydia trachomatis* infection should be performed in the third trimester for women at increased risk (i.e., women under 25 years of age and women who have a new sex partner, more than one sex partner or whose partner has other partners) to prevent maternal postnatal complications and chlamydia infection in the infant. Screening during the first trimester might enable prevention of adverse effects of chlamydia during pregnancy. However, evidence for adverse effects during pregnancy is minimal. If screening is performed only during the first trimester, a longer period exists for acquiring infection before delivery.

- A test for HIV infection should be offered to all pregnant women at the first prenatal visit.

- A test for bacterial vaginosis may be performed early in the second trimester for asymptomatic patients who are at high risk for preterm labor (e.g., those who have a history of a previous preterm delivery). Current evidence does not support universal testing for bacterial vaginosis.

- A Papanicolaou smear should be obtained at the first prenatal visit if none has been documented during the preceding years.

Other Concerns in Pregnant Women

Pregnant women who have either primary genital herpes virus infection, hepatitis B virus infection, primary cytomegalovirus infection, or group B streptococcal infection, and women who have syphilis and who are allergic to penicillin, may need to be referred to an expert for management.

HBsAg-positive pregnant women should be reported to the local and/or state health department to ensure that they are entered into a case-management system and appropriate prophylaxis is provided for their infants. In addition, household and sexual contacts of HBsAg-positive women should be vaccinated.

In the absence of lesions during the third trimester, routine serial cultures for herpes simplex virus are not indicated for women who have a history of recurrent genital herpes. However, obtaining cultures from such women at the time of delivery may be useful in guiding neonatal management. Prophylactic cesarean section is not indicated for women who do not have active genital lesions at the time of delivery.

The presence of genital warts is not an indication for cesarean section. For a more detailed discussion of these guidelines, physicians are referred by the CDC to "Guidelines for Perinatal Care," 3d ed., published by the American Academy of Pediatrics and the American College of Obstetricians and Gynecologists in 1992.

Adolescents

Physicians who provide care for adolescents should be aware of several issues that relate specifically to adolescents. The rates of sexually transmitted diseases are highest among adolescents (e.g., the rate of gonorrhea is highest among females 15 to 19 years of age). Clinic-based studies have demonstrated that the prevalence of chlamydial infections, and possibly of human papillomavirus infections, also is highest in adolescents. In addition, surveillance data indicate that 9 percent of adolescents who have acute hepatitis B virus infection either have had sexual contact with a chronically infected person or with multiple sex partners or gave their sexual preference as homosexual. As part of a comprehensive strategy to eliminate hepatitis B virus transmission in the United States, the Advisory Committee on Immunization Practices has recommended that all children receive hepatitis B vaccine.

Adolescents who are at high risk for sexually transmitted diseases include male homosexuals, sexually active heterosexuals, clients in clinics for sexually transmitted diseases and injecting-drug users. Adolescents less than 15 years of age who are sexually active are at particular risk for infection. Adolescents are at greatest risk for sexually transmitted diseases because they frequently have unprotected intercourse, are biologically more susceptible to infection and face multiple obstacles to use of health care.

Several of these issues can be addressed by clinicians who provide services to adolescents. Clinicians can address the general lack of knowledge and awareness about the risks and consequences of sexually transmitted diseases and offer guidance, constituting true primary prevention, to help adolescents develop healthy sexual behaviors and prevent the establishment of behavior patterns that can undermine sexual health. With some exceptions, all adolescents can consent to the confidential diagnosis and treatment of sexually transmitted diseases. Medical care for sexually transmitted diseases can be provided to adolescents without parental consent or knowledge. Furthermore, in many states, adolescents can consent to counseling and testing for HIV infection. Consent laws for vaccination of adolescents differ by state. Physicians should consider how important confidentiality is to adolescents and should strive to follow policies that comply with state laws to ensure the confidentiality of services provided to adolescents.

The style and content of counseling and health education should be adapted for adolescents. Discussions should be appropriate for the patient's developmental level and should identify risky behaviors, such as sex and drug use. Careful counseling and thorough discussions are especially important for adolescents who may not acknowledge engaging in high-risk behaviors. Care and counseling should be direct and nonjudgmental.

Children

Management of children who have a sexually transmitted disease requires close cooperation between the physician, laboratories and child-protection authorities. Investigations, when indicated, should be initiated promptly. Some diseases (e.g., gonorrhea, syphilis and chlamydia), if acquired after the neonatal period, are almost 100 percent indicative of sexual contact. For other diseases, such as human papillomavirus infection and vaginitis, the association with sexual contact is not as clear.

Sexual Assault and Sexually Transmitted Diseases

The following information has been excerpted from the section of the guidelines on sexual assault and sexually transmitted diseases.

Adults and Adolescents

Trichomoniasis, bacterial vaginosis, chlamydia and gonorrhea are the most frequently diagnosed infections in women who have been sexually assaulted. Because the prevalence of these diseases is substantial among sexually active women, the presence of these infections after an assault does not necessarily signify acquisition during the assault. Chlamydial and gonococcal infections in women are of special concern because of the possibility of ascending infection. In addition, hepatitis B virus infection, if transmitted to a woman during an assault, can be prevented by postexposure administration of hepatitis B vaccine.

Initial Examination

An initial examination should include the following procedures:

- Cultures for *N. gonorrhoeae* and *C. trachomatis* from specimens collected from any sites of penetration or attempted penetration.

- If chlamydial culture is not available, nonculture tests, particularly the nucleic acid amplification tests, are an acceptable substitute. Nucleic acid amplification tests offer advantages of increased sensitivity if confirmation is available. If a nonculture test is used, a positive test result should be verified with a second test based on a different diagnostic principle. Enzyme-linked immunosorbent assay and direct fluorescent antibody are not acceptable alternatives, because false-negative test results occur more often with these nonculture tests, and false-positive test results may occur.

- Wet mount and culture of a vaginal swab specimen for *Trichomonas vaginalis* infection. If vaginal discharge or malodor is evident, the wet mount also should be examined for evidence of bacterial vaginosis and yeast infection.

- Collection of a serum sample for immediate evaluation for HIV, hepatitis B and syphilis.

Follow-Up Examinations

Although it is often difficult for persons to comply with follow-up examinations weeks after an assault, such examinations are essential to detect new infections acquired during or after the assault; to complete hepatitis B immunization, if indicated; and to complete counseling and treatment for other sexually transmitted diseases. For these reasons, it is recommended that assault victims be reevaluated at follow-up examination.

Examination for sexually transmitted diseases should be repeated two weeks after the assault. Because infectious agents acquired through assault may not have produced sufficient concentrations of organisms to result in positive test results at the initial examination, a culture, wet mount and other tests should be repeated at the two-week follow-up visit unless prophylactic treatment has already been provided. Serologic tests for syphilis and HIV infection should be repeated six, 12 and 24 weeks after the assault if initial test results were negative.

Prophylaxis

Many experts recommend routine preventive therapy after a sexual assault. Most patients probably benefit from prophylaxis because the follow-up of patients who have been sexually assaulted can be difficult, and they may be reassured if offered treatment or prophylaxis for possible infection. The following prophylactic regimen is suggested as preventive therapy:

- Postexposure hepatitis B vaccination (without hepatitis B immune globulin) should adequately protect against hepatitis B virus. Hepatitis B vaccine should be given to victims of sexual assault at the time of the initial examination. Follow-up doses of vaccine should be given one to two and four to six months after the first dose.

- An empiric antimicrobial regimen for chlamydia, gonorrhea, trichomonas and bacterial vaginosis should be administered. The recommended regimen is as follows: ceftriaxone, 125 mg intramuscularly in a single dose, plus metronidazole, 2 g orally in a single dose, plus either azithromycin, 1 g orally in a single dose or doxycycline, 100 mg orally twice a day for seven days. Certain patients may require alternative treatments.

The efficacy of these regimens in preventing gonorrhea, bacterial vaginosis or *C. trachomatis* genitourinary infections after sexual assault has not been evaluated. The physician should counsel the patient as to the possible benefits and side effects of these treatment regimens.

Other Considerations

At the initial examination and, if needed, at follow-up examinations, patients should be counseled regarding the following:

- Symptoms of sexually transmitted diseases and the need for immediate examination if symptoms occur.

- Abstinence from sexual intercourse until prophylactic treatment is completed.

Risk of Acquiring HIV Infection

Although HIV-antibody seroconversion has been reported in persons whose only known risk factor was sexual assault or sexual abuse, the risk for acquiring HIV infection through sexual assault is low. The overall probability depends on many factors. These may include the type of sexual intercourse; presence of oral, vaginal or anal trauma; site of exposure to ejaculate; viral load in ejaculate; and presence of a sexually transmitted disease.

In certain circumstances, the likelihood of HIV transmission also may be affected by postexposure therapy for HIV infection with antiretroviral agents. Postexposure therapy with zidovudine has been associated with a reduced risk for HIV infection in a study of health care workers who had percutaneous exposures to HIV-infected blood. However, whether these findings can be extrapolated to other HIV-exposure situations, including sexual assault, is unknown. A recommendation cannot be made regarding the appropriateness of postexposure antiretroviral therapy after sexual exposure to HIV.

Physicians who consider offering postexposure therapy should take into account the likelihood of exposure to HIV, the potential benefits and risks of such therapy, and the interval between the exposure and initiation of therapy. Because timely determination of the assailant's HIV-infection status is not possible in many sexual assaults, the physician should assess the nature of the assault, any available information about HIV-risk behaviors exhibited by persons who are sexual assailants and the local epidemiology of HIV/acquired immunodeficiency syndrome. If antiretroviral postexposure prophylaxis is offered, the following information should be discussed with the patients: the unknown efficacy and known toxicities of antiretrovirals; the critical need for frequent dosing of medications; the close follow-up that is necessary; the importance of strict compliance with the therapy; and the necessity of immediate initiation of treatment for maximal likelihood of effectiveness. If the patient decides to take postexposure therapy, clinical management of the patient should be implemented according to the guidelines for occupational mucous membrane exposure.

Chapter 34

Viral Disease Tests:
A Changing Arena

Improved serology and new molecular techniques are allowing earlier diagnosis of viral infections. This is important news—medications are now available to treat many viral infections and so are tests to monitor the effectiveness of therapy.

Like many primary care physicians, you may not be in the habit of ordering tests to diagnose viral diseases. Until recently, you would have waited as long as several weeks for identification of a virus in tissue culture. In any case, positive test results probably would not have affected management since effective treatments for most viral diseases did not exist.

This picture is changing. New technologies provide rapid test results that sometimes spare patients invasive procedures such as biopsy or inappropriate antibiotic treatment. You may be able to learn in less than 30 minutes whether a patient has a specific infection. Antiviral treatments are now available for a number of illnesses, and more are on the horizon. In fact, the ability to treat patients medically is a major driving force in the refinement of viral diagnostic testing. And the same types of tests that are applied in the diagnostic process may be used to monitor the effectiveness of antiviral therapy. Furthermore, early diagnosis of some viral infections, such as HIV disease and hepatitis C virus (HCV) infection, can lead to decreased transmission when the patient takes preventive measures.

© 1999 Medical Economics Publishing, from *Patient Care*, Feb 28, 1999, Vol.33, Issue 4, Pg.18(1), excerpted from "Viral Disease Tests: A Changing Arena," by Laurie Lewis; reprinted with permission.

Quicker, Safer, Cost-Effective Laboratory Methods

Isolation and identification of a virus in tissue culture is a labor-intensive, time-consuming process requiring well-equipped laboratories staffed by trained technicians. Stringent controls are required to prevent accidental contamination of laboratory workers. When the risk from exposure is extremely serious or when the virus cannot be grown in culture, serologic tests may be used to detect viral antibodies in the patient's blood. Major drawbacks of serologic testing include the window period after infection but before the patient has mounted a measurable antibody response, as well as the inability to distinguish between past and current infections.

Although serologic tests have not been abandoned in viral laboratories, they have taken a secondary role as confirmatory tests. Now tests to screen for viral infections may utilize antigen detection immunologic methods or molecular assays that amplify genetic material from the virus. Several different types of tests may be used to diagnose specific viral disease, and these are much faster than tissue culture because there is no need to wait for the pathogen to grow to measurable numbers.

The new tests tend to be somewhat expensive. A qualitative assay for HCV might cost the patient $90, for example. Nonetheless, the procedures are medically cost-effective. Labor costs are low once the tests become highly automated. More important, the opportunity to provide early, effective treatment means that long-term costs of care may be less in some patients than with the wait-it-out approach typical in the days before the advent of antiviral medications.

Lack of standardization, however, is a potential disadvantage of some of the new diagnostic methods. The FDA has approved only a few molecular diagnostic tests for viral diseases. There are no FDA-approved, commercially available molecular assays for HCV, hepatitis B virus, herpes simplex virus, varicella zoster virus, enterovirus, parvovirus, or other common viral pathogens. Most commercial laboratories develop their own techniques for identifying viruses, and the specificity and sensitivity vary accordingly.

As a physician who orders and receives the results of viral diagnostic tests, you need to be alert to the methods your laboratory uses and how reliable they are. You also need to proceed with caution. For serious illnesses such as HIV and HCV infections, do not rely on a single test result. Repeat a positive test, and if it is still reactive, order a different type of confirmatory test. When a test is negative but the clinical picture is highly suggestive of a particular illness, consider

376

the window for viral detection. Repeat the test after an appropriate interval, or order a more sensitive test.

Diagnostic Tests for Hepatitis C

Hepatitis C, in acute or chronic form, affects some 4 million Americans. The causative virus is most likely to be found in people who received blood transfusions before 1992—when antibody testing of blood donations became standard—and in IV drug users. Tests to detect antibodies to HCV and amplification techniques to identify HCV genetic material are important developments in the management of this infection.

Although only the serologic assays are FDA-approved, a variety of tests are available in local laboratories. Each type of test serves different purposes. Acute hepatitis C often goes undiagnosed because the patient has only mild, nonspecific symptoms. Liver function tests may not be consistently abnormal. A patient who has been infected with HCV may not show a measurable antibody response for as long as 6 months, but the virus may be causing liver damage during this time nonetheless. Furthermore, the patient may be exposing others to the virus, for example, by needle sharing among drug users. The infection becomes chronic in 85% of patients.

If you suspect acute hepatitis C because of the history and clinical or laboratory findings, consider a reverse transcriptase polymerase chain reaction (RT-PCR) or branched chain DNA assay to look for the hepatitis C genome. A single test is not conclusive, however. Repeat testing, including enzyme immunoassay (EIA) to look for HCV antibody, is necessary to confirm the diagnosis.

Most likely, patients will not seek medical care during an acute infection. When you see patients with hepatitis C, the infection usually is chronic. They may not be symptomatic, but you might suspect hepatitis C because of their history. The Centers for Disease Control and Prevention recommends routine testing for HCV in the following:

- Anyone who has ever injected illegal drugs
- Patients who received clotting factor concentrates produced before 1987
- Patients who have received long-term hemodialysis
- Patients with persistently abnormal alanine aminotransferase (ALT) levels

- Recipients of blood transfusions from a donor who subsequently tested positive for HCV

- Recipients of blood transfusions or blood components before July 1992

- Recipients of organ transplants before July 1992

- Health care workers who had needlesticks or mucosal exposure to HCV-positive blood

- Children born to HCV-positive women.

By the time the HCV infection has become chronic, anti-HCV antibody usually can be detected on an ETA, and this should be the initial diagnostic procedure. In high-risk patients and those with clinical or biochemical evidence of liver disease, a positive ETA may be considered diagnostic of chronic hepatitis C.

A supplemental test to confirm the diagnosis, especially in low-risk patients, is the appropriate second step. One test is a recombinant immunoblot assay (RIBA), which detects specific antibodies to HCV. Because this test depends on the same antibodies as the ETA, it frequently is indeterminant. The RT-PCR for HCV RNA is an alternative, less expensive confirmatory test and indicates a current infection if positive. If the RT-PCR or RIBA is positive and the ALT is persistently elevated, the patient should be referred to a gastroenterologist for liver biopsy and possible treatment. All infected patients should be counseled on behavioral changes to avoid disease transmission.

Diagnostic Tests for HIV

The standard of care for diagnosing HIV infection is clear. When you suspect HIV infection, the first test to order is an ETA. A positive antibody assay should be repeated. If the second ETA also is positive, order a Western blot test or immunofluorescence assay to look for antibodies to specific proteins, which will confirm the diagnosis. Both of these serologic tests are highly sensitive and specific. Their main limitation is their inability to detect acute HTV infection. It takes an average of 25 days after infection for detectable antibodies to develop. If you think a patient may be in the very early stages of HTV infection, the most sensitive test is the viral load test, or HIV PCR, although this is not usually recommended as a diagnostic test because of the possibility of false-positive results. The p24 antigen test is no longer recommended for diagnostic purposes.

In the ever-changing arena of HIV management, several developments related to testing merit mention. One is the availability of the rapid HIV test, which people can use at home. It detects antibody to HIV in a blood sample and is as sensitive and specific as the standard ETA. Like the ETA, the rapid test is only a screening test; a positive result requires confirmation by another test. Also, if the test subject has not yet developed antibodies, the result will be a false-negative one.

Although the rapid test was designed for home use by people who wished for greater anonymity than that afforded by a public health clinic or physician's office, clinics and individual physicians also can use the test. Obtaining test results within half an hour, while the patient remains in the office, is a two-edged sword. On the one hand, the patient learns immediately whether the test is positive or negative. On the other hand, counseling may be harder, especially if the patient is shocked by a positive result.

Be certain such patients understand the necessity of confirmatory testing to establish the diagnosis and the importance of precautions to prevent the spread of a possible HIV infection. This information should be communicated both before and after testing to assure that unpleasant news does not limit the patient's understanding of the test results.

The rapid test uses a blood sample. Other tests that analyze urine specimens or oral fluids are coming to market. Although these tests may be easier for people to use at home, confirmatory testing requires an extra step. A Western blot test can be done on the same blood sample as the initially reactive test. With at-home tests, you may have to make an extra effort to assure that patients with positive results return for confirmatory testing.

Another important development in HIV testing is the ability to monitor the effectiveness of treatment. The serologic tests cannot do this; they simply detect antibodies to HIV. But repeated viral load testing with HIV RNA and determination of the CD4+ lymphocyte count can be used to assess how the patient is responding to therapy. If the viral load is increasing, the therapeutic regimen should be changed in conjunction with advice from an HIV specialist.

Diagnostic Tests for Herpes Infections

Herpes infections, if symptomatic, may be diagnosed clinically; blood tests are usually unnecessary. Serologic tests do not indicate whether lesions are caused by herpes simplex I or II, and treatment with antiviral agents is based on clinical findings.

The major breakthrough in diagnostic testing for herpes infections concerns herpes simplex encephalitis. In the past, brain biopsy was necessary to confirm this condition. Now, PCR can detect the viral DNA in spinal fluid obtained via lumbar puncture. Results are available within hours if the test is performed in the hospital laboratory.

Cytomegalovirus is another type of herpes virus for which new diagnostic techniques can make a major difference in outcome. This pathogen, an important cause of neonatal disease and common in immunocompromised adults such as transplant recipients and patients with cancer or AIDS, may take weeks to grow in culture. A shell vial culture, which uses monoclonal antibodies to detect viral antigens, provides results in 18 hours. A rapid antigenic assay on WBCs, although expensive and somewhat subjective, enables prompt antiviral therapy in a seriously ill, hospitalized patient. Furthermore, by measuring the viral load, a quantitative plasma PCR enables the clinician to monitor the effectiveness of the prescribed treatment.

Epstein-Barr virus (EBV), which causes mononucleosis, is a pathogen in the herpes family. Although EBV serology can be done in the diagnostic workup of mononucleosis, the test is expensive and usually is not necessary. The false-negative rate is relatively high in children. A monospot test is generally sufficient to establish the diagnosis, especially if patient characteristics fit the typical clinical pattern for mononucleosis. But if this test is negative or the patient is a child and you suspect an EBV infection on clinical grounds, ordering EBV serology is a logical next step.

Chapter 35

Cervical Cancer Screening for Women Who Have a History of STDs

Women who have a history of STD are at increased risk for cervical cancer, and women attending STD clinics may have other risk factors that place them at even greater risk. Prevalence studies have determined that precursor lesions for cervical cancer occur about five times more frequently among women attending STD clinics than among women attending family planning clinics.

The Pap smear (i.e., cervical smear) is an effective and relatively low-cost screening test for invasive cervical cancer and SIL, the precursors of cervical cancer. Both ACOG and the American Cancer Society (ACS) recommend annual Pap smears for all sexually active women. Although these guidelines take the position that Pap smears can be obtained less frequently in some situations, women with a history of STDs may need more frequent screening because of their increased risk for cervical cancer. Moreover, surveys of women attending STD clinics indicate that many women do not understand the purpose or importance of Pap smears, and almost half of the women who have had a pelvic examination erroneously believe they have had a Pap smear when they actually have not.

Recommendations

At the time of a pelvic examination for STD screening, the health-care provider should inquire about the result of the patient's last Pap smear and discuss the following information with the patient:

Centers for Disease Control and Prevention (CDC). 1998 Guidelines for Treatment of Sexually Transmitted Diseases. *MMWR*, 1998;47(No. RR-1).

- The purpose and importance of a Pap smear;

- Whether a Pap smear was obtained during the clinic visit;

- The need for an annual Pap smear; and

- The names of local providers or referral clinics that can obtain Pap smears and adequately follow up results (i.e., if a Pap smear was not obtained during this examination).

If a woman has not had a Pap smear during the previous 12 months, a Pap smear should be obtained as part of the routine pelvic examination. Health-care providers should be aware that, after a pelvic examination, many women believe they have had a Pap smear when they actually have not, and thus may report having had a recent Pap smear. Therefore, in STD clinics, a Pap smear should be strongly considered during the routine clinical evaluation of women who have not had a normal Pap smear within the preceding 12 months that is documented within the clinic record or linked-system record.

A woman may benefit from receiving printed information about Pap smears and a report containing a statement that a Pap smear was obtained during her clinic visit. If possible, a copy of the Pap smear result should be provided to the patient for her records.

Follow-Up

Clinics and health-care providers who provide Pap smear screening services are encouraged to use cytopathology laboratories that report results using the Bethesda System of classification. If the results of the Pap smear are abnormal, care should be provided according to the Interim Guidelines for Management of Abnormal Cervical Cytology published by the National Cancer Institute Consensus Panel. Appropriate follow-up of Pap smears showing a high-grade SIL always includes referral to a clinician who has the capacity to provide a colposcopic examination of the lower genital tract and, if indicated, colposcopically directed biopsies. For a Pap smear showing low-grade SIL or atypical squamous cells of undetermined significance (ASCUS), follow-up without colposcopy may be acceptable in circumstances when the diagnosis is not qualified further or the cytopathologist favors a reactive process. In general, this would involve repeated Pap smears every 4-6 months for 2 years until the results of three consecutive smears have been negative. If repeated smears show persistent abnormalities, colposcopy and directed biopsy are indicated for low-grade SIL and should be considered for ASCUS. Women with a diagnosis of unqualified ASCUS associated with severe inflammation should at least be reevaluated with a repeat Pap smear after 2-3 months, then repeated Pap smears every 4-6 months for 2 years until the results of three consecutive smears have been negative. If specific infections are identified, the patient should be reevaluated after appropriate treatment for those infections. In all follow-up strategies using repeated Pap smears, the tests not only must be negative but also must be interpreted by the laboratory as "satisfactory for evaluation."

Because many public health clinics, including most STD clinics, cannot provide clinical follow-up of abnormal Pap smears with colposcopy and biopsy, women with Pap smears demonstrating high grade SIL or persistent low-grade SIL or ASCUS usually will need a referral to other local health-care providers or clinics for colposcopy and biopsy. Clinics and health-care providers who offer Pap smear screening services but cannot provide appropriate colposcopic follow-up of abnormal Pap smears should arrange referral services that a) can promptly evaluate and treat patients and b) will report the results of the evaluation to the referring clinician or health-care provider. Clinics and health-care providers should develop protocols that identify women who miss initial appointments (i.e., so that these women can be scheduled for repeat Pap smears), and they should reevaluate such protocols routinely. Pap smear results, type and location of follow-up appointments, and results of follow-up should be clearly documented in the clinic record. The development of colposcopy and biopsy services in local health departments, especially in circumstances where referrals are difficult and follow-up is unlikely, should be considered.

Other Management Considerations

Other considerations in performing Pap smears are as follows:

- The Pap smear is not an effective screening test for STDs.

- If a woman is menstruating, a Pap smear should be postponed, and the woman should be advised to have a Pap smear at the earliest opportunity.

- The presence of a mucopurulent discharge might compromise interpretation of the Pap smear. However, if the woman is unlikely to return for follow-up, a Pap smear can be obtained after careful removal of the discharge with a saline-soaked cotton swab.

- A woman who has external genital warts does not need to have Pap smears more frequently than a woman who does not have warts, unless otherwise indicated.

- In an STD clinic setting or when other cultures or specimens are collected for STD diagnoses, the Pap smear may be obtained last.

- Women who have had a hysterectomy do not require an annual Pap smear unless the hysterectomy was related to cervical cancer or its precursor lesions. In this situation, women should be advised to continue follow-up with the physician(s) who provided health care at the time of the hysterectomy.

- Both health-care providers who receive basic retraining on Pap smear collection and clinics that use simple quality assurance measures obtain fewer unsatisfactory smears.

- Although type-specific HPV testing to identify women at high and low risk for cervical cancer may become clinically relevant in the future, its utility in clinical practice is unclear, and such testing is not recommended.

Special Considerations

Pregnancy

Women who are pregnant should have a Pap smear as part of routine prenatal care. A cytobrush may be used for obtaining Pap smears in pregnant women, although care should be taken not to disrupt the mucous plug.

HIV Infection

Several studies have documented an increased prevalence of SIL in HIV-infected women, and HIV is believed by many experts to hasten the progression of precursor lesions to invasive cervical cancer. The following recommendations for Pap smear screening among HIV-infected women are consistent with other guidelines published by the U.S. Department of Health and Human Services and are based partially on the opinions of experts in the care and management of cervical cancer and HIV infection in women.

After obtaining a complete history of previous cervical disease, HIV-infected women should have a comprehensive gynecologic examination, including a pelvic examination and Pap smear as part of their initial evaluation. A Pap smear should be obtained twice in the first year after diagnosis of HIV infection and, if the results are normal, annually thereafter. If the results of the Pap smear are abnormal, care should be provided according to the Interim Guidelines for Management of Abnormal Cervical Cytology. Women who have a cytological diagnosis of high-grade SIL or squamous cell carcinoma should undergo colposcopy and directed biopsy. HIV infection is not an indication for colposcopy in women who have normal Pap smears.

The 1988 Bethesda System for Reporting Cervical/Vaginal Cytologic Diagnoses introduced the terms "low-grade SIL" and "high-grade SIL". Low-grade SIL encompasses cellular changes associated with HPV and mild dysplasia/cervical intraepithelial neoplasia 1 (CIN 1). High-grade SIL includes moderate dysplasia/CIN 2, severe dysplasia/CIN 3, and carcinoma in situ/CIN 3.

Chapter 36

Diagnosing Oral
Manifestations of STDs

A patient complains of a persistent sore throat and has hemorrhagic spots of 3 to 4 mm in diameter on the oropharynx. Under what circumstances should you include sexually transmitted disease (STD) in the differential diagnosis?

Diagnosis of oral lesions may require more than clinical acumen. Many infectious agents manifest themselves in the oral mucosa and require culture or serologic tests for definitive diagnosis. Both local and systemic infections may present with painful oral hemorrhagic lesions.

A detailed sexual history, which includes oral-genital contact, may expose risk factors for sexually transmitted infections, such as herpes simplex. However, the hemorrhagic lesions described above may just as easily represent other infectious diseases. STDs with similar oral manifestations include secondary syphilis; gonococcal pharyngitis; chlamydial infection; and acute HIV seroconversion[1] or other oral infections seen in HIV-infected persons, such as erythematous candidiasis[2] and Kaposi's sarcoma.

Also, consider infections that are not preferentially transmitted by sexual contact, such as infectious mononucleosis and coxsackievirus infection (hand-foot-and-mouth disease).

Syphilis

Primary oral syphilis is perhaps best known for creating a painless change on the mouth, but many patients have petechial hemorrhage of the soft palate or pharynx. In fact, the most common extragenital site of syphilis is the mouth.[3] Non-tender cervical adenopathy should raise the suspicion of primary oral syphilis; obtain the results of serologic tests (Venereal Disease Research Laboratory [VDRL], rapid plasma reagin [RPR], fluorescent treponemal antibody absorption [FTA-ABS], or microhemagglutination assay-Treponema pallidum [MHA-TP]) to confirm the diagnosis.

A patient with very early primary syphilis (during the first 3 or 4 weeks of infection) may have negative results of VDRL or RPR tests, but the treponemal antigen test results should be positive. Darkfield microscopic examination of lip lesions can also confirm the presence of the spirochete (treponemes other than *T. pallidum* are seen on darkfield examination of other oral lesions).

If left untreated, the disease will progress to the systemic phase of infection: secondary syphilis. Oral lesions in the form of mucous patches may accompany the papular cutaneous rash often seen on the trunk, palms, and soles, or they may be the sole physical finding during this phase.[3]

Gonorrhea

This may present with oral manifestations in up to 20% of cases. Diffuse erythema is more common than discrete lesions, but either may predominate. Oral-genital contact with an infected person is the most common route of infection. Secondary oral infections from lesions of the genital mucosa may also occur.[3] Culture on Thayer-Martin medium is the most cost-effective means of definitive diagnosis.

Chlamydial Infection

Chlamydial pharyngitis may present as a painful or painless mucositis with erythematous or pustular lesions on the oral mucosa. Cervical lymphadenopathy is a common physical finding.[4]

Trichomonal Infection

This may also cause oral symptoms, although diffuse mucosal erythema is more common than discrete lesions.[4] Diagnosis is by wet mount visual identification.

Herpes

Herpes simplex virus (HSV) may manifest itself as intraoral or pharyngeal lesions in addition to the more common labial "cold sores." In general, HSV pharyngitis is quite painful, and intraoral lesions may be extensive. Acyclovir or one of the newer pro-drugs may decrease the duration of symptoms and shedding of the virus.

HIV Infection

Acute HIV seroconversion syndrome has been reported to include oral lesions in up to 26% of symptomatic patients.[5] Fever is the most common symptom, but pharyngitis and other symptoms related to the oral cavity are common and may provide clues to the diagnosis. A detailed history to determine recent exposure and serologic testing for antibody (which may be absent in the acutely ill patient) or for viral RNA are required.

Perhaps in 50% of symptomatic seroconverters who present for treatment, the condition is misdiagnosed, and what may be a crucial window for early therapy—and certainly for early counseling—is missed.

Other Diseases

Oral lesions that occur simultaneously with conjunctivitis, nongonococcal urethritis, and arthritis are the hallmarks of Reiter's syndrome. Other noninfectious but sexually related conditions include the so-called fellatio syndrome of palatal petechiae, erythema, and ecchymoses associated with repetitive negative pressure in the oral cavity.[4]

Several of the previously discussed STDs have serious sequelae if left untreated. If you suspect an STD, obtain adequate cultures and serologic tests to confirm the diagnosis; partners should be counseled and examined. In addition, the health department must be notified of syphilis, gonorrhea, and HIV infection cases.

References

1. McElrath, M.J.; Schacker, T.; Graham, B.S., Primary HIV-1 Infection. *Principles and Practices of Infectious Diseases. Update.* 1997:1-19

2. Laskaris, G., Oral manifestations of infectious diseases. *Dent Clin North Am.* 1996;40:395-423.

3. Siegel, M.A., Syphilis and gonorrhea. *Dent Clin North Am.* 1996;40:369-383.

4. Terezhalmy, G.T.; Naylor, G.D., Oral manifestations of selected sexually related conditions. *Dermatol Clin.* 1996;14:303-317.

5. Kinlock-de Loes, S.; de Saussure, P.; Saurat, J.H., et al., Symptomatic primary infection due to human immunodeficiency virus type 1: review of 31 cases. *Clin Infect Dis.* 1993;17:59-65.

6. Schacker, T.; Colier, A.C.; Hughes, J., et al., Clinical and epidemiologic features of primary HIV infection. *Ann Intern Med.* 1996;125:257-264.

Chapter 37

Confidential Versus Anonymous Testing for HIV

Reporting of HIV cases by individual states in the U.S. does not appear to have any consistent effect on testing rates.

The need for anonymous HIV testing continues to be a source of debate, according to two articles published in the October 28, 1998, issue of *The Journal of the American Medical Association* (*JAMA*, 1998;280:1416-1420).

The first study found that anonymous testing contributes to early HIV testing and medical care, while the other study found no decline in HIV tests when the sites changed to confidential reporting.

Andrew B. Bindman, MD, University of California, San Francisco, and colleagues evaluated whether anonymous HIV testing was associated with earlier HIV testing and HIV related medical care than confidential HIV testing. They found that people who used anonymous HIV testing services got tested earlier and received medical care earlier than those who used confidential services.

The difference between anonymous and confidential testing is that in the latter, the person's name is linked to the blood specimen being tested and the test result is recorded in his or her confidential medical chart. In anonymous testing the patient's name is replaced by an identifier (usually a number) and the results are not recorded in a medical chart linked to the patient's name.

The average time between learning they were HIV positive and the diagnosis of AIDS was 1,246 days for those who used anonymous testing compared to 718 days for those who used confidential testing. People who tested anonymously experienced an average of 918 days in HIV related care before being diagnosed with AIDS. Confidential testers had 531 days of HIV related care before AIDS diagnosis.

According to the researchers, "After adjustment for the subject's age, sex, race/ethnicity, education, income, insurance status, HIV exposure group, whether the respondent had a regular source of care or symptoms at the time of the HIV test, and state residence, anonymous testing remained significantly associated with earlier entry to medical care."

As a result of this earlier testing and care, people tested anonymously received the potential benefits of a significantly longer period of HIV related medical care compared with those tested confidentially, the authors reported.

"A question can be raised whether the benefit we observed for anonymous testing is attributable to the availability of this type of testing or to characteristics of persons tested anonymously that make them seek earlier testing and care," wrote Bindman et al. "For example, among HIV exposure groups, men who have sex with men (MSM) are more likely to seek anonymous testing. From a policy perspective, the question is whether the same persons who seek early HIV testing at anonymous sites would do so at confidential sites if anonymous testing sites were eliminated."

Bindman's group concluded, "To achieve the public health goal of providing early access to HIV testing and HIV related medical care, public health departments should maintain and in some instances enhance the broad availability of anonymous testing options."

In a related article, Allyn K. Nakashima, MD, and colleagues from the U.S. Centers for Disease Control and Prevention (CDC), Atlanta, Georgia, described the trends in the use of HIV testing services at publicly-funded HIV counseling and testing sites in six states after the sites implemented confidential HIV reporting by risk group.

The CDC researchers found no significant declines in the total number of HIV tests provided. Increases occurred in Nebraska (15.8 percent), Nevada (48.4 percent), New Jersey (21.3 percent), and Tennessee (62.8 percent); decreases occurred in Louisiana (10.5 percent) and Michigan (2.0 percent). Of these, a statistically significant difference in the before-and-after trends was found in Nevada, New Jersey, and Tennessee, Nakashima et al. reported. Though they did not find a consistent increase in all the states, the researchers did find some trends in testing behavior.

"In all areas, testing of at-risk heterosexuals increased in the year after HIV reporting was implemented (Louisiana, 10.5 percent; Michigan, 225.1 percent; Nebraska, 5.7 percent; Nevada, 303.3 percent; New Jersey, 462.9 percent; Tennessee, 603.8 percent).

"Declines in testing occurred among men who have sex with men in Louisiana (4.3 percent) and Tennessee (4.1 percent) after HIV reporting; testing increased for this group in Michigan (5.3 percent), Nebraska (19.6 percent), Nevada (12.5 percent), and New Jersey (22.4 percent). Among injection drug users, testing declined in Louisiana (15 percent), Michigan (34.3 percent), and New Jersey (0.6 percent), and increased in Nebraska (1.7 percent), and Nevada (18.9 percent), and Tennessee (16.6 percent)."

They continued: "Anonymous testing was available in four of the states in our study. Reports have suggested that the introduction of anonymous testing increases testing in high-risk populations and the elimination of it decreases testing in these groups. In Nevada and Tennessee, where anonymous testing was not available, overall testing increased after HIV reporting; however, a small decline in testing occurred among MSMs in Tennessee. If there had been no access to anonymous testing in the other states, more declines in testing after HIV reporting policies might have been seen."

Nakashima et al. concluded, "With the changing trends in clinical AIDS incidence (6 percent between 1995 and 1996) and AIDS deaths (23 percent between 1995 and 1996) brought about by improved therapies, information on HIV infected, non-AIDS cases obtained through HIV case reporting will be needed for monitoring, planning, and allocation of resources for prevention and clinical services. As states implement confidential HIV reporting policies, these data indicate that the impact of surveillance on those seeking HIV testing will be small and should not hinder HIV prevention efforts."

Chapter 38

Testing Yourself for HIV

AIDS is a serious disease that can be fatal. You can determine if you are infected with the Human Immunodeficiency Virus-1 (HIV-1), the virus that causes AIDS, by taking a test for the presence of antibodies to the virus.

The tests that are approved by the United States Food and Drug Administration (FDA) for detecting whether or not you are infected with HIV are available through your doctor or at clinics. However, there is one HIV-1 Home Collection Test System that is currently approved by the FDA in which a sample for testing is collected in the privacy of your home and then sent to a laboratory for analysis. The "Home Access Express HIV-1 Test System" manufactured by Home Access Health Corporation is the only HIV-1 Home Collection Test System approved by FDA and legally sold in the United States.

Be aware that there are a number of different HIV home test systems and kits that are being marketed on the Internet and through magazine or newspaper promotions that claim to detect antibodies to HIV in blood or saliva samples and provide results in the home in 15 minutes or less. The FDA has NOT APPROVED these rapid HIV-1 home test kits being promoted on the Internet for use and marketing in the United States. Some of the HIV home test kits falsely claim to be approved by the FDA or manufactured in a FDA approved/registered/licensed facility. All HIV home sample collection kits approved to date

1999 U.S. Food and Drug Administration (FDA)/Center for Biologics Evaluation and Research.

by FDA require laboratory analysis and provide counseling for the consumer.

FDA warned consumers about an unapproved, fraudulently marketed home-use HIV test system labeled "Lei-Home Access HIV test" distributed by Lei-Home Access Care located in Sunnyvale, California in a press release issued on September 26, 1997. The "Lei-Home Access HIV test" was advertised on the Internet as the "Personal HIV Test Kit" and was offered for sale through several Central Valley pharmacies. After an extensive investigation by FDA, the businessman responsible for distributing this fraudulent HIV test kit was recently sentenced to over 5 years in prison for selling the medically useless HIV test kits to consumers in the United States.

The Center for Biologics Evaluation and Research is working with FDA's Office of Regulatory Affairs and Office of Criminal Investigations in investigating firms and persons involved in the sale, distribution, and manufacture of unapproved HIV home test kits in the United States.

The following Questions & Answers may help to explain how HIV-1 home tests differ, and how to select a test that you can trust.

Q. How many different kits are available, and how do they work?

A. There are more than a dozen different HIV home test kits being advertised on the market today. Only the Home Access test system is FDA approved and legally marketed in the United States. Because the Home Access test consists of multiple components, including materials for specimen collection, a mailing envelope to send the specimen to a laboratory for analysis, and includes pre- and post-test counseling, it is considered a testing system.

This approved system uses a simple finger prick process for home blood collection which results in dried blood spots on special paper. The dried blood spots are mailed to a laboratory with a confidential and anonymous personal identification number (PIN), and analyzed by trained clinicians in a certified medical laboratory using the same procedures that are used for samples taken in a doctor's office. The results are obtained by the purchaser through a toll free telephone number using the PIN, and post-test counseling is provided by telephone when results are obtained.

The advertisers of the unapproved HIV home test kits claim that the presence of a visual indicator, such as a red dot, within 5 to 15 minutes of taking the test shows a positive result for HIV infection. These unapproved test kits use a simple finger prick process for home blood collection or a special sponge device for saliva collection. The blood or saliva sample is then added to a plastic testing device containing a special type of paper. A developing solution is added to determine if the sample is positive for HIV. The samples are not sent to a laboratory for professional analysis. Although this approach may seem faster and simpler, it may provide a less accurate result than can be achieved using an approved test, which is analyzed under more controlled conditions than is possible in the home.

Q. How reliable are the unapproved HIV home test kits?

A. Diagnostic testing depends on precise science. Unapproved HIV home test kits do not come with any guarantee of the accuracy of the test, or the sensitivity of the reagents used in the analysis. Nor do they have a documented history of delivering dependable results. Proper training to interpret results is not provided with the kits, and they do not have a validated record of precision. This means that they may not be as accurate and that they may yield inconsistent results. Users can get a positive result when they are, in fact, not infected (called a false positive), or the test may indicate that a person is not infected with the virus, when, in fact, they are (called a false negative).

Both of these outcomes can have grave consequences in terms of mental anguish, access to proper medical treatment, and on future transmission of the disease. None of the unapproved tests have undergone the intense scrutiny and validation required for FDA marketing approval. Although unapproved tests might be promoted as sensitive and reliable, the consumer has no guarantee that the results produced by the test are, in fact, accurate. Even if they have been tested by independent laboratories, they have not been analyzed and validated by the FDA to assure that the test results were correct and reliable.

FDA is unaware of any data to confirm the reliability or accuracy of the process used in the unapproved HIV home test kits.

Q. How reliable are approved HIV test systems?

A. Approved HIV test systems, on the other hand, have undergone extensive study and review by the manufacturer of the product to ensure that they work, that the results they provide are specific, meaning that they will accurately detect antibodies to the HIV-1 virus that causes AIDS, and that they are sensitive, meaning that they can detect even low levels of these antibodies, indicating that someone has been exposed to HIV-1.

Clinical studies have shown that the approved HIV test system is able to correctly identify 100% of known positive blood samples, and 99.5% of HIV-1 negative blood samples. In addition, manufacturer's tests on the approved HIV test system have been carefully reviewed by the FDA to assure that the tests conducted were themselves adequate to demonstrate that the system is capable of yielding accurate, dependable results. FDA review also assures that the system contains adequate directions for proper use, and that the quality standards will be monitored to ensure that each kit is as consistently accurate and sensitive.

Q. What about counseling?

A. The unapproved HIV home test kits do not provide direct counseling to help the user understand results, answer questions about the test or about HIV infection, or to discuss available options.

The approved HIV test system has a built in mechanism for pre- and post-test counseling provided by the manufacturer. Counseling is an important part of HIV testing. It is anonymous and confidential. Counseling, which uses both printed material, and telephone interaction, not only provides the user with an interpretation of what positive or negative results really mean, but provides information on how to keep from getting infected if you are negative, and how to prevent transmission of disease if you find you are infected. Counseling also provides you with information about treatment options if you are infected, and can even provide referrals to doctors that treat HIV-infected individuals in your area.

Q. Are approved HIV test systems really confidential?

A. The approved HIV home test system is anonymous. It can be purchased anonymously at pharmacies, or by mail order from the manufacturers. The mail-in system uses a confidential code number that is unrelated to the identity of the buyer or user.

Although some states require that new cases of HIV infection be reported to the health department, only the number of cases detected with home test systems can be reported. The identity of the user remains anonymous.

The number of cases reported allows local or state public health officials to assess the extent of infection to properly budget, plan and administer programs for people with HIV. The lack of reporting of the number of new cases in a geographic area also means that adequate services for people with HIV infection may not be available in your area.

Q. Is one test better than another?

A. Since the approved HIV home test system has been independently tested, validated, and approved by the FDA for marketing, the consumer can feel confident that the approved HIV test system will provide the most accurate results available from an HIV-1 home test. In addition, the user is provided with counseling and referrals if needed. Use of an approved HIV test system also assures that accurate numbers of infection are reported to public health departments so that adequate services can be provided.

Q. Are there other ways I can be tested for infection with HIV-1?

A. There are several kinds of tests available through your doctor to determine if you are infected with HIV-1, the virus that causes AIDS. In addition to blood tests, there is a test that uses oral fluid, collected from between the cheek and gum of the mouth, and a urine test. All of these tests have been thoroughly tested and reviewed, and provide the highest possible level of confidence in determining HIV infection. All are collected in the doctor's office, and analyzed in a medical laboratory. Only a doctor or clinic can administer these tests.

So, ask yourself what is the best choice for you:

- An HIV home test system that has been approved by the FDA for marketing after extensive review and in which you can feel confident about the results?

OR

- An HIV home test kit that has not even been reviewed by the FDA and may not provide accurate results about whether you are HIV positive or negative?

Is it worth your time, money, mental anguish and your life to gamble on an unapproved HIV home test kit? Only you can answer that question.

If you are in doubt about whether an HIV home test kit you are considering using is approved, or if you have other questions related to HIV home test kits, you may call the HIV/AIDS Program of the

FDA, in the Office of Special Health Issues for further information about this topic. The Office can be reached at 301-827-4460.

Part Five

Issues Related to Youth and Adolescents

Chapter 39

Growing Pains: Adolescents and STDs

One of the fastest-growing AIDS populations in the United States is teenagers: in the first six months of 1995, AIDS cases in 13- to 19-year-olds increased 524 percent compared with all of 1994, according to the Centers for Disease Control and Prevention.

Most of this increase occurred among gay teenagers, reflecting the coming of age of these boys within a population that has always been at high risk.

The overall picture of AIDS in adolescents, however, differs in some striking ways when compared with the pattern in adults: a greater percentage of teenagers with AIDS are female (35 percent vs. 14 percent of adults with AIDS), are African American or Hispanic (63 percent vs. 51 percent), and were infected with HIV through heterosexual contact (20 percent vs. 8 percent).

The accumulation of incurable sexually transmitted infections in a population over time is analagous to a faucet dripping water into a beaker. Each infection is like a single waterdrop. Not only do the incurable infections—herpes simplex virus (HSV), human papillomavirus infection (HPV), and human immunodeficiency virus (HIV)—accumulate, so do untreated infections such as chlamydial infection. As the beaker fills up, the individual's chances of encountering an infected partner increase.

To understand these differences and curb the swelling number of AIDS cases in teenagers, the unique aspects of adolescents that bear

1996 National Institute of Allergy and Infectious Diseases (NIAID).

on the acquisition of HIV and other STDs—their behavior, their biology, and the social milieu of their lives—must receive attention, argues Penny J. Hitchcock, D.V.M., chief of NIAID's Sexually Transmitted Diseases Branch, in a recent article in *AIDS Patient Care*.

"There is an important link between STDs and HIV and yet this connection in adolescents has not been well studied," says Dr. Hitchcock. This chapter defines the problem so we can develop a rational research agenda in response. "About one-fourth of the nearly 12 million new cases of STDs in the United States each year occur in teenagers. The possibility that adolescent populations and STDs (chlamydial infection and genital herpes) could provide the messenger and the opportunity for HIV infection to become more broadly distributed in the

Table 39.1 Potential Risk Factors or Markers of Std Risk: Factors That Increase Risk for Adolescents

Infectivity Rate	Rate of Partner Change and Partner Characteristics	Duration of Infection
Infectivity of organism	Number of partners	Infecting organism
Genetic susceptibility	Type of partner	Host response
Sexual practices	Age	Health care behaviors:
Age	Age at first intercourse	Routine screening
Age at first intercourse	Gender	Early diagnosis and treatment
Gender		Treatment compliance
Contraceptive method		Partner notification
Circumcision status		Vaccine compliance
Alcohol use		
Drug use: IV and other		
Smoking		
Co-infections (STDs)		
Intravaginal or intra-anal preparations		

population is raised in studies of adolescent populations that are geographically and socially juxtaposed to high-risk populations," she writes.

Behavioral studies, she says, indicate the magnitude of the risk to adolescents of STDs. According to reports she cites:

- more than half of women and nearly three-fourths of men have had sexual intercourse by their eighteenth birthday,

- sexual activity among teens is increasing, and

- teens are inconsistent users of condoms.

In addition, today's teens generally begin having sexual intercourse at an early age, so their lifetime number of sex partners will be large, Dr. Hitchcock contends, increasing their risk for all STDs. One-third of 20-year-olds already have had three to five sexual partners.

Several biological factors, Dr. Hitchcock notes, influence the infectivity rate for STDs/HIV among adolescents. The hormonal changes of puberty and hormonal contraceptives increase the area on the cervix where gonorrhea and chlamydia infections become established. In addition, fluctuating hormone levels may increase the risk of STD infection because of changes in the character or amount of mucus, or changes in acidity and alkalinity. Also, the practice of anal intercourse by some adolescents as a method of birth control or to preserve virginity increases their susceptibility to HIV infection.

Aside from these behavioral and biological factors, the duration of infection is an important variable in the spread of STDs/HIV among adolescents. "Of the seven infections that are solely or primary sexually transmitted, four are treatable/curable bacterial infections (chlamydial infection, gonorrhea, syphilis, and chancroid), one is a treatable/curable parasitic disease (trichomoniasis), and three are incurable viral infections (human papillomavirus infection, genital herpes, and HIV infection). For the most part, all of these infections can and do manifest without symptoms," Dr. Hitchcock writes.

As a result, people who acquire STDs as adolescents can be a continued source of infection for their sexual partners for decades. Complicating matters are socioeconomic factors, such as the lack of access to and cost of health care, policies of parental and partner notification, and failure to accept and comply with treatment regimens, which also influence the persistence of STDs.

"Whether we will be able to address aggressively and effectively the implicit research and program needs and opportunities that must be met in order to prevent the spread of STDs and HIV infection into adolescent populations remains to be seen," writes Dr. Hitchcock. Making medical researchers aware of the complexity of the situation and the need for multidisciplinary research, she says, is the first step.

A monograph on adolescents and STDs, the result of a collaborative process between NIAID and the Rockefeller Foundation, is scheduled for publication in 1997. It will present both biomedical and behavioral perspectives from multidisciplinary teams of scientists. Topics include the nature of the problem, tools for intervention, diagnostic and treatment measures, and research recommendations.

Chapter 40

Facts of Life Versus Facts of Love

When David Sherrer talks to teenagers about sexual abstinence, he likes to poke fun at himself and the awkwardness of the topic. "So I laugh, I talk about great sex and I tell this group of 15-year-olds that me and my wife—we have great sex," he says. "You can just hear a few of them groaning, 'Uuuhhhhh!'"

Sherrer who heads the Denver-based abstinence-counseling organization Worth Waiting For, believes that in the back of their minds, teenagers want to know that 40-year-olds are sexually active and that they can have honest, open—even enjoyable—discussions with adults about sex. The part-time lecturer and abstinence activist says a light-hearted approach is more effective than fear-provoking rhetoric, as long as the discussion leader turns the corner and emphasizes the benefits of waiting to have sex until after marriage—what he considers "the best choice."

This version of the timeworn talk about the birds and the bees may sound a tad unorthodox, but it's typical of a new approach that some are using to persuade teenagers that sex in the nineties requires special consideration. It's also a sign that the premarital abstinence movement is growing, gaining new momentum with changing dynamics.

Sherrer was one of approximately 300 leaders of abstinence programs who met in Washington in late July for the National Leadership Summit on Abstinence. There, chastity advocates from across the country discussed new education strategies, the medical risks of casual sex and inspiring messages from those who have toiled on the abstinence-education trail. The summit, sponsored by the Austin, Texas-based Medical Institute for Sexual Health, or MISH, was heralded as a national planning session for a "new sexual revolution"—one that would change the ideas and behaviors of the last 20 to 30 years.

Many of the attendees of the two-day event had struggled to establish programs in schools across the country offering abstinence as the only foolproof way to curb teen pregnancy and the personal and societal problems that accompany it. In 1997, Congress gave these organizations something to celebrate—a $50 million-a-year federal grant program states can use for abstinence education. All of the 50 states applied for the grants, which the federal Maternal and Child Health Bureau will oversee. Initial state plans included curriculum programs for children under 14, media campaigns and state and regional abstinence conferences and mentoring programs.

The support of the Republican-led Congress signaled a long-sought victory for the abstinence movement. On the first day of the summit, Rep. Tom Coburn, a Republican from Oklahoma who is a practicing obstetrician and abstinence advocate, said that some 20 to 30 members of Congress were strongly behind the movement. "There is no question about it. The tide is turning," he said.

With congressional and financial backing the abstinence coalition, once almost entirely a creature of religious organizations, is beginning to diversify. MISH, the 5-year-old medical educational nonprofit which sponsored the summit, is a perfect example of a group offering a new perspective on one of the oldest ethical issues. Joe McIlhaney Jr., the president and founder of MISH, says his organization provides medical research to the movement, helping to bridge a scientific chasm—one that left character-based abstinence programs stymied by attacks.

The organization was founded to confront the worldwide epidemic of sexually transmitted diseases, or STDs, and nonmarital pregnancy. As a doctor specializing in in-vitro fertilization, McIlhaney was alarmed to see so many women whose sterility was directly linked to STDs they had acquired as young people. The last patient he treated at his clinic was a 42-year-old woman with numerous partners in her sexual history. When she was 38, she married and struggled to have a child of her own. She then realized that she had been infected by one of the people in her past. "No one had mentioned that possibility to her," says McIlhaney.

Too often, McIlhaney believes, the very real risk of sterility associated with casual sex is swept under the rug. He believes that teen sexual activity should be considered in the same way people have begun to view children's use of tobacco. "Our whole society has decided that it's not healthy for teens to smoke in spite of the fact that smoking does not generally hurt teens until 20 or 30 years down the road," he says. "We're saying that sexual activity for singles, especially teens, gets them infected with disease, can cause pregnancies—things that will damage their life today and in their future."

To grab the media's attention, staffers at MISH decided to place a condom on their summit materials with the words "Is this enough?" printed in bold lettering underneath. McIlhaney says many people, including physicians, are not fully aware of how ineffective condoms are in preventing STDs. "Most have never heard that condoms give almost no protection against the sexual transmission of human papilloma virus—the cause of genital warts. It's the most common sexually transmitted disease and it causes almost all cervical cancers. Most women have not heard about studies that show even if they use condoms they still are just as likely to be sterile later on in life as if they had not." Each year, more women in America die of cervical cancer (nearly 5,000) than of AIDs-related disease.

Although most of the people who attended the summit are leaders of faith-based organizations, they welcome the statistical ammunition MISH has provided. "For many parents, abstaining from sex is a medical-safety issue. They want their children to survive as far as their fertility is concerned and as far as cancer is concerned," says McIlhaney Still, most of the participants at the summit hold convictions stemming from a belief that waiting to have sex is not only safe physically and emotionally, but safe and appropriate spiritually as well.

"For me, it does seem like a spiritual decision not to have sex," says Sherrer. "To dance around the spiritual issues, which our schools make us do all the time, leaves out a huge, huge issue that kids are facing. So it's nice to have the backing of the medical community. But I want to talk more than just about the facts of life, I want to talk about the facts of love."

Just what does it take to reach teens these days? Sherrer says it's all about relationships—making seminars enjoyable enough that teens will invite their friends to the next one. On a daily basis, Sherrer has worked to respond to two basic criticisms of the abstinence movement:

1. that supporters are naive to think that children are capable of waiting to have sex, and

2. that people who counsel the young against premarital sex are killjoys and puritans who rely too heavily on guilt and fear.

"They say, 'You always shake your finger,'" he explains. "Why would anybody want to listen to you guys? You're such a downer. You're miserable to be around.'" To combat these stereotypes, abstinence leaders work honestly to report heart-wrenching and heartwarming stories with which teens can identify. "They look at me and say, 'You're just some white dumpy bald male, you're married—you couldn't get it if you wanted to,'" Sherrer says, chuckling. "You need to find a way to communicate with passion. You can decide to go ahead and be confrontational without being condemnational."

Most difficult of all, abstinence advocates say, is competing with a culture dominated by television and the lifestyles it promotes. "What images of marriage do our children see?" asked media critic Michael Medved as the summit's lunchtime speaker. "The Simpsons, the Bundys (of Married ... With Children), Roseanne ....?" Instead, young people need to know that "a life of sanity and fulfillment sexually is possible. It happens."

Chapter 41

Adolescence and Abstinence

Adolescents should be encouraged to delay sexual behaviors until they are physically, cognitively, and emotionally ready for mature sexual relationships and their consequences. Comprehensive sexuality education programs offer them a wide range of information while abstinence-only programs focus exclusively on abstinence until marriage. This Fact Sheet presents current statistics on adolescence and abstinence as well as research on both education approaches.

More than half of teenagers are virgins until they are at least 17 years of age.[1] By the time they reach the age of 20, 20 percent of boys and 24 percent of girls have not had sexual intercourse.[2] The largest study of adult sexual behavior found that only 6.9 percent of men and 21 percent of women aged 18 to 59 had their first intercourse on their wedding night.[3] Many virgins are sexually involved. In one study of urban students in the ninth through the twelfth grades, 47 percent were virgins. More than a third of virgin male and female adolescents had engaged in some form of heterosexual genital sexual activity in the past year:

- 29 percent of virgins had engaged in masturbation of a partner of the opposite gender.

- 31 percent had been masturbated by a partner of the opposite gender.

- 9 percent had engaged in fellatio with ejaculation with a partner of the opposite gender.

- 10 percent had engaged in cunnilingus with a partner of the opposite gender.

- 1 percent had engaged in anal intercourse with a partner of the opposite gender.[4]

Comprehensive Sexuality Education Can Help Postpone Intercourse

Helping adolescents to postpone sexual intercourse until they are ready for mature relationships is a key goal of comprehensive sexuality education.[5] Sexuality educators have always included information about abstinence in sexuality education courses.

Interventions that are effective in encouraging teenagers to postpone sexual intercourse help young people to develop the interpersonal skills they need to resist premature sexual involvement. Effective programs include a strong abstinence message as well as information about contraception and safer sex. For interventions to be most effective, teenagers need to be exposed to these programs before initiating intercourse.[6]

In a 1993 study, SIECUS found that state curricula emphasize abstinence. Abstinence was among the topics most often covered in state curricula and guidelines along with families, decision-making, and sexually transmitted diseases and HIV. The topics least likely covered included sexual identity and orientation, shared sexual behavior, sexual response, masturbation, and abortion.[7]

Sexuality education does not encourage teens to start having sexual intercourse, increase the frequency of intercourse, or increase the number of sexual partners.[8]

Teenagers who start having intercourse following a sexuality education program are more likely to use contraception that those who have not participated in a program.[9]

Abstinence-Only Education

To date, six studies of abstinence-only programs have been published. None of these studies found consistent and significant program effects on delaying the onset of intercourse, and at least one study provided strong evidence that the program did not delay the onset of intercourse. Thus, the weight of evidence indicates that these abstinence-only programs do not delay the onset of intercourse.[10]

A study of 7,326 seventh and eighth graders in California who participated in an abstinence-only program found that the program did not have a measurable impact upon either sexual or contraceptive behaviors.[11]

Nearly two-thirds of teenagers think teaching "Just Say No" is an ineffective deterrent to teenage sexual activity.[12]

The National Institutes of Health's Consensus Panel on AIDS said in February 1997 that the abstinence-only approach to sexuality education "places policy in direct conflict with science and ignores overwhelming evidence that other programs are effective."[13]

References

1. Alan Guttmacher Institute, Sex and America's Teenagers (New York: The Alan Guttmacher Institute, 1994), p. 19.

2. *Ibid*, pp. 22-3.

3. E. Laumann, et al, The Social Organization of Sexuality— Sexual Practices in the United States (Chicago: The University of Chicago Press, 1994).

4. M. A. Schuster, et al, "The Sexual Practices of Adolescent Virgins: Genital Sexual Activities of High School Students Who Have Never Had Vaginal Intercourse," *American Journal of Public Health*, 86, No.11 (1996), pp. 1570-76.

5. Sexuality Information and Education Council of the United States (SIECUS), *Guidelines for Comprehensive Sexuality Education, 2nd Edition* (New York: SIECUS, 1996).

6. D. Kirby, *No Easy Answers: Research Findings on Programs to Reduce Teen Pregnancy* (Washington, DC: The National Campaign to Prevent Teen Pregnancy, 1997), p. 25.

7. Sexuality Information and Education Council of the United States (SIECUS), *Unfinished Business: A SIECUS Assessment of State Sexuality Education Programs* (New York: SIECUS, 1993), p. 18.

8. J. J. Frost and J. D. Forrest, "Understanding the Impact of Effective Teenage Pregnancy Prevention Programs," Family Planning Perspectives, 27, no. 5 (1995), pp. 188-96; D. Kirby, et al, "School-Based Programs to Reduce Sexual Risk Behaviors: A Review of Effectiveness," *Public Health Reports*, 190,

no. 3 (1997), pp. 339-60; A. Grunseit and S. Kippax (1993); D. Kirby (1997), p.25.

9. A.Grunseit and S. Kippax, Effects of Sex Education on Young People's Sexual Behavior (Geneva: World Health Organization, 1993), pp. 5-6.

10. D. Kirby (1997), p. 25.

11. H. H. Cagampang, R. P. Barth, M. Korpi, and D. Kirby, "Education Now and Babies Later (ENABL): Life History of a Campaign to Postpone Sexual Involvement," *Family Planning Perspectives*, 29, no. 3 (1997), pp. 109-14.

12. Roper Starch Worldwide, Teens Talk About Sex: Adolescent Sexuality in the 90s (New York: Sexuality Information and Education Council of the United States, 1994), p. 18.

13. National Institutes of Health, Consensus Development Conference Statement, Feb. 11-13, 1997.

Chapter 42

Abstinence and Safer Sex: Risk-Reduction Interventions for African-American Adolescents

This was a prospective, randomized trial to compare abstinence and safer sex interventions with a control group in reducing behaviors that place adolescents at risk for sexually transmitted diseases and HIV infection. This study also evaluated relative effectiveness of adult and peer group leaders of different genders in delivering the interventions.

Six hundred and fifty-nine African-American adolescents with a mean age of 11.8 years attending the sixth or seventh grade in three middle schools serving low-income communities in Philadelphia were recruited through announcements in assemblies, classrooms, and the cafeteria and in letters to parents and guardians. The recruitment statement indicated that the project was designed to reduce health problems such as cardiovascular diseases, cancer, and AIDS. After stratification by gender and age, subjects were randomly assigned to one of the three intervention groups, which met for two 4-hour sessions on consecutive Saturdays and covered eight 1-hour modules.

The abstinence group included information on HIV and sexually transmitted diseases (STDs) and acknowledged that condoms can reduce pregnancy, STDs, and HIV but emphasized the need for abstinence to provide absolute protection. This intervention also placed emphasis on the beliefs that abstinence can prevent pregnancy, STDs, and HIV as well as increase the likelihood of attaining future goals.

Finally, this intervention stressed development of skills and self-efficacy in negotiating abstinence and resisting peer pressure to have sexual intercourse. The safer sex group included information that abstinence was the "best choice" in preventing negative outcomes from sexual activity; however, this group emphasized the need to use condoms if one was sexually active.

Topics covered included knowledge of HIV and STDs, enhancement of hedonistic beliefs regarding condom use as it relates to sexual pleasure, and exercises to increase skills and self-efficacy to use condoms and negotiate condom use. The control group focused on non-HIV/nonsexuality health issues, including healthy dietary practices, aerobic exercise, breast and testicular self-examination, and cigarette smoking, to reduce behaviors related to cardiovascular disease, stroke, and cancer. Each group had educational and entertaining exercises, which included videos, games, discussion, and skill building.

Subjects completed confidential questionnaires before and after the intervention and again at 3, 6, and 12 months after the intervention. These questionnaires measured self-reported sexual behaviors in the previous 3 months including condom use, as well as behavioral beliefs based on the theory of reasoned action, planned behavior, and social cognitive theory. Condom availability beliefs, as well as condom use technical skills, impulse control, negotiation, self-efficacy, prevention beliefs, intentions to use condoms, and knowledge about use were measured. In addition, the questionnaire probed beliefs about abstinence preventing pregnancy and AIDS, about enhancing attainment of future career goals, about attitudes and intentions to have sexual intercourse, and about HIV risk reduction knowledge. Finally, health promotion knowledge about topics presented to the control group was assessed, and respondents were asked how much they liked the intervention and the facilitator.

The adult and peer facilitators were trained before the interventions and after being stratified by age and gender, were randomly assigned to one of the interventions. The sessions were monitored during the intervention, facilitators recorded which activities were completed, and they were instructed on the importance of following the intervention manual.

There were very high follow-up rates in this study with 97% completing the 3-month follow-up, 94% completing the 6-month, and 93% completing the 12-month follow-up. There was no significant difference among retention rates for the three intervention groups. Subjects were paid for completing each aspect of the study. The significant differences in preintervention variables between those who returned and those who did not were that those who returned at 3 months had higher scores on condom prevention beliefs and those who returned at 6 months had higher abstinence prevention beliefs as well as lower condom use knowledge. There were no differences between outcomes based on the gender of the facilitator or on whether the group was adult or peer led.

The surveys completed immediately after the interventions showed that subjects in the abstinence group had stronger beliefs that abstinence would prevent pregnancy and AIDS, were less likely to plan to have intercourse in the next 3 months, and had less favorable attitudes toward intercourse than the other two groups. Those in the abstinence group compared with the control group were also more likely to believe that abstinence would help them achieve future goals. (This was not the case for the abstinence-safe sex comparison.) Adolescents in the safe sex group had better condom use knowledge; were more likely to believe that condoms prevent pregnancy, STDs, and HIV and would not interfere with sexual enjoyment; and were more likely to believe that they would have condoms available than subjects in the other two intervention groups. Subjects in the safe sex group scored better on impulse control for condom use and self-efficacy than the control group. Overall HIV knowledge was better for both the abstinence and safe sex groups than the control group, and the safe sex group scored the best.

Results from the 3-month follow-up showed that subjects in the abstinence group were less likely to report sexual intercourse as compared with the control group (odds ratio 0.45) while subjects in the safer sex group were more likely to report consistent condom use than the control group or abstinence group and to have fewer days/times of unprotected sex than the control group. For adolescents who had never been sexually active before the intervention, subjects in the abstinence group were less likely to report sexual activity at 3 months as compared with the control group, although there was no effect on unprotected sexual intercourse for this group from any of the interventions.

Among subjects who had been sexually active before the study, those in the safer sex group had less unprotected sex than the control or abstinence group.

At the 6-month follow-up, the safer sex group had fewer days of reported sexual intercourse and were more likely to use condoms than the control group. There were no differences in likelihood of sexual intercourse when the abstinence group was compared with the control group. Among those who had been sexually active before the study and were in the safer sex group, there was less reported intercourse than in either the abstinence or control group and less unprotected intercourse than in the control group. There were no significant differences for those who had not been sexually active before the study.

Finally at the 12-month follow-up, subjects in the safer sex and abstinence group were more likely to use condoms than the control group. As was the case at the 3- and 6-month follow-ups, there were no differences in likelihood of sexual intercourse when the abstinence group was compared with the control group. Among those who had been previously sexually active, subjects in the safer sex group had less frequency of intercourse and unprotected sex than those in the control or abstinence groups. Again there were no differences for subjects who had not been sexually active before the intervention.

In summary: Although the abstinence intervention showed immediate effects on intentions to remain abstinent and increased self-reported abstinence at 3 months, this effect was not sustained at the 6- and 12-month follow-ups. The safer sex intervention, on the other hand, increased self-reported condom use at 3, 6, and 12 months. For those adolescents who had prior sexual experience, the safer sex intervention was even more effective showing less intercourse on long-term follow-up at 6 and 12 months than in the other two intervention groups and more condom use at all time points than in the control group.

Commentary: Understanding how to effectively reach adolescents and decrease the risk associated with unprotected sexual activity is crucial since adolescents have the highest rate of STD of any sexually active age group and the United States has the highest teen pregnancy rate in the Western World. Many young adults with AIDS are believed to have contracted HIV infection during adolescence. Preventing acquisition of HIV infection during adolescence is an important public health concern. The latest data from the 1997 Youth Risk Behavior Survey (YRBS) showed a decline in sexual activity among adolescents. The YRBS data are encouraging, and studies such as this one give clues about how to approach adolescents on this difficult topic. This study also provides concrete information for the debate over abstinence only vs. safer sex education. Since federal funds have been allocated for programs that deal only with abstinence, it is important to review studies such as this one, which suggests that abstinence only may not be the best approach in the long run.

This well-designed study provided a head-to-head comparison of abstinence and safe sex interventions with a control group. The results show that the more well-rounded safer sex intervention provided a sustained decrease in unprotected sex by increasing self-reported condom use. The results were even more dramatic for those with previous sexual experience who also demonstrated sustained decrease in frequency of sexual intercourse, which did not occur in the abstinence group. Despite the apparent immediate effect of increasing abstinence in the abstinence intervention group, the inability to sustain this effect raises questions about this one-sided approach. This is one more study showing that well-rounded sex education can lead to behavior that should reduce the negative consequences for adolescent who choose to be sexually active.

It is interesting that the safe sex intervention appeared to be more effective for adolescents who reported previous sexual activity. Perhaps adolescents who had previous experience with situations involving negotiation of condom use and the decision to become sexually active were able to better incorporate the intervention because of these previous experiences. Certainly in terms of psychosocial development, adolescents in this age group are just beginning to develop abstract thought. Concrete thinkers have more difficulty understanding situations that are not part of their previous experience. Part of the challenge of working with adolescents is trying to change behavior in a group who feel invulnerable to harm and engage in risk-taking behavior as part of the normal developmental process. Further investigation into the differences between these groups taking into account developmental milestones may help in the design of programs to delay the initiation of sexual activity.

This study also shows that peers can be as effective as experienced adults in the role of group facilitators and that the gender of the facilitator is not crucial. The importance of the peer group in influencing behavior, especially in middle adolescence, is well known. Peers may play an important role in delivering information to adolescents.

Although the results of this study cannot be generalized to all adolescents, it provides a framework for approaching adolescents that can be repeated in other groups from varied socioeconomic and ethnic/racial backgrounds.

Chapter 43

The Sports Physical: A Good Time for Hepatitis B Shots

The start of school signals another round of preparticipation physical examinations for athletes. Because the preparticipation exam is the only regular contact many teens have with the medical system,[1] it can be an opportune time to cover routine health matters such as assessing a student's hepatitis B immunization status.

Many teenagers have not received hepatitis B vaccinations because the universal immunization recommendation was not in place when they were younger. In 1991 the Advisory Committee on Immunization Practices of the Centers for Disease Control and Prevention (CDC) recommended infant immunization as a means of eradicating hepatitis B.[2] In January 1996, the group amended the schedule to include hepatitis B vaccination for 11- and 12-year-olds who were not immunized as infants.[3]

Because of their changing behaviors, young people entering their teens have a higher risk of contracting hepatitis B, a fairly common liver disease spread through contact with blood, saliva, or semen. Most at risk are those who are sexually active, share personal items like razors and toothbrushes, use intravenous drugs, or get tattoos or body piercings with unsterile needles. The CDC estimates there are 1 million carriers of hepatitis B in the United States. The risk for spreading hepatitis B through sports contact, however, is tiny in comparison with the risk in off-the-field activities.[4] Among sports, contact and collision sports carry the highest risk, but only one case of sports-related hepatitis B transmission has been reported in the medical literature—among sumo wrestlers in Japan.[5]

Certain barriers could limit the use of the preparticipation exam to help stop hepatitis B. First, immunization requires three intramuscular injections, with the second and third doses administered 1 and 6 months after the first. Will teens return for follow-up shots? Second, there are no firm guidelines on reviewing a student's hepatitis B immunization status at the preparticipation exam, says pediatrician Suzanne M. Tanner, MD, assistant professor of pediatrics at the University of Colorado Health Sciences Center in Denver and editorial board member of The Physician and Sportsmedicine. "There's a debate about whether to immunize all teens or only high-risk ones," she says.

When middle school students in San Francisco were offered hepatitis B vaccinations at school, more than 95% of those who received the first dose completed the series. At first, students were rewarded with school items and a dance. However, a questionnaire revealed that the desire to be protected from hepatitis B outweighed gifts and dances as motivators.[6] School district nurse Lynda Boyer-Chu, RN, MPH, who coordinated the demonstration project, said that she believes the high completion rate was due to the school-based population, which created a captive audience. Unless schools provide all three shots on site, she suggests giving athletes the first shot at a primary care physician's office to allow tracking of return visits for the second and third shots. Athletes who receive the first dose from an unfamiliar team physician or clinic may be less likely to get the remaining two shots, she says.

Another obstacle is the cost of the vaccine, which is $25 to $55 a dose. "Everybody wants to immunize children against hepatitis B. What people struggle with is who pays," says Gregory L. Landry, MD, a professor of pediatrics at the University of Wisconsin Medical School and an editorial board member of *The Physician and Sportsmedicine*. Landry says he feels uncomfortable telling financially strapped schools that all athletes must be immunized.

The two hepatitis B vaccines available contain no live viruses and carry few side effects. More than 6,000 immunizations were given in the San Francisco school study, and just two mild allergic reactions occurred, says Boyer-Chu.

References

1. Krowchuk, D.P.; Krowchuk, H.V.; Hunter, D.M., et al: Parents' knowledge of the purposes and content of preparticipation

physical examinations. *Arch Pediatr Adolesc Med* 1995;149(6):653-657.

2. Advisory Committee on Immunization Practices: Hepatitis B virus: a comprehensive strategy for eliminating transmission in the United States through universal childhood vaccination: recommendations of the Immunization Practices Advisory Committee. *MMWR* 1991;40(RR-13):1-19.

3. Centers for Disease Control and Prevention: Recommended childhood immunization schedule, United States, January-June 1996. *MMWR* 1996;44(51 and 52):940-943.

4. Mast, E.E.; Goodman, R.A.; Bond, W.W., et al: Transmission of blood-borne pathogens during sports: risk and prevention. *Ann Intern Med* 1995;122(4):283-285.

5. Kashiwagi, S.; Hayashi, J.; Ikematsu, H., et al: An outbreak of hepatitis B in members of a high school sumo wrestling club. *JAMA* 1982;248(2):213-214.

6. Centers for Disease Control and Prevention: Hepatitis B vaccination of adolescents: California, Louisiana, and Oregon, 1992-1994. *MMWR* 1994;43(33):605-609.

Part Six

Other Issues Related to Sexually Transmitted Diseases

Chapter 44

STDs and Pregnancy

Women who are pregnant can become infected with the same sexually transmitted diseases (STDs) as women who are not pregnant. Pregnancy does not provide women or their babies any protection against STDs. In fact, the consequences of an STD can be significantly more serious—even life threatening—for a woman and her baby if the woman becomes infected with an STD while she is pregnant. As the list of diseases known to be sexually transmitted continues to grow, it is increasingly important that women be aware of the harmful effects of these diseases and know how to protect themselves and their children against infection.

How can STDs affect a woman during pregnancy?

STDs can have many of the same consequences for pregnant women as for women who are not pregnant. STDs can cause cervical and other cancers, chronic hepatitis, cirrhosis, and other complications. Many STDs are silent—or present without symptoms—in women.

Among the additional consequences pregnant women may suffer from STDs are early onset of labor, premature rupture of the membranes surrounding the baby in the uterus, and uterine infection after delivery.

1997 Centers for Disease Control and Prevention (CDC), National Center for HIV, STD & TB Prevention.

427

How can a pregnant woman's baby become infected?

STDs can be transmitted from a pregnant woman to the fetus, newborn, or infant before, during, or after birth. Some STDs (like syphilis) cross the placenta and infect the fetus during its development. Other STDs (like gonorrhea, chlamydia, hepatitis B, and genital herpes) are transmitted from the mother to the infant as the infant passes through the birth canal. HIV infection can cross the placenta during pregnancy, infect the newborn during the birth process, and, unlike other STDs, infect an infant as a result of breast-feeding.

How can STDs affect the fetus or newborn?

Harmful effects on the baby may include stillbirth, low birth weight, conjunctivitis (eye infection), pneumonia, neonatal sepsis (infection in the blood stream), neurologic damage (such as brain damage or motor disorder), congenital abnormalities (including blindness, deafness, or other organ damage), acute hepatitis, meningitis, chronic liver disease, and cirrhosis. Some of these consequences may be apparent at birth; others may not be detected until months or even years later.

Table 44.1. Estimated Number of Pregnant Women in the U.S., Per Year

STDs	Estimated Number of Pregnant Women
Bacterial vaginosis	800,000
Herpes simplex	800,000
Chlamydia	200,000
Trichomoniasis	80,000
Gonorrhea	40,000
Hepatitis B	40,000
HIV	8,000
Syphilis	8,000

(Source: Goldenberg et al., 1997)

How common are STDs among pregnant women in the U.S.?

Some STDs, such as genital herpes and bacterial vaginosis, are quite common among pregnant women in this country. Other STDs, notably HIV and syphilis, are much less common in pregnant women. Table 44.1 shows the estimated number of pregnant women in the U.S., per year with specific STDs.

Should pregnant women be tested for STDs?

STDs affect women of every socioeconomic and educational level, age, race, ethnicity, and religion. The CDC STD Treatment Guidelines (1997) recommend that pregnant women be screened for the following STDs:

- Chlamydia
- Gonorrhea
- Hepatitis B
- HIV
- Syphilis

Pregnant women should request these tests specifically because some doctors do not routinely perform them. New and increasingly accurate tests continue to become available. Even if a woman has been tested in the past, she should be tested again when she becomes pregnant.

Can STDs be treated during pregnancy?

Bacterial STDs (like chlamydia, gonorrhea, and syphilis) can be treated and cured with antibiotics during pregnancy. There is no cure for viral STDs such as genital herpes and HIV, but antiviral medication for herpes and HIV may reduce symptoms in the pregnant woman. In addition, the risk of passing HIV infection from mother to baby is dramatically reduced by treatment. For women who have active genital herpes lesions at the time of delivery, a cesarean section may be performed to protect the newborn against infection.

How can pregnant women protect themselves against infection?

Although a woman may be monogamous during her pregnancy, she can remain at risk of STDs if her partner is not monogamous. For this reason, she may want to consider consistent and correct use of latex condoms for every act of intercourse. Protection is critical throughout a woman's pregnancy, including the last trimester when active infection can present a great threat to the health of a woman and her baby.

Where can I get more information?

CDC National STD Hotline 1-800-227-8922

National AIDS/HIV Hotline 1-800-342-AIDS

References

Goldenberg, R.L.; Andrews, W.W.; Yuan, A.C.; MacKay, H.T.; St. Louis ME, 1997. Sexually transmitted diseases and adverse outcomes of pregnancy. In: *Clinics in Perinatology: Infections in Perinatology,* 24(1):23-41.

Institute of Medicine, 1997. The Hidden Epidemic: Confronting Sexually Transmitted Diseases. Eng, T.R.; Butler, W.T., eds. *Washington: National Academy Press.*

Chapter 45

HIV and Breastfeeding

It's one of the few bright spots to emerge from the AIDS epidemic: With zidovudine therapy, mother-to-infant transmission of HIV occurs in fewer than 10% of pregnancies.

More than 6,500 HIV-infected women gave birth in the United States in 1993. Based on a generally accepted 25% vertical transmission rate, an estimated 1,630 of those infants were HIV-positive.[1]

The increasing incidence of HIV infection among women of child-bearing age has made HIV infection a leading cause of death in young children. In 1992, HIV infection became the seventh leading cause of death in children 1-4 years old in this country. And in 1991, it was the second leading cause of death among black children aged 1-4 years in New Jersey, Massachusetts, New York, and Florida and among Hispanic children in this age-group in New York.[2]

Nearly 90% of cumulative AIDS cases reported among children and virtually all new HIV infections among children in the United States are attributable to perinatal transmission of HIV. An increasing proportion of perinatally acquired AIDS cases has been reported among children whose mothers acquired HIV infection through heterosexual contact with an infected partner whose infection status and risk factors were unknown to her. While HIV infection can and does occur in utero, a substantial number of infants acquire the infection during the peripartum period. Consequently, interventions initiated shortly before and during delivery may be particularly important.

Risk Factors

HIV vertical transmission rates of 14-40% have been reported. Maternal factors that may possibly heighten the risk include other sexually transmitted diseases, a low CD4 cell count, advanced or long-standing HIV disease or AIDS, seroconversion during pregnancy, low vitamin A levels, breastfeeding, premature birth, prolonged rupture of membranes, and chorioamnionitis.

A new study has documented that the risk of transmission is higher when the mother's plasma HIV-1 RNA level (vital load) exceeds 50,000 copies/[micro]L at delivery. Although this study confirmed the excellent protective effects of zidovudine (AZT), the results suggested that the drug is less effective in women with very high viral loads or AZT-resistant HIV.[3]

Breastfeeding by mothers with infection established before pregnancy increases the risk of vertical transmission by 14%.[4] When a mother develops primary HIV infection while breast-feeding, the risk of transmission rises to 29%. Some studies have reported transmission rates to be higher during vaginal delivery than Cesarean section. Nonetheless, the increased risk of transmission is not enough to offset the general risks associated with cesarean sections, and surgery is not performed unless other indications exist.[5] This issue remains under investigation, however.

AZT

Maternal AZT therapy during pregnancy has been shown to reduce the HIV transmission rate by two thirds—from 25% to 8% without any adverse consequences for mother or child. The long-term ramifications are unknown, however.[6] The Centers for Disease Control and Prevention now recommends that all HIV infected pregnant women receive AZT during pregnancy regardless of CD4 cell count, even if they are already receiving didanosine (ddI), zalcitabine (ddC), or other prophylactic or therapeutic agents.[7]

For pregnant women, the AZT regimen generally consists of an antepartum dosage of 100 mg po five times daily—beginning between 14 and 34 weeks of gestation—and an intrapartum dosage of 2 mg/kg IV over a one-hour period, then 1 mg/kg/h until delivery. Newborns receive 2 mg/kg of AZT syrup po q6h within 12 hours after birth and continuing for six weeks.

Other measures under study to reduce the risk of perinatal HIV transmission include:

- Administration of HIV immune globulin to infected pregnant women and their infants

- Boosting maternal and infant immune responses through vaccination. (In HIV-infected children, bacillus Calmette-Guerin vaccine is usually withheld in areas of low tuberculosis prevalence, and inactivated poliovirus vaccine is preferred to live poliovirus vaccine.)

- Virucidal cleansing of the birth canal before and during labor and delivery

- Modified and shortened antiretroviral regimens and therapy with antiretrovirals other than AZT

- Cesarean section delivery

- Vitamin A supplementation in women with very severe vitamin A deficiency.

Timing and Diagnosis

We cannot determine conclusively in utero if a fetus is infected. We can't even tell conclusively in all cases at birth. HIV antibody tests of the newborn reflect maternal HIV status because of antibodies that cross the placenta. More sophisticated tests can diagnose HIV at birth, but about 50% of HIV-positive babies are infected during the last two months of pregnancy, and the other 50% are infected during the birth process. Infection status isn't usually determined conclusively until about 3 months of age at the earliest.[8]

A diagnosis of HIV infection in infants is made after detecting either the virus in culture, the HIV genome by polymerase chain reaction (PCR), the viral antigen, or persistent HIV antibody beyond the age of 18 months. The sensitivity of viral culture and PCR is only about 40% at birth but rises sharply after one week in infants who are not breastfed. The sensitivity of PCR and viral culture increases little after one month, when the sensitivity of viral culture is about 90% and the sensitivity of PCR is perhaps higher. Diagnosis is confirmed by positive results with two separate blood samples, using one or a combination of tests (viral culture, PCR, or p24 antigen).

Signs, Symptoms, and Disease Course

HIV signs and symptoms are rarely present at birth but develop over subsequent months or years. HIV infection progresses rapidly to AIDS or death in the first year in about 25% of infected children. The remainder of infected children experience slower disease progression, sometimes surviving childhood into adolescence.

Nonetheless, rapid disease progression is more common in children than in adults. This may be because of the immaturity of their immune systems at the time of acquisition, the infecting dose of the virus, or the route of infection. In addition, the limited ability of neonatal T cells to produce cytokines, such as interferon gamma, interleukin-3, interleukin-4, and tumor necrosis factor, may limit development of appropriate humoral and cellular responses. Infants with HIV infection are also exposed to primary infection with opportunistic organisms, which differs from the reactivation of such infections that occurs in adults.

References

1. Davis, S.F.; Byers, R.H. Jr.; Lindegren, M.L., et al: Prevalence and incidence of vertically acquired HIV infection in the United States. *JAMA* 1995;274:952-955.

2. U.S. Department of Health and Human Services: U.S. Public Health Service recommendations for human immunodeficiency virus counseling and voluntary testing for pregnant women. *MMWR* 1995; 44(RR-7):1-15.

3. Dickover, R.E.; Garratty, E.M.; Herman, S.A., et al: Identification of levels of maternal HIV-1 RNA associated with risk of perinatal transmission: Effect of maternal zidovudine treatment on viral load. *JAMA* 1996; 275:599-605.

4. Dunn, D.T.; Newell, M.L.; Ades, A.E., et al; Risk of human immunodeficiency virus type 1 transmission through breastfeeding. *Lancet* 1992;340:585-588.

5. Peckham, C.; Gibb, D.: Mother-to-child transmission of the human immunodeficiency virus. *N Engl J Med* 1995; 333:298-302.

6. Connor, E.M.; Sperling, R.S.; Gelber, R., et al: Reduction of maternal-infant transmission of human immunodeficiency

virus type 1 with zidovudine treatment. *N Engl J Med* 1994; 331:1173-1180.

7. Matheson, P.B.; Abrams, E.J.; Thomas, P.A., et al: Efficacy of antenatal zidovudine in reducing perinatal transmission of human immunodeficiency virus type 1. *J Infect Dis* 1995; 172:353-358.

8. Rouzioux, C.; Costagliola, D.; Burgard, M., et al: Estimated timing of mother-to-child human immunodeficiency virus type 1 (HIV-1) transmission by use of a Markov model. *Am J Epidemiol* 1995; 142:1330-1337.

Suggested Reading

American Academy of Pediatrics, Committee on Pediatric AIDS: Human milk, breastfeeding, and transmission of human immunodeficiency virus in the United States. *Pediatrics* 1995; 96:977-979.

Centers for Disease Control and Prevention: Recommendations of the U.S. Public Health Service Task Force on the use of zidovudine to reduce perinatal transmission of human immunodeficiency virus. *MMWR* 1994; 43:(RR-11):1-20.

Grubman, S.; Simonds, R.J.: Preventing Pneumocystis carinii pneumonia in human immunodeficiency virus-infected children: New guidelines for prophylaxis. *Pediatr Infect Dis J* 1996; 15:165-168.

Mayaux, M.J.; Burgard, M.; Teglas, J.P., et al: Neonatal characteristics in rapidly progressive perinatally acquired HIV-1 disease. *JAMA* 1996; 275:606-610.

Mofenson, L.M.: A critical review of studies evaluating the relationship of mode of delivery to perinatal transmission of human immunodeficiancy virus. *Pediatr Infect Dis J* 1995; 14:169-177.

Nduati, R.W.; John, G.C.; Richardson, B.A., et al: Human immunodeficiency virus type 1-infected cells in breast milk: Association with immunceuppression and vitamin A deficiency, *J Infect Dis* 1995; 172:1461-1468.

Nelson, R.P.; Price, L.J.; Halsey, A.B., et al: Diagnosis of pediatric human immunodeficiency virus infection by means of a commercially available polymerase chain reaction gene amplification. *Arch Pediatr Adolesc Med* 1996; 150:40-45.

Sperling, R.S.; Stratton, P.; O'Sullivan, M.J., et al: A survey of zidovudine use in pregnant women with human immunodeficiency virus infection. *N Engl J Med* 1992; 326:857-861.

Chapter 46

Domestic Violence and Sexually Transmitted Diseases

Current public health practice concerning the provision of prenatal care services emphasizes the need to address a wide variety of medical and behavioral risk factors when assessing women's clinical histories, factors that may affect the course of their pregnancy and birth outcomes.[1] Recent attention has focused on including domestic violence, both physical and sexual violence, among these risk factors.[2] Domestic violence is a concern not only because of the direct injury it may inflict but also because it may result in other health problems, such as sexually transmitted diseases (STDs).

STDs comprise a significant public health threat to women in general given the high prevalence of these infections and their potentially serious health consequences and sequelae (for example, pelvic inflammatory disease, cancer of the genital tract, infertility, ectopic pregnancy, and poor birth outcomes). In 1995, more than 600,000 STD cases were reported among females in the U.S., with chlamydia being the most common, followed by gonorrhea.[3] In light of these concerns, there have been calls for greater emphasis on STD prevention strategies that target women.[4]

One of the most commonly recommended methods of STD prevention, the use of condoms during sex,[5] requires male cooperation. Clear and open communication between women and their male partners

1999 U.S. Government Printing Office, from *Public Health Reports*, May 1999, Vol.114, Issue 3, Pg.262, by Sandra L. Martin; Louis S. Matza; Lawrence L. Kupper; James C. Thomas; Matthew Daly; Suzanne Cloutier.

regarding sexual practices (sometimes termed "sexual negotiation") increases the probability of condom use.[6] Condom use is more common among couples in which women feel comfortable discussing sexual matters with their partners.[7] However, traditional gender role standards that define socially appropriate female behavior[8] may impede sexual negotiation so that some women feel uncomfortable requesting (or requiring) that their male partners use condoms.[9] Although the meanings ascribed to condom use and to male reactions to female suggestions of condom use are likely to vary, some of the social norms surrounding sexual behaviors cross many cultural boundaries; such norms may include the beliefs that women should not be assertive in sexual situations, women should emphasize their male partners' pleasure during sex rather than their own safety,[10] and women should not ask their partners about their STD histories or risky behaviors that may have put them (and now the women) at risk for acquiring infections.[11]

Women are even less willing or able to negotiate protective practices in the context of relationships in which they feel less powerful than their male partners. Studies of female sex workers indicate that at least some prostitutes feel that their past use of condoms, or suggestions of condom use, resulted in abusive experiences; consequently, they may be less likely to request the use of condoms, enhancing their risk for acquiring or transmitting STDs.[12,13] Studies of married women and women in relatively permanent relationships have found mixed results concerning whether women fear violent reactions from their partners in response to the suggestion to use a condom.[14,16]

The large number of women who are victims of domestic violence each year may be especially unlikely (or unable) to negotiate safer sex practices with their partners due to the extreme imbalances of power in their relationships. Some research suggests that abuse victims fear that safer sex negotiation with their partners would lead to intensification of the violence already present in their relationships, resulting in less condom use.[17]

Despite the evidence that some women are reluctant or unable to negotiate safer sex practices with male partners due to fear of violent reactions and that abused women may be less likely than other women to use condoms, there has been little research concerning associations between women's experiences of partner violence and women's experiences of STD infections. A study of prenatal care patients in Boston found that women who had suffered abuse during pregnancy (defined as physical or sexual violence or both) were twice as likely as non-abused women to have experienced an STD during their lifetime;[18] however, the potentially differential effects of sexual abuse and non-sexual physical abuse on STD risk were not examined. A Norwegian investigation compared the reported medical histories of 66 physically abused women (recruited from both the emergency department of a local hospital and a local battered women's shelter) with those of 114 non-abused women (recruited from a city population register)[19] and found that abused women were more likely than non-abused women to have suffered from pelvic inflammatory disease (PID), a condition often resulting from an STD infection. A study that examined a variety of health issues among 115 residents of battered women's shelters across the state of Michigan found that approximately 7% of the women who had been sexually abused by their husbands or other partners reported contracting an STD as a result of this abuse.[20] Although these studies suggest links between women's experiences of abuse and their experiences of STDs, each of these previous investigations has suffered from methodological shortcomings (for example, not differentiating between sexual abuse and non-sexual physical abuse, not recruiting representative samples, or not controlling for important confounding variables).

Pregnant women are one group in which it is especially important to examine potential associations between violence and STDs because of the high prevalence of domestic violence among women of reproductive age and because STDs may affect the health of both the woman and the fetus. In addition, the vast majority of pregnant women become pregnant by engaging in "unsafe sex" (not using condoms during intercourse), thereby enhancing their likelihood of acquiring and transmitting STDs. Therefore, the study reported here extends past research by examining a relatively large sample of prenatal care patients to explore the associations between women's experiences of sexual and physical abuse and their STD histories, controlling for potentially confounding factors.

Methods

Study setting and sample. This study was undertaken as part of an evaluation of a prenatal care program in a large health department in North Carolina. All women seen for prenatal care over an approximately eight-month period from October 1992 through May 1993 were eligible for the study. Complete information was available for 774 (92%) of 843 women assessed during this time period; these 774 women comprised the study sample.

Assessment. Prenatal patients of the health department were routinely interviewed (usually by a nurse or social worker) using a structured procedure to determine whether the patients were in need of specialized services.

Each woman's experience of sexual abuse was assessed by asking whether she was ever forced to have sexual activities with anyone, and each woman's experience of non-sexual physical abuse was assessed by asking whether she had ever been hit, slapped, kicked, or otherwise physically hurt by anyone. As part of the routine assessment, all abused women were asked about their social relationships with the perpetrators of the violence.

Women's STD histories were assessed during the interviews by asking the women if they had ever been diagnosed with an STD; they were prompted with a list of specific infections (chlamydia, genital warts, gonorrhea, herpes, syphilis, trichomoniasis, HIV). Those who reported having had an STD were asked to identify the type of STD. The women's use of substances was assessed by asking about their use during the previous year of alcoholic beverages (interviewers asked specifically about consumption of beer, wine, and liquor) and illegal drugs (interviewers asked about a number of specific types of drugs, for example, marijuana, cocaine, "crack," heroin, PCP, psychedelics, and inhalants). Women were also asked about cigarette smoking during the previous year.

We classified women's use of alcohol into three categories (heavy drinkers, moderate drinkers, and non-drinkers) based on their self-reported alcohol consumption patterns during the previous year. We classified women as "heavy drinkers" if they reported usually having six or more alcoholic drinks per drinking session or two to five drinks (or more) per drinking session with these sessions occurring once a week or more. We classified all others who reported any consumption of alcoholic beverages during the previous year as "moderate drinkers."

We classified women as users of illicit drugs if they reported using one or more illicit drugs in the previous year. We classified women as cigarette smokers if they reported usually smoking one or more cigarettes per day in the previous year.

All collected information was entered into the patient's chart, and treatment plans were developed and implemented. Later, patient names were removed and the assessment information was passed to the quality assurance evaluation team.

Statistical analysis. We used descriptive statistics (including proportions, means, and standard deviations) to examine the women's

STD histories, experiences of sexual and physical abuse, substance use behaviors in the past year, and sociodemographic characteristics. We also looked at bivariate associations between the women's STD histories and these other variables.

Using unconditional logistic regression analysis[21] and SAS software, we modeled each woman's STD status (a positive STD history vs. a negative STD history) as a function of the woman's experience of violence (whether the woman had experienced sexual abuse or physical abuse), controlling for use of illicit drugs, alcohol, and tobacco; previous children; educational level; marital status; younger vs. older age; and self-reported ethnicity. The strengths of associations are reported here as odds ratios (ORs) with 95% confidence intervals (CIs).

We included ethnicity as a variable because of the possibility that in this group of low-income women, there may have been differences in cultural norms that influenced the outcome of the analysis; for example, women belonging to different ethnic groups may have differed in their likelihood of revealing a history of abuse or STDs.

Institutional Review Board approval. The overall evaluation research protocol, of which this study was a part, was reviewed and approved by the Committee on Human Subjects Institutional Review Board of the School of Public Health at the University of North Carolina at Chapel Hill.

Results

More than a quarter of the 774 women (28% [220/774]) reporting being victims of some type of abuse: 97 women (12%) reported having experienced both sexual and physical abuse, and 123 women (16%) reported having experienced non-sexual physical abuse but not sexual abuse. It is noteworthy that all of the women who had been sexually abused had also been physically abused.

The most common perpetrators of sexual violence were the women's husbands, boyfriends, and male friends (67%); less commonly reported were the women's relatives (17%), multiple perpetrators (15%), and strangers (1%). The women's husbands, boyfriends, and male friends also were the most common perpetrators of non-sexual physical violence (82%), with less common perpetrators being the women's relatives (13% of women) and multiple perpetrators (5%).

Thirty percent of the women reported having been infected with at least one type of STD. The most common STD infections were chlamydia and gonorrhea. None of the women reported being infected with HIV.

Logistic regression analysis. After controlling for the substance use-related and sociodemographic factors, we found that sexually abused women were more likely than non-victims to report having been infected with an STD (OR = 2.25, 95% CI 1.37, 3.69). Furthermore, a higher percentage of physically abused women than of non-victims reported having had STDs, although the association between physical abuse and STDs was only of borderline statistical significance (OR = 1.54, 95% CI 0.97, 2.45).

Women who were moderate drinkers were more likely than non-drinkers to report having experienced an STD (OR = 1.78, 95% CI 1.22, 2.61), and heavy alcohol use showed a borderline statistically significant positive association with STD infection. Women who used illicit drugs were more likely to report having experienced an STD than non-drug-using women (OR = 1.70, 95% CI 1.03, 2.80). In addition, African American women were more likely to report having experienced one or more STDs than other women (OR = 3.50, 95% CI 2.32, 5.28).

Discussion

Our results agree with those of other studies in finding that many prenatal care patients have experienced STDs (most commonly chlamydia and gonorrhea)[18] and that many have suffered physical or sexual violence, often at the hands of their intimate partners.[22] Women who were both sexually and physically abused were more likely than non-abused women to have experienced an STD, and physical abuse showed an association of borderline statistical significance with STDs, findings consistent with the limited empirical information available from past studies concerning this association.[18,19] In addition, these findings are unique in showing that, among prenatal care patients, the association between having experienced both types of abuse and STDs is stronger than the association between non-sexual physical abuse and STDs and that these associations were found even after we controlled for potentially confounding factors, including substance use.

Although these research findings suggest that women in abusive situations, especially sexually abusive situations, are more likely than other women to suffer from STDs, the reasons why this may be true are still open to question. The methodology used in this study cannot establish whether the STD of an abused women was transmitted to her during a sexually abusive act, or even whether the woman acquired the STD from her abuser. However, other research suggests that male abusers tend to be sexually active with multiple partners, thereby enhancing their own risk of contracting STDs and transmitting them to the woman they are abusing.[23] An alternative explanation of this study's findings could be that women who suffer physical and sexual abuse are more likely than other women to engage in sexual activities with multiple partners, resulting in their increased risk of STD infection. The methodological constraints of this study still leave questions concerning the exact nature of the association between abuse and STDs.

The links between violence and STDs among prenatal care patients have implications for public health practice. First, providers of prenatal care should assure that all pregnant women are routinely screened for both STDs and exposure to violence and that identified women are provided with the appropriate treatment or other interventions. Toward this end, providers of care for pregnant women, for STD patients, and for victims of violence (such as the staff of domestic violence programs and battered women's shelters) should strengthen their working relationships with each other. Second, providers of care to women in violent relationships should be sensitive to the potentially dangerous implications posed to these women by STD prevention measures such as condom use and partner notification.

This study found that several factors, in addition to violence, were associated with STD infection. In particular, STDs were significantly more common among women who drank moderate amounts of alcohol than among non-drinkers and more common among users than non-users of illicit drugs. The data also showed a relationship of borderline statistical significance (probably not reaching statistical significance due to the relatively small sample of heavy drinkers) between heavy drinking and STDs.

The results of this study must be viewed in light of its methodologic limitations. First, the analysis reported here was part of a larger investigation designed to examine the effectiveness of a prenatal care clinic, not to specifically examine links between violence and STDs. All of the study information was drawn from the women's clinical interview responses and therefore may be subject to various forms of recall and response bias, especially given that both abuse and STDs are socially stigmatized experiences that women may hesitate to report. Thus, this study would have benefited from additional confirmatory information regarding the violence in the women's lives, for example, from medical records or police reports. In addition, it would have been helpful to supplement self-reported STD histories with information from medical records and lab findings. Furthermore, the battery of questions used to assess violence could have been more extensive, including questions on additional forms of abuse such as psychological abuse and fear of harm.

Second, although this study did find a positive association between violence and STDs, it must be kept in mind that this study was cross-sectional in nature and relied upon prevalence data. Therefore, we cannot be sure whether the violence-STD association reported here reflects a causal relationship. We encourage future researchers to employ longitudinal study designs through which they may clearly describe the patterns of both violent events and STD occurrences within women's lives.

Finally, since the study focused on prenatal care patients of a North Carolina health department (a group of pregnant, relatively young, poor women), it is unclear whether these findings are generalizable to other populations of women.

Violence in women's lives is an understudied public health problem that has many implications for the well being of women and their families. Health care providers, researchers, legal professionals, and others concerned with women's issues should work together to prevent domestic abuse and to offer therapeutic health, social, and legal services to victims of violence.

This study was supported by the Center for Health Promotion and Disease Prevention, University of North Carolina at Chapel Hill; by the Chancellor's Office of the University of North Carolina at Chapel Hill; in part by the Alcohol and Drug Section, Division of Mental Health, Developmental Disability, and Substance Abuse Services, North Carolina Department of Human Resources; and by Grant # MCJ-107 from the Maternal and Child Health Bureau of the U.S. Department of Health and Human Services.

The authors thank the staff of the Wake County (NC) Department of Health for their assistance and Melissa Hays, MS, Brian Killgallen, MS, Melissa McPheeters, MPH, and Sherry Rhodes of the University of North Carolina at Chapel Hill for analytic and technical support.

References

1. Bennett, T.; Kotelchuck, M. Mothers and infants. In: Kotch, J.B., editor. Maternal and child health: programs, problems, and policy in public health. Gaithersburg (MD): Aspen Publishers; 1997. p. 85-114.

2. Committee on Technical Bulletins of the American College of Obstetricians and Gynecologists. ACOG Technical Bulletin: domestic violence. *Int J Gynaecol Obstet* 1995;51:161-70.

3. Centers for Disease Control and Prevention, Division of STD Prevention (US). Sexually transmitted disease surveillance, 1995. Atlanta: Department of Health and Human Services; 1996.

4. Stein, Z.A. More on women and the prevention of HIV infection [editorial]. *Am J Public Health* 1995;85:1485-8.

5. Cates, W.; Stewart, F.H.; Trussell, J. The quest for women's prophylactic methods—hopes vs. science. *Am J Public Health* 1992;82:1479-82.

6. Oakley, D.; Bogue, E.L. Quality of condom use as reported by female clients of a family planning clinic. *Am J Public Health* 1995;85:1526-30.

7. Weisman, C.S.; Plichta, S.; Nathanson, C.A.; Ensminger, M.; Robinson, J.C. Consistency of condom use for disease prevention among adolescent users of oral contraceptives. *Fam Plann Perspect* 1991;23:71-4.

8. Carovano, K. More than mother and whores: redefining the AIDS prevention needs of women. *Int J Health Serv* 1989:21:131-42.

9. Weiss, E.; Gupta, G.R.; Whelan, D. Violence and HIV prevention for women. Presented at the National Council for International Health Conference; 1995 Jun 26; Arlington, VA.

10. Maxwell, C.; Boyle, M. Risky heterosexual practices amongst women over 30: gender, power and long-term relationships. *AIDS Care* 1995;7:277-93.

11. Sheahan, S.L.; Coons, S.J.; Seabolt, J.P.; Churchill, L.; Dale, T. Sexual behavior, communication, and chlamydial infections among college women. *Health Care Women Int* 1994;15:275-86.

12. Karim, Q.A.; Karim, S.S.A.; Soldan, K.; Zondi, M. Reducing the risk of HIV infection among South African sex workers: socioeconomic and gender barriers. *Am J Public Health* 1995;85:1521-5.

13. Vanwesenbeeck, I.; Zessen, G.V.; Graaf, R.D.; Straver, C.J. Contextual and interactional factors influencing condom use

in heterosexual prostitution contacts. *Patient Education and Counseling* 1994;24:307-22.

14. Heise, L.; Morre, K.; Toubia, N. Sexual coercion and reproductive health. New York: Population Council; 1995.

15. Adbool, Karim Q.; Morar, N. Determinants of a woman's ability to adopt HIV protective behaviour in Natal/Kwazulu, South Africa: a community based approach. *Women and AIDS Program Research Report Series.* Washington DC: International Center for Research on Women; 1995.

16. Wyatt, G.E.; Tucker, M.B.; Eldermire, D.; Bain, B.; Le Franc, E.; Simeon, D.; Chambers, C. Female low income workers and AIDS in Jamaica. *Women and AIDS Program Research Report Series.* Washington DC: International Center for Research on Women; 1995.

17. Wingood, G.M.; DiClemente, J. The effects of an abusive primary partner on the condom use and sexual negotiation practices of African-American women. *Am J Public Health* 1997:87:1016-18.

18. Amaro, H.; Fried, L.E.; Cabral, H.; Zuckerman, B. Violence during pregnancy and substance use. *Am J Public Health* 1990;80:575-9.

19. Schei, B. Physically abusive spouse—a risk factor of pelvic inflammatory disease? *Scand J Prim Health Care* 1991;9:41-5.

20. Campbell, J.C.; Alford, P. The dark consequences of marital rape. *AM J Nurs* 1989;89:946-9.

21. Hosmer, D.W.; Lemeshow, S. Applied logistic regression. New York: Wiley; 1989.

22. Gazmararian, J.A.; Lazorick, S.; Spitz, A.M.; Ballard, T.J.; Saltzman, L.E.; Marks, J.S. Prevalence of violence against pregnant women. *JAMA* 1996;275:1915-20.

23. Martin, S.L.; Kilgallen, B.; Tsui, A.O.; Maitra, K.; Singh, K.K.; Kupper, L.L. Domestic violence: associations with reproductive health in Northern India. Presented at the Annual Meeting of the American Public Health Association; 1998 Nov 16; Washington DC.

Chapter 47

Occupational Exposure to HIV

The Public Health Service recently updated its recommendations for chemoprophylaxis after exposure to HIV. These recommendations correlate the use of antiretroviral agents with the risk of infection, which is determined by evaluating the exposure and the potential for transmission from the source patient.

Information on the treatment for patients infected with HIV has changed rapidly over the past several years, and recommendations for the prevention of HIV transmission after occupational exposures are no exception. In May 1998, updated recommendations on the prevention of occupational transmission of HIV were published as a result of new information, Food and Drug Administration approval of new antiretroviral agents, and a meeting of experts convened by the Centers for Disease Control and Prevention.

Presented here are the Public Health Service recommendations for the use of these antiretroviral agents for postexposure prophylaxis (PEP). The Public Health Service recommendations for PEP are intended to provide guidance to physicians. They can be modified by local experts on a case-by-case basis. When possible, expert consultation is recommended.

Epidemiology of Occupational Exposures

Transmission of bloodborne pathogens is an occupational hazard for healthcare workers. Nationally, as of June 30, 1997, 52 healthcare workers became infected with HIV as a result of an occupational exposure. Twenty-four of these workers developed AIDS. The 52 healthcare workers include 21 nurses, 19 laboratory technicians, 6 physicians, 2 surgical technicians, 1 dialysis technician, 1 housekeeper/maintenance worker, 1 health aide/attendant, and 1 respiratory therapist.[2]

The most common route of exposure for occupational HIV transmission is percutaneous (needlestick or other penetrating sharps-related event). Forty-five of the seroconversions occurred as a result of a percutaneous exposure, five occurred through a mucocutaneous exposure (mucous membrane and/or skin exposure), one occurred through a combined percutaneous and mucocutaneous exposure, and one route of exposure was unknown. Forty-six employees were exposed to HIV-infected blood, three were exposed to concentrated virus in the laboratory, one was exposed to visibly bloody body fluid, and one was exposed to an unspecified fluid. The objects involved in the percutaneous exposures include a hollow-bore needle (41), a broken glass vial (2), a scalpel (1), and an unknown sharp object.[2]

Workplace Safety: How to Protect Yourself

Workplace safety includes the incorporation of infection control precautions, also known as standard precautions, into daily practice to prevent exposure to blood. These precautions include the appropriate use of personal protective equipment (e.g., gloves, eye protection, gowns) when contact with blood and other body fluids is anticipated. Needlestick and other sharps injuries may be prevented by changes in technique that eliminate the need for needles/sharps and/or by the use of safer devices. Needles should not be bent, recapped, or broken. Needles/sharps should be placed in a puncture resistant container to minimize the risk of exposure.[3,4]

The Occupational Safety and Health Administration requires that primary methods to decrease occupational risk include engineering controls.[5] A six-hospital study conducted by the CDC indicated that safety devices for phlebotomy, such as vacuum-tube blood collection devices and winged steel needles, significantly reduced the risk of percutaneous injury.[6]

New technology to obtain specimens for HIV testing may also decrease the risk of occupational exposure. An oral test kit received FDA approval in 1996 and a urine test was approved in 1998. These tests obviate the need to draw blood to test for HIV. Because no phlebotomy is required, and the patient can obtain the specimen, the risk of occupational exposure during specimen collection is less than with obtaining the classic blood specimen.[7]

What Is an Occupational Exposure?

An occupational exposure is defined as skin, eye, mucous membrane, or parenteral contact with blood or other potentially infectious material. Parenteral contact includes piercing mucous membranes or the skin barrier through such events as a needlestick, human bite, cut, or abrasion. Blood is defined as human blood, human blood components, and products made from human blood. The other potentially infectious materials include the following human body fluids: semen, vaginal secretions, amniotic fluid, cerebrospinal fluid, synovial fluid, pleural fluid, peritoneal fluid, pericardial fluid, saliva in dental procedures, any body fluid that is visibly contaminated with blood, and all body fluids in situations where it is difficult or impossible to differentiate between body fluids. Any unfixed tissue or organ (other than intact skin) from a human (living or dead); HIV-containing cell or tissue cultures, organ cultures, and culture medium or other solutions; and blood, organs, or other tissues from experimental animals with HIV-infection are also included in the category of other potentially infectious material.[5]

What Is the Risk of Occupational Exposures?

The CDC has been tracking occupational exposure to HIV. The average risk of HIV infection from all types of percutaneous exposures to HIV-infected blood is 0.3%.[8] The CDC conducted a case-control study to determine the risk of HIV infection from different types of percutaneous exposures. This case-control study showed that the risk of HIV infection exceeded 0.3% for exposures that involved one of the following: (1) a deep injury to the healthcare worker, (2) visible blood on the device that caused the injury, (3) if the device had been placed in the source patient's vascular system (e.g., a needle used for phlebotomy), or (4) if the source patient died as a result of AIDS within 60 days after exposure.[9]

The increased risk associated with these scenarios may be related to exposure to larger volumes of blood or to blood containing a higher titer of the HIV virus. However, the utility of viral load measurements from the source patient to estimate the risk of transmission based on the vital titer is unknown. Plasma vital load reflects only the level of cell-free virus in the blood. It does not reflect the level of cell-associated virus in the blood or the amount of virus present in compartments, such as lymphatic tissue. HIV transmission from persons with a viral load below detectable limits has been reported in the seroconversion of one healthcare worker and in instances of mother-to-infant transmission.[1,10,11]

The average risk of HIV infection after a mucous membrane or skin exposure is less than the risk associated with a percutaneous exposure. The average risk of HIV infection after a mucous membrane exposure is 0.1%. The average risk of HIV infection after a skin exposure is less than 0.1%. The risk for skin exposure may be increased if skin contact is prolonged, contact involves an extensive area of the skin, the integrity of the skin is not intact, and/or if the exposure involves a higher titer of HIV.[1]

Follow-Up for Occupational Exposures

Employers need to provide healthcare workers with a system for prompt evaluation, counseling, and follow-up after an occupational exposure that may place the employee at risk for HIV infection. First aid should be administered immediately after an exposure. Puncture wounds and other cut injuries should be washed with soap and water. Exposure to oral and nasal mucosa should be decontaminated by flushing with water. Eyes should be irrigated with clean water and saline or sterile irrigants designed for flushing eyes. The exposure should be reported to the person or department (e.g., employee health, infection control) responsible for managing exposures.

Workers with occupational exposures to HIV should receive follow-up counseling and medical evaluation. HIV antibody tests should be performed at baseline and periodically for at least 6 months after exposure (e.g., 6 weeks, 12 weeks, and 6 months). The employee should be counseled on precautions to prevent secondary transmission of HIV.[12]

In some instances, appropriate postexposure management also includes the use of antiretroviral agents for PEP. If PEP is used, drug toxicity monitoring should be included in the medical management and follow-up of the employee. Although it is the employer's responsibility to offer PEP when it is appropriate, the employee can refuse it.

Postexposure Prophylaxis: Does it Work?

A multi-national study found that PEP with zidovudine (AZT, ZDV) may reduce the risk of HIV infection. The use of zidovudine PEP was shown to decrease the risk of HIV infection after a percutaneous exposure by 81%.[13] However, as with chemoprophylaxis measures for other infectious diseases, failures have occurred with zidovudine PEP.[5] The reason(s) zidovudine PEP failed to prevent HIV infection in at least 14 cases is not known; however, in one case, the virus was noted to be partially resistant to zidovudine.

Recommendations for PEP have changed with the development and FDA approval of new antiretroviral agents, but other aspects of postexposure management (e.g., reporting exposures, counseling, and testing of both the exposed healthcare worker and source patient) have not changed.[9]

When Should PEP Start?

When PEP is indicated, it should be initiated promptly, preferably within 1-2 hours after the exposure. There are several reasons why PEP may not be started immediately, such as when an employee refuses the therapy. The interval after which PEP is not effective is unknown, however. Initiating PEP after a longer interval (e.g., 1-2 weeks) may be considered for exposures that represent an increased risk of transmission. Even if infection is not prevented, early treatment of HIV infection may be beneficial.[1] The optimal duration of PEP is uncertain. The Public Health Services recommend 4 weeks of PEP because 4 weeks of zidovudine appeared protective in certain studies.[1,8]

The Recommendations

Although these recommendations represent the most recent Public Health Service recommendations for PEP, they are always subject to change, PEP is not recommended for all types of occupational exposure to HIV because most occupational exposures do not result in HIV transmission. For many types of exposure, the risk of serious side effects may exceed the risk of HIV infection. Exposures with a lower risk of infection may not warrant the potential side effects of these agents. When discussing the use of PEP, the employee should be informed that: (1) knowledge about the efficacy and toxicity of PEP is limited; (2) for agents other than zidovudine, data are limited regarding toxicity in persons who are not HIV infected or who are pregnant; and (3) the employee can decline PEP.[1]

The Risk from Exposure

The first factor to consider is the exposure itself. Situations that pose a risk for bloodborne transmission and require further evaluation are:

1. Exposures to blood, fluid containing visible blood, or other potentially infectious fluid or tissue through a percutaneous injury or through contact with a mucous membrane.

2. Any direct contact (i.e., personal protective equipment either was not used or was ineffective in protecting skin or mucous membranes) with concentrated HIV in a research laboratory or production facility is considered an exposure that requires clinical evaluation to assess the need for PEP.[1]

3. For skin exposures, follow-up is indicated if it involves direct contact with a body fluid listed previously and if there is evidence of compromised skin integrity (e.g., dermatitis, abrasion, or open wound). However, if contact is prolonged or involves a large area of intact skin, postexposure follow-up may be considered on a case-by-case basis or when it is requested by the healthcare worker.[1]

4. For human bites, the clinical evaluation must consider possible exposure of both the bite recipient and the person who inflicted the bite. HIV transmission has rarely been reported by this route. If a bite results in blood exposure to either person involved, postexposure follow-up, including consideration of PEP, should be provided.[1]

Risk from the Source Patient

The second component in assessing the risk of transmission is to evaluate the source of the occupational exposure. The source person should be evaluated for risk of HIV infection. This can be done through information available on the medical record at the time of the exposure (e.g., laboratory test results, admitting diagnosis, or medical history). Certain pieces of information from the source person may suggest or rule out possible HIV infection, such as prior HIV test results, results of past immunologic testing (e.g., CD4+ T-cell count), clinical symptoms (e.g., acute syndrome suggestive of HIV infection or undiagnosed immunodeficiency disease), and a history of possible HIV exposure (e.g., injection drug use, sexual contact with a known HIV-positive partner, unprotected sexual contact with multiple partners, or receipt of blood products prior to 1985).[1]

If the source is known to be infected with HIV, available information about the source's stage of infection (including asymptomatic or AIDS, CD4+ T-cell count, and viral load test results) as well as current and previous antiretroviral therapy should be considered when selecting PEP regimen. However, when PEP is indicated, it should not be delayed while this information on infection status is being gathered. if necessary, changes in the PEP regimen can be made after it has been started.[1]

If the HIV status of the source person is unknown, the source person should be informed of the incident. If consent is obtained, testing should be done with appropriate pre- and post-test counseling. Confidentiality regarding the HIV status of the source person should be maintained at all times.[1]

If the source agrees to HIV testing, the testing should be done as soon as possible. Physicians and infection control practitioners may request information from the laboratory regarding the most appropriate FDA-approved HIV antibody test to expedite these results. An FDA-approved rapid HIV antibody test should be considered for use in these situations, especially if enzyme immunoassay testing cannot be completed within 24-48 hours.[1]

If the source is HIV-seronegative and has no clinical evidence of AIDS or symptoms of HIV infection, no further testing of the source is indicated. It is unclear whether follow-up testing of a source who engaged in a high-risk behavior within the last 3 to 6 months is useful in the postexposure management of healthcare workers. Healthcare workers who become infected generally seroconvert before repeat testing of the source would normally be performed.[1]

If the exposure source is unknown, information about where and under what circumstances the exposure occurred should be assessed epidemiologically for the risk of transmission. Certain situations may suggest an increased or decreased risk of transmission. The prevalence of HIV in the population group (e.g., institution or community) is important. For example, an exposure that occurs in a geographic area where injection drug use is common or on an AIDS unit in a healthcare facility would be considered to have an epidemiologically increased risk for transmission than in a nursing home for the elderly where no known HIV-infected residents are present. Decisions regarding appropriate management should be individualized based on the risk assessment.[1]

HIV testing of needles or other instruments associated with an exposure, regardless of whether the source is known, is not recommended. The reliability and interpretation of findings in such circumstances are unknown.[1]

Medications Used for PEP

After an occupational exposure, PEP should be recommended based on the risk presented by the exposure and information about the source. Most HIV exposures will warrant only a basic two-drug regimen, using two nucleoside reverse transcriptase inhibitors, usually zidovudine and lamivudine (3TC). The addition of a third drug as part of an expanded regimen, usually a protease inhibitor such as indinavir (IDV) or nelfinavir (NEL), should be considered for exposures that pose an increased risk of transmission or where resistance to other drugs used for PEP is known or suspected. Whenever possible, the regimens should be implemented in consultation with experts in antiretroviral therapy and HIV transmission.

Zidovudine should be considered for all PEP regimens because it is the only agent for which data support the efficacy of PEP in a clinical setting. Lamivudine should usually be added to a regimen that includes zidovudine because it increases antiretroviral activity and activity against many zidovudine-resistant strains. A protease inhibitor should be added to the treatment regimen for exposures with a high risk of transmission. However, individual clinicians may prefer other combinations of drugs based on local knowledge and experience in treating HIV disease.[1]

Currently, the FDA has approved zidovudine, lamivudine, indinavir, and nelfinavir for the treatment of HIV infection, but not for PEP. However, physicians may prescribe any FDA-approved medication when, in their professional judgment, use of the medication is clinically indicated.

Monitoring and Side Effects

If PEP is used, drug toxicity monitoring needs to be performed. This should include a complete blood count and renal and hepatic chemical function tests at baseline and 2 weeks after starting PEP. Monitoring for hyperglycemia should be included for PEP regimens that include a protease inhibitor. If indinavir is included, monitoring for crystalluria, hematuria, hemolytic anemia, and hepatitis should also be performed. If subjective or objective toxicity is noted, dose reduction or drug substitution should be considered with expert consultation. Further diagnostic studies may be indicated. Healthcare workers who become infected with HIV should be counseled on and receive the appropriate medical care.

Side effects may make it difficult to remain on PEP. Preliminary information from healthcare workers taking zidovudine and lamivudine for PEP, with or without a protease inhibitor, suggests that 50-90% report subjective side effects. These side effects caused 24-36% of healthcare workers to stop PEP. Common symptoms associated with these medications are headache, malaise, fatigue, or insomnia. However, more serious side effects including kidney stones, hepatitis, and pancytopenia have been reported with combination PEP. In general, the frequency of these side effects has not been greater when these agents have been used in combination. The symptoms can frequently be managed without changing the regimen by prescribing antimotility, anti-emetic, or other medications that target specific symptoms. In other situations, modifying the dose interval (i.e., taking a lower dose more frequently during the day, as recommended by the manufacturer), may make it easier for people to stay on PEP.

All of the FDA-approved protease inhibitors have potentially serious drug interactions. Therefore, it is extremely important for healthcare workers to let their physicians know about all medications before a protease inhibitor is prescribed.

Voluntary Registry for PEP

Currently, only limited data are available on the side effects and toxicity of antiretroviral agents in people who are not HIV-infected. To learn more about the safety and outcomes associated with PEP, healthcare providers are encouraged to enroll all workers who receive PEP in a voluntary, anonymous registry. The registry is a collaborative effort among the CDC, Glaxo Wellcome Inc., and Merck and Co., Inc. The specific information requested in the registry includes the exposure, the antiretroviral agents being taken, abnormal laboratory findings, and physical symptoms associated with using these antiretroviral agents. Healthcare workers and providers can learn more about the registry by calling 1-888-PEP4HIV (1-888-737-4448).

Additional Information on Healthcare Worker Occupational Exposure

Information on HIV PEP is available from multiple sources. These include[9]:

1. The CDC's Web site at http://www.cdc.gov

2. The CDC's fax information service at 1-401-332-4565

3. The National AIDS Clearinghouse at 1-800-458-5231

4. The HIV/AIDS Treatment Information Service at 1-800-448-0440.

Clinicians can seek consultation on HIV PEP from the National Clinicians Postexposure Hotline at 1-888-448-4911.[1]

References

1. Centers for Disease Control and Prevention. Public Health Service guidelines for the management of healthcare worker exposures to HIV and recommendations for postexposure prophylaxis. *MMWR*. 1998; 47(RR-7):1-33.

2. Centers for Disease Control and Prevention. HIV/AIDS Surveillance Report. 1997;7(9): 15.

3. Hospital Infection Control Practices Advisory Committee, Centers for Disease Control and Prevention. Guideline for isolation precautions in hospitals, Part II. Recommendations for isolation precautions in hospitals. *Am J Infect Control*. 1996;24: 32-45.

4. Garner, J.S. Guideline for isolation precautions in hospitals. *Infect Control Hosp Epidemiol*. 1996;17:53-80.

5. Occupational Safety and Health Administration. Occupational exposure to bloodborne pathogens: Final rule. *Federal Register 1991* ;56:64004-64182.

6. Centers for Disease Control and Prevention. Evaluation of safety devices for preventing percutaneous injuries among healthcare workers during phlebotomy procedures: Minneapolis-St. Paul, New York City, and San Francisco, 1993-1995. *MMWR*. 1997;46:21-25.

7. Gallo, D.; George, J.R.; Fitchen, J.H.; Goldstein, A.S.; Hindahl, M.S. Evaluation of a system using oral mucosal transudate for HIV-1 antibody screening and confirmatory testing. *JAMA*. 1997;277:254-258.

8. Tokars, J.I.; Marcus, R.; Culver, D.H., et al. Surveillance of HIV infection and zidovudine use among healthcare workers after occupational exposure to HIV infected blood. *Ann Intern Med*. 1993;118:913-919.

9. Centers for Disease Control and Prevention. Case-control study of HIV seroconversion in healthcare workers after percutaneous exposure to HIV-infected blood: France, United Kingdom, and United States, January 1988-August 1994. *MMWR*. 1995; 44:929-933.

10. Sperling, R.S.; Shapiro, D.E.; Coombs, R.W., et al. Maternal viral load, zidovudine treatment, and the risk of transmission of human immunodeficiency virus type 1 from mother to infant. *N Engl J Med*. 1996;335: 1621-1629.

11. Ippolito, G.; Puro, V.; De Carli, G., The Italian Study Group on Occupational Risk of HIV Infection. The risk of occupational human immunodeficiency virus infection in healthcare workers. *Arch Intern Med*. 1993; 153:1451-1458.

12. Centers for Disease Control and Prevention. Public Health Service statement on management of occupational exposure to human immunodeficiency virus, including considerations regarding zidovudine post exposure use. *MMWR*. 1990;39(RR-1): 1-14.

13. Cardo, D.M.; Culver, D.H.; Cieselski, C.A., et al. A case-control study of HIV seroconversion in healthcare workers after percutaneous exposure. *N Engl J Med*. 1997; 337:1485-1490.

Chapter 48

"My Needle Stick"— A Nurse's Experience

From my earliest years, I was fascinated with nursing. Because one of my four sisters was born with spina bifida, hospital visits and operations were commonplace or my family. Studying nursing was a natural choice for me.

In 1992, I graduated with a BSN from York College of Pennsylvania. Deeply interested in critical care nursing, I jumped at an offer to work in the intensive care unit (ICU) of the Community Hospital of Lancaster (Pa.). Located in the heart of a rural area famous for its Amish community, the 206-bed facility was like home to me, especially because it was where I'd interned.

In May 1992, when I'd just turned 23, 1 began my career. Excited and confident, I felt prepared to meet the challenges of professional nursing. But nothing could have prepared me for what was to come.

In Harm's Way

On September 9, 1992, 1 was working the evening shift in the ICU when my supervisor was called to another unit. Then we suddenly received an admission from the outpatient clinic—an unusual admission route for us. What's more, we had no information on the patient, except that he was admitted for probable pneumonia. I worked with the clinic's nursing assistant and our day-shift supervisor to undress him, attach cardiac monitoring leads, and administer oxygen. The patient was semiconscious, withdrawn, and silent. Following procedure, I then prepared to insert an 18-gauge intravenous (I.V.) catheter. This was nothing new for me—I'd started more than 100 I.V. lines.

I found a good vein, cleaned the area, put on gloves, warned the patient, and inserted the needle and catheter. Then I began to withdraw the needle from the catheter. As I pulled it free, the patient suddenly moved his arm, knocking mine. The bloody, exposed needle I held in my right hand sank into my left palm.

I was alarmed but took time to finish connecting the intermittent-infusion device. At that point, I was more concerned about losing the I.V. site or allowing blood to escape than the needle stick.

I walked to the sink, took off my gloves-and saw blood. I washed my hands with soap and water and asked the day-shift supervisor what to do. It was my first needlestick injury.

Immediately, we began documenting the event, and I went to the emergency department (ED) for evaluation. About an hour later, my worst fears were confirmed: The patient was in the final stages of acquired immunodeficiency syndrome (AIDS). The ED physicians said my chances of seroconverting were about 0.4%, or 1 in 250. Those odds sounded okay to me. At the time, the physicians were much more concerned about potential exposure to hepatitis B and C. I hadn't yet completed my hepatitis B vaccination series and we didn't have recent lab tests on this patient.

I filled out various forms, got a baseline human immunodeficiency virus (HIV) test, and went back to work. A little shaken, I called my best friend and told her what had happened. She reminded me that the odds were in my favor. That evening I cried, but only a little.

Strange Symptoms

Later that week, my baseline test results showed I was HIV-negative. Maggie Huber, our employee health/infection-control nurse, said I should be retested at 6 weeks, 3 months, 6 months, and optionally at 1 year.

Meanwhile, colleagues stepped forward to comfort me, some telling me stories of their own exposures. A few confided that they'd skipped the 6-month or 1-year follow-up test; others said they'd never even reported their needle sticks.

Three weeks after the incident, I developed a sore throat, fever, and rash. The general practitioner I visited prescribed topical ointment and ordered tests for hepatitis, which came back negative.

The rash and other symptoms cleared up quickly. Feeling fine, I went back to work. Eight weeks after the needle stick, I developed abdominal pain, nausea, and vomiting. I was admitted to the hospital for an appendectomy. But my appendix was free from disease. The diagnosis? Extensive mesenteric lymphadenopathy, swelling of abdominal lymph nodes. I was worried about this finding, but my caregivers reassured me that the condition was probably related to a self-limiting virus, not my needle stick.

Meanwhile, my 6-week test came back HIV-negative. So after recovering from surgery, I again went back to my job. The pain and other symptoms resolved.

Having begun to put the needle stick behind me, I was thriving at work. What's more, my personal life had blossomed: I'd fallen in love with an air force sergeant named Tony. He knew that I'd been exposed to HIV through a needle stick and that all my tests had come back negative. He also understood that I needed several more tests to be absolutely sure I hadn't seroconverted.

When my 3-month test came back HIV-negative, we celebrated. We figured the remaining tests were just a formality. A few months later, Tony asked me to marry him, and I said yes.

Five Fateful Words

On April 7, 1993, 1 week after our engagement, I walked into the employee-health office to find out about my 6-month test. I took one look at Maggie's face and we both began to cry. "Lynda," she said, "you are HIV-positive." Those five words rang in my ears like a death sentence.

I don't remember much else about that day. I remember crying, feeling alone, and worrying that my fiancé would leave me. I felt suffocated, confused, and in a state of shock.

Since that day, my life has changed dramatically. I no longer work at the Community Hospital of Lancaster, having left in April 1994 on full disability. I'm not involved in direct patient care. Instead, I limit my dreams to those I can accomplish within a reasonable period.

I now fight chronic fatigue, night sweats, cervical dysplasia, hepatitis, fungal infections, and peripheral neuropathy. I've had three lengthy hospital stays, numerous invasive tests, and far too many blood draws. I've had therapy with many antiviral drugs, including a protease inhibitor.

I've officially crossed the boundary between "them" and "us." Now I'm truly an HIV-positive woman who depends on colleagues to care for me. I fear the possibility of debilitation and death before I reach my 40th birthday.

Days of Joy

Despite the trauma of HIV infection, however, I've had days of joy. One was May 13, 1994, when I married Tony, who has stood by me through it all and remains HIV-negative. Another was the day 2 years later when we finalized the adoption of our son, David. A third came this past Christmas, when we welcomed Ashley, only 4 days old, into our home.

For nurses and other health care professionals, my story highlights the need for continual education and awareness about occupational exposure to bloodborne pathogens from needle sticks. Over 800,000 accidental needle sticks occur in U.S. hospitals each year. Those involving patients infected with HIV or hepatitis pose the greatest danger when:

- the needles are hollow-bore, which can hold significant quantities of blood
- the needles have been placed directly into a vein or
- the injury is a deep puncture
- the source patient is in the end stage of disease.

Using these criteria, my chances of HIV seroconversion were much higher than 0.4%. My injury met all of these high-risk criteria; the source patient died 2 weeks after my needle stick.

The riskiest devices are I.V. catheter and blood-drawing devices. By using protected devices such as selfsheathing or retractable systems, you can reduce exposure—and thus transmission—80% to 90% of the time.

I suffered a needle-stick injury despite having followed all the recommended procedures for I.V. insertion. Even if I'd known the patient was HIV-positive, I wouldn't have done a thing differently. But I believe that if I'd been using a protected device, my injury would never have happened. To advocate for use of these devices, which are now widely available, I've founded the National Campaign for Health Care Worker Safety.

Dreams of the Future

Today, I've put aside my dream of advancing in nursing. Now I dream instead of creating safer workplaces where needle-stick injuries no longer occur. I also dream of the day when all people with HIV receive the compassion and support that I have. And I pray for an affordable, accessible AIDS cure for everyone.

Until then, I'll spread the message about safe devices to all who will listen. I'll hold my children tight and carefully choose the dreams I hold dear. And I'll kiss my husband tenderly and wish that everyone could have that kind of love to sustain them through the toughest of times.

The National Campaign for Health Care

Worker Safety: Setting a Higher Standard

The campaign's goals are to:

* generate awareness of the life-threatening risks associated with accidental needle sticks

* inform the health care industry about protected I.V. catheters and blood-drawing devices

* obtain a written commitment from every U.S. health care facility to use safer devices.

Launched in February 1996, the campaign plans to distribute a health care worker safety packet to all U.S. health care facilities. The packet includes a needle-stick fact sheet, descriptions of safety devices, a *New York Times* article about the campaign, a certificate that describes the dangers of occupational exposure to bloodborne pathogens, and a pledge of intent that the institution will begin using protected I.V. catherers and blood-drawing devices within 1 year of signing.

Part Seven

Additional Help and Information

Chapter 49

Glossary of Related Terms

A

Abdomen: The part of the body that contains the stomach, intestines, liver, reproductive organs, and other organs.

Abstinence: Refraining from sexual intercourse.

Acute: Refers to intense, short-term symptoms or illnesses that either resolve or evolve into long-lasting, chronic disease manifestations.

Acyclovir (Zovirax): An antiviral drug used in the treatment of herpes simplex virus 1 (fever blisters, cold sores), herpes simplex virus 2 (genital herpes) and herpes zoster (shingles). Acyclovir comes in the form of pills, ointment or injection. The drug functions as a nucleoside analog, but must be converted to an active (phosphated) form by the thymidine kinase enzyme produced only by cells infected by certain herpes viruses, including varicella zoster virus (shingles) and herpes simplex-1 and -2. Acyclovir causes few side effects—occasionally nausea, diarrhea or headaches. It is now available in a generic form.

AIDS (Acquired Immunodeficiency Syndrome): The late stage of the illness triggered by infection with human immunodeficiency virus (HIV). According to the official definition published by the CDC, a person receives an AIDS diagnosis when he or she has a CD4 (helper T-cell) count of less that 200 and/or certain opportunistic infections common with advanced immune deficiency.

AIDS Clinical Trials Group (ACTG): A network of medical centers around the country in which federally-funded clinical trials are conducted to test the safety and effectiveness of experimental treatments for AIDS and HIV infection. ACTG studies are sponsored by the National Institute of Allergy and Infectious Diseases (NIAID).

AIDS Dementia Complex: A frequent cerebral condition in people with AIDS that results in the loss of cognitive capacity, affecting the ability to function in a social or occupational setting. Its cause has not been determined exactly, but may result from HIV infection of cells in the brain or an inflammatory reaction to such infection.

Alternative Medicine: A catch-all phrase for a long list of treatments or medicinal systems including traditional systems such as Chinese medicine, homeopathy, various herbals and other miscellaneous treatments that have not been accepted by the mainstream, or Western, medical establishment. Alternative medicine is also referred to as complementary medicine. The designation "alternative medicine" is not equivalent to "holistic medicine," which is a more narrow term.

Antibody: A disease-fighting protein in the blood created by the immune system, also known as immunoglobulin. Antibodies coat, mark for immune destruction or render harmless foreign particles like bacteria, viruses or harmful toxins. Antibodies also tag infected cells, making them vulnerable to attack by the immune system. Each antibody attaches itself to a single specific chemical sequence on an antigen. Elements of the body's immune response, these substances circulate in the blood and in other bodily fluids to fight disease-causing microbes.

Antigen: A foreign substance, usually protein, such as a fragment of a virus or bacteria that stimulates an immune response with antibodies or other defenses. An antigen contains several subunits called epitopes that are targets of specific antibodies and cytotoxic T-lymphocytes.

Antiretroviral: A substance that stops or suppresses the activity of a retrovirus such as HIV. AZT, ddC, ddI and d4T are examples of antiretroviral drugs.

Asymptomatic: Without signs or symptoms of disease or illness.

Asymptomatic transmission of herpes: The spread of virus from one person to another during a period of asymptomatic shedding, i.e., the body sheds virus in the absence of symptoms.

Atrophy: A wasting or shrinking of cells, tissue, organs or muscle.

Autoinoculation of herpes simplex virus (HSV): The spread of HSV from one part of the body to another. This can result when a person with active herpes deposits a significant amount of virus onto some other vulnerable part of the body—most often a mucous membrane.

AZT (Retrovir, Zidovudine): A nucleoside analog used to slow replication of HIV. AZT is approved for the initial treatment of HIV infection. AZT is increasingly administered in combination with other antiviral drugs, especially 3TC (a combination that is under consideration by the FDA as another initial treatment regimen for HIV) as well as ddC (an FDA-approved combination for persons with progressive disease and CD4 cell counts below 300). Possible side effects include bone marrow suppression leading to anemia, leukopenia or neutropenia nausea, muscle weakness and headaches.

B

Bacterial STDs: Such as syphilis, gonorrhea and chlamydia respond effectively to antibiotic treatment, yet they remain epidemic in the population.

Bacterial Vaginosis (BV): The most prevalent cause of vaginal symptoms among women of childbearing age, BV, previously called nonspecific vaginitis, is characterized by a strong fishy odor and a gray, watery discharge.

Balanitis: Inflammation of the glans penis or clitoris.

Balanoposthitis: Inflammation of the glans penis and overlying prepuce.

B-Cell (B-Lymphocyte): A type of lymphocyte that is a precursor to plasma cells. During infections, individual B-cell clones multiply and are transformed into plasma cells, which produce large amounts of antibodies against a particular antigen on a foreign microbe. This transformation occurs through interaction with the appropriate CD4 T-helper cells.

bDNA (branched DNA): A test developed by the Chiron Corp. for measuring the amount of HIV (as well as other viruses) in blood plasma. The test uses a signal amplification technique, which creates a luminescent signal whose brightness depends on the viral RNA present. Test results are calibrated in numbers of virus particle equivalents per milliliter of plasma. bDNA is similar in results but not in technique to the PCR test.

Benign: Not cancerous; does not invade nearby tissue or spread to other parts of the body.

Bioavailability: The extent to which an oral medication is absorbed in the digestive tract and reaches the bloodstream.

Biological therapy: Treatment to stimulate or restore the ability of the immune system to fight infection and disease. Also called immunotherapy.

Biopsy: The removal of a sample of tissue that is then examined under a microscope to check for cancer cells.

Burkitt's Lymphoma: A cancerous tumor, frequently involving jaw bones, ovaries and abnormal lymph nodes. The disease is common in Africa and has been associated with Epstein-Barr virus.

C

Cancer: A term for diseases in which abnormal cells divide without control. Cancer cells can invade nearby tissues and can spread through the bloodstream and lymphatic system to other parts of the body.

Candida: A group of yeast-like fungi, in particular Candida albicans, that infect the mouth as well as other mucous membranes in the esophagus, intestines, vagina, throat and lungs. Oral or recurrent vaginal candida infection is an early sign of immune system deterioration.

Candidiasis: An infection due to candida yeast. The symptoms of oral candidiasis (thrush) and vaginal candidiasis (formerly called monilia) include pain, itching, redness and white patches in their respective sites. Some common treatments are clotrimazole, nystatin and miconazole.

Cauterization: The use of heat to destroy abnormal cells. Also called diathermy or electrodiathermy.

CD4: The protein structure on the surface of a human cell that allows HIV to attach, enter, and thus infect a cell. CD4 receptors are present on CD4 cells (helper T-cells), macrophages and dendritic cells, among others. Normally, CD4 acts as an accessory molecule, forming part of larger structures (such as the T-cell receptor) through which T-cells and other cells signal each other.

CD4 Cell: A type of T-cell involved in protecting against viral, fungal and protozoal infections. The CD4 cell modulates the immune response to an infection through a complex series of interactions with antigen presenting cells (macrophages, dendritic cells and B cells) and other types of lymphocytes (B-cells and CD8 cells). Other names for CD4 cell are T-helper cell or helper T-cell.

CD4 Cell Count: The most commonly used surrogate marker for assessing the state of the immune system. As CD4 cell count declines, the risk of developing opportunistic infections increases. The normal range for CD4 cell counts is 500 to 1500 per cubic millimeter of blood. CD4 count should be rechecked at least every six to twelve months if CD4s are greater than 500/mm3. If the count is lower, testing every three months is advised.

Cell culture: A diagnostic test for many kinds of viruses. In a cell culture for HSV, a swab of the patient's herpes lesion is placed in a dish containing normal skin cells to see if HSV will grow.

Cellular immune response: The portion of the body's immune response that involves T-lymphocytes or other cells designed to fight an "antigen" or invading microbe.

Centers for Disease Control and Prevention (CDC): The federal public health agency serving as the center for preventing, tracking, controlling and investigating the epidemiology of AIDS and other diseases.

Cervical Dysplasia: An abnormal tissue growth on the cervix, which may progress to cancer if not treated in time. Cervical dysplasia is detected through a Pap Smear.

Cervical Intraepithelial Neoplasia: A general term for the growth of abnormal cells on the surface of the cervix. Numbers from 1 to 3 may be used to describe how much of the cervix contains abnormal cells. Also called CIN.

Cervix: The lower, cylindrical end of the uterus that forms a narrow canal connecting the upper (uterus) and lower (vagina) parts of a women's reproductive tract.

Chancroid: A highly contagious sexually transmitted disease caused by the Hemophilus ducreyi bacterium. It appears as a pimple, chancre, sore or ulcer on the skin of the genitals. The lesion appears after an incubation period of three to five days and may facilitate the transmission of HIV.

Chlamydia: The fastest-spreading STD in the U.S., chlamydia infects as many as four million men and women each year. As many as 85 percent of cases in women and 40 percent of cases in men are symptomless. If undetected and untreated, chlamydia can lead to serious complications in women. Each year, chlamydia causes as many as half of the one million cases of pelvic inflammatory disease (PID), an infection of the female reproductive organs that can cause infertility and ectopic pregnancy. Infants born to mothers with chlamydia may be infected with chlamydial conjunctivitis or pneumonia. When symptoms are present, they usually appear within one to three weeks after sex with an infected partner. Symptoms include abnormal genital discharge and burning during urination. Women may experience lower abdominal pain if PID develops as a result of the chlamydia infection. Men may suffer swelling or pain in the testicles.

Clinical Trial: A study done to test an experimental medicine in human beings to see if it is safe and effective.

CMV (Cytomegalovirus): A herpes infection that causes serious illness in people with AIDS. CMV can develop in any part of the body but most often appears in the retina of the eye, the nervous system, the colon or the esophagus.

Cold sores: Otherwise known as "fever blisters" and herpes type-1 infection.

Condom: Male: A cover for the penis, worn during sex to prevent STDs and pregnancy. There is now a "female condom" that lines the vagina, which is worn by the woman during sex for similar protection. Condoms are highly effective at preventing STDs and pregnancy if used consistently and correctly.

Condyloma Acuminatum: A projecting warty growth on the external genitals or the anus caused by infection with certain types of the human papillomavirus (HPV). It is usually a benign or non-cancerous growth. Condyloma acuminatum is also referred to as genital warts or verruca acuminata.

Conization: Surgery to remove a cone-shaped piece of tissue from the cervix and cervical canal. Conization may be used to diagnose or treat a cervical condition. Also called cone biopsy.

Cryosurgery: Treatment performed with an instrument that freezes and destroys abnormal tissue.

Cyst: A sac or capsule filled with fluid.

Cystoscopy: A procedure in which the doctor inserts a lighted instrument into the urethra (the tube leading from the bladder to the outside of the body) to look at the bladder.

D

Dermatitis: Inflammation of the skin.

Diathermy: The use of heat to destroy abnormal cells. Also called cauterization or electrodiathermy.

Dilation and curettage: A minor operation in which the cervix is dilated (expanded) so that the cervical canal and tissue from the uterine lining can be scaped with a spoon-shaped instrument called a curette. Also called a D and C.

Disseminated infection: A herpes infection that spreads over a wider than usual area of the body, frequently afflicting internal organs.

Douching: Using water or a medicated solution to clean the vagina and cervix.

Dyspareunia: The medical term for painful sex.

Dysplasia: Abnormal changes or growth of cells and tissues.

Dysuria: Painful or difficult urination. Dysuria may be due to a STD.

E

Efficacy: Strength, effectiveness. The ability of a drug to control or cure an illness. Efficacy should be distinguished from activity, which is limited to a drug's immediate effects on the microbe triggering the disease.

ELISA (Enzyme-Linked ImmunoSorbent Assay): A diagnostic test utilizing an enzyme-labeled immunoreactant (antigen or antibody) and an immunosorbent (antigen or antibody bound to a solid support). The most common test used to detect the presence of HIV antibodies in the blood, which are indicative of ongoing HIV infection. One type of ELISA is the preliminary test for HIV antibodies (to detect HIV infection). A positive ELISA test result must be confirmed by another test called a Western Blot.

Endocervical curettage: The removal of tissue from the inside of the cervix using a spoon-shaped instrument called a curette.

Endometrium: The mucous membrane that lines the uterus.

Enzyme: A cellular protein whose shape allows it to hold together several other molecules in close proximity to each other. Enzymes in this way are able to induce chemical reactions in other substances with little expenditure of energy and without being changed itself.

Epidemiology: The branch of medical science that studies the incidence, distribution and control of disease in a population.

Epithelial: Refers to the cell linings covering most internal and external surfaces of the body and its organs.

Epstein-Barr Virus (EBV): A member of the herpesvirus family that causes one of two kinds of mononucleosis (the other is caused by CMV). It infects the nose and throat and is contagious. It lies dormant in the lymph glands and has been associated with Burkitt's lymphoma and oral hairy leukoplakia.

F

Fallopian tubes: Tubes on each side of the uterus through which an egg moves from the ovaries to the uterus.

Famciclovir (Famvir): A prodrug for an acyclovir-like active compound. It has especially high bioavailability and is an approved therapy for shingles. It also is under investigation for herpes simplex-2 (genital herpes).

FDA: The Food and Drug Administration, an agency of the United States Department of Health and Human Services that regulates the testing of experimental drugs and approves new medical products for marketing based on evidence of safety and efficacy.

First episode of herpes: The body's first encounter with a particular type of herpes simplex, an event that often produces marked symptoms. There are two types of "first episodes." A primary first episode describes the symptoms that appear in the person who has never been infected with either herpes simplex virus type 1 (HSV-1) or HSV-2 before. It's sometimes called a "true primary." A nonprimary first episode describes the symptoms that occur in the person who has been infected first with one type of HSV and then later infected with the second. For example, a person who is infected with HSV-1 and then years later infected with HSV-2 can be said to have a "first episode" of HSV-2 when he or she first has symptoms.

Fomite: An object, such as a towel, bicycle seat, or an article of clothing, that is not in itself harmful, but is able to harbor pathogenic microorganisms and thus may serve as an agent of transmission for an infection. Many people think fomites can spread STDs, but there are very few documented cases of fomite transmission of any STD.

Fungal Infection: A range of distinct diseases caused by fungi. Candidiasis, cryptococcosis and histoplasmosis are examples of AIDS-related fungal infections.

G

Ganglion: A knot-like grouping of the nerves that serve a particular part of the body.

Genital Ulcer Disease (GUD): Ulcerative lesions on the genitals, usually caused by a sexually transmitted condition such as herpes, syphilis or chancroid. The presence of genital ulcers may increase the risk of transmitting HIV.

Gonorrhea: An estimated 1.1 million American men and women each year contract gonorrhea. Many people who are infected show no signs of the disease. When symptoms are present, they are similar to those of chlamydia infections. They usually appear two to five days after sex with an infected partner and include burning during urination and discharge from the penis or vagina. Like chlamydia symptoms, gonorrhea symptoms can be so mild that they go unnoticed, particularly in women. Also like chlamydia, gonorrhea may cause pelvic inflammatory disease if left untreated, resulting in infertility or ectopic pregnancy. Gonorrhea can cause serious infections in infants who contract the disease from an infected mother during delivery. Complications of gonorrhea include arthritis.

Granuloma Inguinale: A sexually transmitted disease caused by *Calymmatobacterium granulomatis*. Causes ulcerated granulomatous lesions that occur in the inguinal regions and the genitalia.

Gynecologic oncologists: Doctors who specialize in treating cancers of the female reproductive organs.

Gynecology: The branch of medicine that involves care of the female reproductive system and breasts.

H

Hepatitis: Inflammation of the liver caused by microbes or chemicals. Often accompanied by jaundice, enlarged liver, fever, fatigue and nausea and high levels of liver enzymes in the blood.

Hepatitis A: A self-limiting virus-induced liver disease. Hepatitis A is acquired through ingesting fecally contaminated water or food or engaging in sexual practices involving anal contact. Injection drug users who share unclean needles also are at risk.

Hepatitis B: A virus-induced liver disease that infects approximately 200,000 Americans each year. The hepatitis B virus is found in blood, semen, vaginal secretions and saliva. This highly contagious virus is spread through sexual contact, sharing contaminated drug needles, blood transfusions, and piercing the skin with contaminated instruments. Many people with hepatitis B have no symptoms; others experience fever, headaches, muscle aches, fatigue, loss of appetite, vomiting and diarrhea. Hepatitis B may damage the liver, putting people at risk for cirrhosis and liver cancer. Most infections clear up by themselves within four to eight weeks. Some individuals (about 10% of the cases), however, become chronically infected. Hepatitis B is the only STD for which there is a vaccine. Although many public health officials recommend the vaccine for children, adolescents and young adults, it is not widely administered, due in part to the stigmatization of STDs and the cost of the three-part vaccine.

Hepatitis C: Another virus-induced liver disease. It appears to be more common among heterosexuals and injection drug users than hepatitis B.

Herpes: While "genital herpes" can cause symptoms in a variety of sites below the waist, the term is used to denote all HSV infection that is latent in the sacral ganglion, at the base of the spine. An estimated 40 million Americans have genital herpes, with 500,000 new cases each year. Approximately two-thirds of people who are infected do not know they have genital herpes, either because they have no symptoms or because their symptoms are so mild they go unnoticed. Symptoms of the first infection usually appear one to 26 days after exposure and last two to three weeks. Symptoms in the genital area include an itching or burning sensation, discharge and blisters or painful open sores. They are sometimes accompanied by flu-like symptoms such as swollen glands and fever. After the first infection, the virus can reactivate and cause new outbreaks of sores. The frequency and severity of recurrences vary from person to person.

Herpes encephalitis: A rare, severe illness that occurs when the brain becomes infected with HSV.

Herpes gladiatorum: The presence of herpes lesions on the body caused by HSV infection that is transmitted usually through the abrasion of skin in a contact sport, such as wrestling.

Herpes whitlow: The presence of herpes lesions on the fingers or toes.

Herpesvirus: Any one of eight known members of the human herpesvirus family that include: herpes simplex type 1 (HSV-1), herpes simplex type 2 (HSV-2), cytomegalovirus (CMV), Epstein-Barr virus (EBV), varicella zoster virus (VZV), human herpes virus type 6 (HHV-6), human herpes virus type 7 (HHV-7), and human herpes virus type 8 (HHV-8). Herpes simplex virus 1 (HSV-1) can cause painful "cold sores" or "fever blisters" on the lips, in the mouth or around the eyes; herpes simplex 2 (HSV-2) is usually transmitted sexually and generally causes lesions in the genital area or the anus.

HHV-6: A newly observed agent found in the blood cells (T lymphocytes) of a few patients with a variety of diseases affecting the immune system. This virus causes roseola infantum, a common childhood infection children under 4. Symptoms of roseola infantum include high fever and listlessness followed by a rash.

HHV-7: This virus has been identified in the laboratory, but has not been associated with any diseases to date. It infects T-cells, and genetically resembles HHV-6.

HHV-8: A recently recognized virus that has notable homology with several known herpesviruses. Detection of HHV-8 in peripheral blood mononuclear cells or HHV-8 antibody seroconversion is associated with an increased risk of developing Kaposi's sarcoma.

HIV/AIDS (Human Immunodeficiency Virus/Acquired Immune Deficiency Syndrome): The virus is spread through the blood, semen and vaginal secretions of an HIV-infected person. Both men and women can pass HIV to a sex partner. The virus can also be passed from person to person through sharing needles. HIV-infected women can pass the virus to their babies during pregnancy and childbirth. Some people contracted the virus through blood products before a successful screening process was begun in 1985. There is no evidence that HIV can spread through other body fluids such as saliva, feces, urine, tears and sweat. Currently, there is no way to get rid of the virus once a person is infected. However, medications can slow the damage that HIV causes to the immune system.

HIV-1: Human immunodeficiency virus type 1, the retrovirus recognized as the agent that induces AIDS.

HIV-2: Human immunodeficiency virus type 2, a virus closely related to HIV-1 that also leads to immune suppression. HIV-2 is not as virulent as HIV-1 and is epidemic only in West Africa.

Holistic (Wholistic) Medicine: Various systems of health protection and restoration, both traditional and modern, that are reputedly based on the body's natural healing powers, the various ways the different tissues affect each other and the influence of the external environment.

Hormone: An active chemical substance formed in the glands and carried in the blood to other parts of the body where it stimulates or suppresses cell and tissue activity.

HPV (Human PapillomaVirus): Human papillomavirus is one of the most common STDs. An estimated 40 million Americans are infected with HPV, with 1 million new cases each year. HPV is the name of a group of viruses that includes more than 80 different types. Certain types of HPV cause warts on the hands or feet, while others can cause genital warts on the vulva, vagina, anus, cervix, penis or scrotum. These may be raised or flat, single or multiple, small or large. Some cluster together; some can't be seen by the naked eye (subclinical infection). Often flesh-colored and painless, genital warts only rarely cause symptoms such as itching, pain or bleeding. HPV and genital warts are usually spread by direct, skin-to-skin contact during sex. Warts might appear within several weeks after sex with an infected person, they might take months to appear or they might never appear. Very little is known about the transmission of subclinical HPV infection. Other types of HPV (not the types that cause genital warts) are strongly linked to cervical cancer. Yearly Pap smears are recommended to detect the abnormal cell growth caused by HPV that may progress to cervical cancer. If detected in time, the progression of cervical HPV can be stopped, and even cervical cancer can usually be treated successfully.

HSV: Abbreviation for herpes simplex virus. HSV-1 denotes herpes simplex type 1, the usual cause of herpes around the mouth or face ("cold sores," "fever blisters"); HSV-2 denotes herpes simplex type 2, the usual cause of recurrent genital herpes.

Hysterectomy: An operation in which the uterus and cervix are removed.

Hysteroscopy: A surgical procedure in which a slender, light-transmitting telescope, the hysteroscope, is used to view the inside of the uterus or perform surgery.

I

Immune Deficiency: A breakdown or inability of certain parts of the immune system to function, thus making a person susceptible to certain diseases that they would have not contracted with a healthy immune system. Immune deficiencies may be temporary or permanent and be triggered by genetic mutation, therapy with immune-suppressive drugs (as during organ transplants) or an infection such as HIV.

Immune System: The body's complicated natural defense against disruption caused by invading microbes and cancers. There are two aspects of the immune system's response to disease: innate and acquired. The innate part of the response is mobilized very quickly in response to infection and does not depend on recognizing specific proteins or antigens foreign to an individual's normal tissue. It includes complement, macrophages, dendritic cells and granulocytes. The acquired, or learned, immune response arises when dendritic cells and macrophages present pieces of antigen to lymphocytes, which are genetically programmed to recognize very specific amino acid sequences. The ultimate result is the creation of cloned populations of antibody-producing B-cells and cytotoxic T-lymphocytes primed to respond to a unique pathogen.

Immunity: Protection against disease. Immunity can be achieved for hepatitis B through vaccination. Vaccines which can provide immunity from herpes and HPV are being tested.

Immunocompetent: Refers to an immune system capable of developing a normal protective response when confronted with invading microbes or cancer.

Immunocompromised: Refers to an immune system in which the response to infections and tumors is subnormal.

Immunosuppression: Weakening of the immune response that occurs with HIV infection as well as with some antiviral or anticancer treatments.

Immunotherapy: Treatment aimed at reconstituting an impaired immune system. Examples of experimental immunotherapies for AIDS include passive hyperimmune therapy (PHT), IL-2 and therapeutic vaccines.

Interferon: A type of biological therapy, treatment that can improve the body's natural response to disease. It slows the rate of growth and division of cancer cells, causing them to become sluggish and die.

In Vitro: Refers to laboratory experiments conducted in cell cultures grown in an artificial environment, for example in a test tube or culture plate.

J

Jargon: The technical or specialized language used in a profession or other field of activity. Health care providers often use medical jargon when discussing STDs. We hope this Sexual Health Glossary will make your conversations with your provider more productive.

K

Kaposi's Sarcoma (KS): An AIDS-defining illness consisting of individual cancerous lesions caused by an overgrowth of blood vessels.

KS typically appears as pink or purple painless spots or nodules on the surface of the skin or oral cavity. KS also can occur internally, especially in the intestines, lymph nodes and lungs, and in this case is life-threatening. There has been considerable speculation that KS is not a spontaneous cancer but is sparked by a virus. A species of herpes virus similar to Epstein-Barr virus is currently under extensive investigation. Up to now, KS has been treated with alpha interferon, radiation therapy (outside the oral cavity) and various systemic and intralesional cancer chemotherapies. KS frequently occurs in immuno-compromised patients, such as those with AIDS.

Killer Cell: A generalized name for immune system cells that kill cancerous and virus-infected cells. Among the killer cells are killer T-cells (cytotoxic T-lymphocytes), NK (natural killer) cells and K-cells.

L

Laparoscopy: A surgical procedure in which a slender, light-transmitting telescope, the laparoscope, is used to view the pelvic organs or perform surgery.

Laparotomy: A surgical procedure in which an incision is made in the abdomen.

Latency: The phenomenon by which disease (such as HSV or HPV) can hide away in the nerve roots in an inactive state, only to reactivate and cause viral shedding or symptoms again.

Lesion: A very general term denoting any abnormality on the surface of the body, whether on the skin or on a mucous membrane. Includes sores, wounds, injuries, pimples, tumors, on the skin or elsewhere.

Long-Term Nonprogressor: An individual who has been infected with HIV for at least seven to twelve years (different authors use different timespans) and yet retains a CD4 cell count within the normal range.

Lubricant: A slippery substance. Can be oil- or water-based. A vaginal lubricant may be helpful for women who feel pain during intercourse because of vaginal dryness. If using a lubricant with latex condoms, use one that is water-based, as oil can weaken the latex.

Lymph: The almost colorless fluid that travels through the lymphatic system and carries cells that help fight infections and other diseases.

Lymph Node (Lymph Gland): Small bean-shaped organs made up mostly of lymphocytes, lymph fluid and connective tissue. Clusters of lymph nodes are widely distributed in the body and are essential to the functioning of the immune system. They are connected with each other and other lymphoid tissue by the lymphatic vessels.

Lymphadenopathy: Swelling or enlargement of the lymph nodes due to infection or cancer. The swollen nodes may be palpable or visible from outside the body.

Lymphocyte: White blood cells that mature and reside in the lymphoid organs and are responsible for the acquired immune response. The two major types of lymphocytes are T-cells and B-cells.

M

MAC (Mycobacterium Avium Complex): A serious opportunistic infection caused by two similar bacteria (Mycobacterium avium and Mycobacterium intercellulare) found in the soil and dust particles. In AIDS, MAC can spread through the bloodstream to infect lymph nodes, bone marrow, liver, spleen, spinal fluid, lungs and intestinal tract. Typical symptoms of MAC include night sweats, weight loss, fever, fatigue, diarrhea and enlarged spleen. MAC is usually found in people with CD4 counts below 100. MAC is also called MAI.

Maintenance Therapy: Extended drug therapy, usually at a diminished dose, administered after a disease has been brought under control. Maintenance therapy is utilized when a complete cure is not possible, and a disease is likely to recur if therapy is halted.

Malabsorption: Inability of the intestines to absorb food, drug or any substance needed to maintain good health.

Mammogram: An X-ray of the breast, used to detect breast cancer.

Manifestation: The outward sign that an illness is present: a symptom or condition.

Memory T-Cell: A T-cell that bears receptors for a specific foreign antigen encountered during a prior infection or vaccination. After an infection or a vaccination, some of the T-cells that participated in the response remain as memory T-cells, which can rapidly mobilize and clone themselves should the same antigen be re-encountered during a second infection at a later time.

Menarche: The time in a young woman's life when menstrual periods begin.

Menopause: The time in a women's life when menstrual periods stop. Also called the "change of life."

Menstruation: The periodic discharge of bloody fluid from the uterus occurring at more or less regular intervals during the life of a woman from age of puberty to menopause.

Microbe: A microscopic living organism, such as a bacteria, fungus, protozoa or virus. Moisture barrier: A material, usually latex, used during sexual activity to prevent sexual fluids or blood from passing between people. In addition to condoms for sexual intercourse, moisture barriers for oral sex include household plastic wrap or "dams," such as the SheerGlyde Dam.

Molluscum Contagiosum: A skin condition caused by a pox virus infection, distinguished by small dome-shaped papules (bumps) on the face, upper trunk or extremities. Current treatment is mainly cosmetic. It often involves application of liquid nitrogen to the papules as a means of excising them.

Myopathy: Progressive muscle weakness. Myopathy may arise as a toxic reaction to AZT or as a consequence of HIV infection itself.

N

Neoplasia: Abnormal new growth of cells.

NGU (NonGonococcal Urethritis): Urethritis, manifested by urethral discharge, painful urination, or itching at the end of the urethra, is the response of the urethra to inflammation NOT due to gonococcal infection.

NIAID (National Institute of Allergy and Infectious Diseases): The federal agency that is responsible for a great deal of the government-sponsored AIDS research. NIAID is a branch of the NIH.

NIH (National Institutes of Health): The federal agency responsible for overseeing government-sponsored biomedical research. It is divided into 24 institutes and research centers.

Nucleoside Analog: A type of antiviral drug, such as AZT, ddI, ddC or d4T, whose makeup constitutes a defective version of a natural nucleoside. Nucleoside analogs may take the place of the natural nucleosides, blocking the completion of a viral DNA chain during infection of a new cell by HIV. The HIV enzyme reverse transcriptase is more likely to incorporate nucleoside analogs into the DNA it is constructing than is the DNA polymerase normally used for DNA creation in cell nuclei.

O

Obstetrician-Gynecologist: A physician with special skills, training and education in women's health.

Obstetrics: The branch of medicine that involves care of a woman during pregnancy, during labor and delivery, and after childbirth.

Ocular herpes: Herpes infection in the eyes.

Opportunistic Infections (OI): Infections that occur in persons with weak immune systems due to AIDS, cancer or immunosuppressive drugs such as corticosteroids or chemotherapy. PCP, toxoplasmosis and cytomegalovirus are all examples of OIs.

Oral-facial herpes: The presence of latent herpes simplex infection in the trigeminal ganglion, at the top of the spine. When reactiviated, oral-facial herpes can cause symptoms anywhere on mouth or face: typically cold sores on the lips. Recurrent oral-facial herpes is largely caused by HSV-1.

Oral Hairy Leukoplakia (OHL): A whitish lesion that appears on the side of the tongue and inside cheeks. The lesion appears raised, with a ribbed or "hairy" surface. OHL occurs mainly in people with declining immunity and may be caused by Epstein-Barr virus infection.

P

Pap Test: A way to examine cells collected from the cervix and vagina. This test can show the presence of infection, inflammation, abnormal cells, or cancer. Also called a Pap smear.

Papillomavirus: The virus group that includes the cause of genital warts or condylomata.

Pathologist: A doctor who identifies diseases by studying cells and tissues under a microscope.

PCR (Polymerase Chain Reaction) Test: A very sensitive test that measures the presence or amount of RNA or DNA of a specific organism or virus (for example, HIV or CMV) in the blood or tissue.

Pelvic Inflammatory Disease (PID): A gynecological condition caused by an infection (usually sexually transmitted) that spreads from the vagina to the upper parts of a women's reproductive tract in the pelvic cavity. PID takes different courses in different women, but can cause abscesses and constant pain almost anywhere in the genital tract. If left untreated, it can cause infertility or more frequent periods. Severe cases may even spread to the liver and kidneys causing dangerous internal bleeding, lung failure and death.

Perinatal Transmission: Transmission of a pathogen, such as HIV, from mother to baby during birth.

Peripheral Neuropathy: A condition characterized by sensory loss, pain, muscle weakness and wasting of muscle in the hands or legs and feet. It may start with burning or tingling sensations or numbness in the toes and fingers. In severe cases, paralysis may result. Peripheral neuropathy may arise from an HIV-related condition or be the side effect of certain drugs.

Peyronie's disease: A disease of unknown cause in which there are strands of dense fibrous tissue surrounding the corpus cavernosum of the penis, causing deformity and painful erection. Also known as penile fibromatosis.

PID (Pelvic Inflammatory Disease): A serious infection of the upper genital tract in women. It often damages the fallopian tubes, making it difficult or impossible for a woman to have children. Often there are no symptoms. If there are symptoms, they may include dull pain or tenderness in the lower abdomen, abnormal periods, abnormal vaginal discharge, nausea and/or vomiting, fever and chills.

Placebo: A comparison substance against which experimental drugs are sometimes compared. A placebo may be either a standard treatment or an inactive substance. In placebo-controlled trials the control group takes placebo, while the test group takes an experimental drug. Many such studies are also double-blinded, which means that neither doctors nor patients know who is receiving drug or placebo.

Precancerous: Not cancerous, but may become cancerous with time.

Prevention: Not having sex (abstinence) is the best way to prevent STDs.

Primary HIV Infection: The flu-like syndrome that occurs immediately after a person contracts HIV. This initial infection precedes seroconversion and is characterized by fever, sore throat, headache, skin rash and swollen glands. Also called acute infection.

Prodrome: An early warning symptom of illness. (i.e., prodrome for a genital herpes outbreak often involves an aching, burning, itching, or tingling sensation in the genital area, buttocks, or legs).

Prognosis: The probable outcome or future course of disease in a patient; the chance of recovery.

Protease: An enzyme that triggers the breakdown of proteins. HIV's protease enzyme breaks apart long strands of viral protein into the separate proteins making up viral core. The enzyme acts as new virus particles are budding off a cell membrane.

Protease Inhibitor: A drug that binds to and blocks HIV protease from working, thus preventing the production of new infectious viral particles.

R

Rash: A general term applied to any eruption of the skin, especially those pertaining to communicable diseases. A rash is usually a shade of red, which varies with disease and is usually temporary.

Rectum: The last 6 to 8 inches of the large intestine. The rectum stores solid waste until it leaves the body through the anus.

Recurrence: The return of symptoms after a remission (time without symptoms). An example of this is outbreaks of herpes after periods of time without herpes lesions.

Reiter's syndrome: A group of symptoms which appear as a complication of nonspecific urethritis. Symptoms include urethritis, arthritis, and conjunctivitis.

Reproductive system: In women, the organs that are directly involved in producing eggs and in conceiving and carrying babies.

Resectoscope: A slender telescope with an electrical wire loop or rollerball tip used to remove or destroy tissue inside the uterus.

Retrovirus: A type of virus that, when not infecting a cell, stores its genetic information on a single-stranded DNA. HIV is an example of a retrovirus. After a retrovirus penetrates a cell, it constructs a DNA version of its genes using a special enzyme, reverse transcriptase. This DNA then becomes part of the cell's genetic material.

Reverse Transcriptase (RT): A viral enzyme that constructs DNA from an RNA template, which is an essential step in the life-cycle of a retrovirus such as HIV.

Risk factor: Something that increases the chance of developing a disease.

Roseola: Skin condition marked by red spots of varying sizes on the skin. Measles or German measles.

S

Schiller Test: A test in which iodine is applied to the cervix. The iodine colors healthy cells brown; abnormal cells remain unstained, usually appearing white or yellow.

Seroconversion: Development of detectable antibodies to HIV in the blood serum as a result of infection. It may take several months or more after HIV transmission for antibodies to the virus to develop. After antibodies to HIV appear in the blood, a person will test positive in the standard ELISA test for HIV.

Serology: A test that identifies the antibodies in serum (a clear fluid that is a component of the blood).

Seroprevalence: For HIV, the rate at which a given population tests positive on the ELISA test for HIV antibodies. The seroprevalence rate is nearly the same as the rate of HIV infection in a given population, leaving out mainly those who were recently infected.

Serostatus: The condition of having or not having detectable antibodies to a particular microbe in the blood as a result of infection: for example, HSV-1, HSV-2, or HIV. One may have either a positive or negative serostatus.

Shingles: A skin condition caused by reactivation of a Varicella zoster virus (VZV) infection, usually acquired in childhood (when it appears as chicken pox). It consists of painful, inflammatory blisters on the skin that follow the path of individual peripheral nerves. The blisters generally dry and scab, leaving minor scarring. Standard treatment is with famciclovir or acyclovir.

Side Effects: Problems that occur when treatment affects healthy cells. For example, common side effects of cancer treatment are fatigue, nausea, vomiting, decreased blood cell counts, hair loss, and mouth sores.

Spermicide: An agent which kills spermatozoa.

Staging: Doing exams and tests to learn the extent of the cancer, especially whether it has spread from its original site to other parts of the body.

STD (Sexually Transmitted Disease): Any infection that is acquired through sexual contact in a substantial number of cases.

Stomatitis: Inflammation of the mucous membranes in the mouth.

Surrogate Marker: A laboratory measurement of biological activity within the body that indirectly indicates the effect of treatment on disease state. CD4 cell counts and viral load are examples of surrogate markers in HIV infection.

Symptomatic reactivation: The presence of lesions or any other symptoms caused by reactivation of HSV; a "recurrence."

Syphilis: There are an estimated 120,000 new cases of syphilis in the U.S. each year. Syphilis progresses in three stages, with the earliest symptoms appearing in 10 days to three weeks after sex with an infected partner. A painless sore (chancre) may appear on the genitals or in the vagina. Second-stage symptoms include a skin rash and flu-like symptoms. The infection remains even after these symptoms disappear. If left untreated, syphilis lapses into the latent stage, during which it is not contagious and has no symptoms. About one-third of people who reach this stage will develop the severe complications of late, or tertiary, syphilis, which can result in mental illness, blindness, heart disease and death.

Systemic: Concerning or affecting the body as a whole. A systemic therapy is one that the entire body is exposed to, rather than just the target tissues affected by a disease.

T

T-Cell (T-Lymphocyte): Any lymphocyte that matures in the thymus.

Teratogenicity: The ability to cause defects in a developing fetus. This is distinct from mutagenicity, which causes genetic mutations in sperms, eggs or other cells. Teratogenicity is a potential side effect of many drugs, such as thalidomide.

Testosterone: A naturally occurring male hormone. When administered as a drug it can cause gain in lean body mass, increased sex drive and possibly aggressive behavior. Many men with HIV have low testosterone levels.

Therapeutic Vaccine: An injected therapy consisting of synthetic HIV antigen that is administered to people who already have HIV. It is supposed to heighten and broaden the immune response to HIV, helping to halt disease progression.

Toxoplasmosis: A disease caused by the protozoa *Toxoplasma gondii*. Toxoplasmosis can affect a number of organs, but it most commonly causes encephalitis (brain inflammation).

Transmission: The spread of disease, including a sexually transmitted disease, from one person to another.

Trichomoniasis: An infection with a flagellated protozoan, *Trichomonas vaginalis*. When symptomatic, the infection results in vaginitis in women and urethritis in men. There are an estimated 3 million new cases of trichomoniasis each year. Many infected persons, however, remain asymptomatic.

Trigger (factor): Any biologic or behavioral event that influences latent HSV to reactivate.

U

Ultrasonography: A test in which sound waves (called ultrasound) are bounced off tissues and the echoes are converted into a picture (sonogram).

Ultrasound: A test in which sound waves are used to examine internal structures. During pregnancy, it can be used to examine the fetus.

Ureaplasma: A genus of bacteria found in the human genitourinary tract, occasionally in the pharynx and rectum. In males, they are associated with nongonococcal urethritis (NGU) and prostatitis; in females, with genitourinary tract infections and reproductive failure.

Urethritis: Inflammation of the urethra. STDs, if they are symptomatic, often cause urethritis.

Uterus: The small, hollow pear-shaped organ in a woman's pelvis. This is the organ in which an unborn child develops. Also called the womb.

V

Vaccine: A suspension of infectious agents or some part of them, given for the purpose of establishing resistance to an infectious disease. It stimulates development of specific defensive mechanisms in the body which result in more or less permanent protection against a disease.

Vagina: The muscular canal between the uterus and the outside of the body.

Vaginitis: Inflammation of the female vagina.

Varicella Zoster Virus (VZV): The cause of chicken pox in children. Its reactivation in adults causes shingles.

Viral Load: The number of viral particles (usually HIV) in a sample of blood plasma. HIV viral load is increasingly employed as a surrogate marker for disease progression. It is measured by PCR and bDNA tests and is expressed in number of HIV copies or equivalents per milliliter.

Viral STDs: Viral STDs, including genital herpes, human papillomavirus (HPV), hepatitis B, and HIV (the cause of AIDS): are as yet incurable.

Viruses: Small living particles (much smaller than bacteria) that can infect cells and change how the cells function. Infection with a virus can cause a person to develop symptoms. A virus is a noncellular entity composed merely of genetic material (DNA or RNA) surrounded by a protein envelope. Viruses can reproduce only within living cells into which they inject their genetic material. The viral genes then subvert an infected cell's normal chemical processes to create new virus particles, usually killing the cell in the process. The disease and symptoms that are caused depend on the type of virus and the type of cells that are infected.

W

Wart: A raised growth on the surface of the skin or other organ.

Wasting Syndrome: A condition characterized by loss of ten percent of normal weight without obvious cause. The weight loss is largely the result of depletion of the protein in lean body mass and represents a metabolic derangement frequent during AIDS.

Western Blot: A test for detecting the specific antibodies to HIV in a person's blood. It commonly is used to double-check positive ELISA tests. A western blot test is more reliable that the ELISA, but it is harder to do and costs more money.

Whitlow: Herpes infection on the fingers or toes.

Womb: The uterus.

Wrestler's herpes: The presence of herpes lesions on the body caused by HSV infection that is usually transmitted through the abrasion of skin during a contact sport, such as wrestling. Also known as herpes gladitorum.

X

X chromosome: The chromosome that determines that female sex characteristics will develop in an individual. In the normal female there are two X chromosomes and in the male only one.

Xeroderma: roughness and dryness of the skin, mild ichthyosis, *X. pigmentosum*, Kaposi's Sarcoma.

Y

Y chromosome: One of a pair of chromosomes (X and Y) which is present in fetuses which have male sexual characteristics.

Z

Zoster: Acute inflammatory disease with vesicles grouped in the course of cutaneous nerves, as in herpes zoster.

Chapter 50

Resources for STD Information

Alan Guttmacher Institute
120 Wall Street, 21st floor
New York, NY 10005
Phone: (212) 248-1111
Fax: (212) 248-1951

or

1120 Connecticut Avenue, N.W.
Suite 460
Washington, D.C. 20036
Phone: (202) 296-4012
Fax: (202) 223-5756
E-mail: info@agi-usa.org
Website: http://www.agi-usa.org

Numerous materials available including articles, brochures and comprehensive information on sexual behavior, birth, pregnancy prevention and contraception, and STDs.

Website covers multiple topics in sexual health.

American Medical Women's Association
801 North Fairfax Street
Suite 400
Alexandria, VA 22314
Phone: (703) 838-0500
Website: http://www.amwa-doc.org

Offers a wide range of materials on women's health topics, a comprehensive list of recommended books for the public and profession, and position papers on health issues, including reproductive health, osteoporosis, and menopause.

American Social Health Association
P.O. Box 13827
Research Triangle Park, NC 27709
Toll Free: (800) 277-8922
Phone: (919) 361-8400
Fax: (919) 361-8425
Website: http://www.ashastd.org

Free and confidential written STD information from Web site on variety of topics including genital herpes, and HPV.

Education materials on prevention of STDs and their harmful consequences to individuals, families, and communities.

Information about hotlines and public advocacy groups are available.

Association of Reproductive Health Professionals
2401 Pennsylvania Ave NW
Suite 350
Washington, D.C. 20037
Phone: (202) 466-3825
Fax: (202) 466-3826
Email: arhp@aol.com
Website: http://www.arhp.org

Provides information about HIV/AIDS prevention and options for birth control and STD prevention.

Educational materials available on family planning, contraceptives, and other reproductive health issues, including STDs, HIV, urogenital disorders, menopause, sexual health and infertility.

CME-accredited programs available to professionals.

Centers for Disease Control and Prevention
National Center for HIV, STD & TB Prevention
1600 Clifton Road NE
Atlanta, GA 30333
Website: http://www.cdc.gov/nchstp/od/nchstp.html

Brochures, pamphlets and other aids available on the prevention of STDs, including HIV, complications of these diseases, infertility, adverse outcomes of pregnancy, and reproductive tract cancer.

Web site lists national STD prevention training centers.

Family Health International
P.O. Box 13950
Research Triangle Park, NC 27709
Phone: (919) 544-7040
Fax: (919) 544-7261
Website: http://www.fhi.org

Brochures, pamphlets, and booklets are available on AIDS/HIV, STDs, family planning, reproductive health and women's studies.

Web pages available in English, Spanish, French, and Russian.

Comprehensive list of links to other Web sites on reproductive health.

National Institute of Allergy and Infectious Diseases
National Institutes of Health
NIAID Office of Communications
Building 31, Room 7A-50
31 Center Drive MSC 2520
Bethesda, MD 20892-2520 USA
Phone: (301) 402-1663
Fax: (301) 907-0878
E-mail: ocpostoffice@flash.niaid.nih.gov
Website: http://www.niaid.nih.gov

Provides information on a wide variety of topics including STDs, HIV/ AIDS.

Brochures and written materials available.

Extensive links to other Web sites for authoritative information.

National Women's Health Resource Center
120 Albany St., Suite 820
New Brunswick, NJ 08901
Phone: (877) 986-9472
Fax: (732) 249-4671
Website: http://www.healthywomen.org

Information available on contraception options, STDs, adolescent sexual health, hormone replacement therapy fact sheets, breast cancer, breast health.

Newsletter may be purchased.

Planned Parenthood Federation of America
810 Seventh Ave
New York, NY 10019
Phone: (800) 829-7732
Chapter locations: 800-230-PLAN
Website: http://www.plannedparenthood.org

Publications available from local chapters to public on contraception and STDs.

Information is free or at nominal charge.

Toll-free numbers to make appointments at clinic sites are available on the Web site.

Sexuality Information and Education Council of the United States
130 West 42nd St
Suite 350
New York, NY 10036
Phone: (212) 819-9770
Fax: (212) 819-9776
Website: http://www.siecus.org

Publications focus on comprehensive sexuality, with information available for young, middle-aged and older adults.

Fact sheets on STDs.

Information available on sexual education in public schools.

Hotlines

ASHA Resource Center
(800) 230-6039

CDC National STD Hotline
(800) 227-8922
(Mon-Fri, 8am-11pm, EST)

Provides anonymous, confidential information on sexually transmitted diseases (STD) and how to prevent them. Also, provides referrals to clinical and other services.

National Herpes Hotline
(919) 361-8488

National HIV/AIDS Hotline
(800) 342-AIDS

WebLink Resources

American Social Health Association
http://www.ashastd.org

Institute of Medicine
The Hidden Epidemic: Confronting STDs
http://books.nap.edu/html/epidemic/

National STD/HIV Prevention Training Center Network
http://www.stdptc.uc.edu

Index

Index

Page numbers followed by 'n' indicate a footnote. Page numbers in *italics* indicate a table or illustration.

A

cardiovascular syphilis 283
  see also syphilis
Carpenter, Betsy 142n
Carson, Sylvia 204n
cauterization, defined 471
CBC *see* complete blood count
CD4 cells 37, 152–53, 379, 453
  count, defined 471
  defined 471
  pediatric HIV infection 187
CDC *see* Centers for Disease Control
  and Prevention
cefotetan 258
cefoxitin 258, 260
ceftriaxone 89, 93, 258, 260, 261, 320
  syphilis treatment 280, 290
cell culture, defined 471
cellular immune response, defined 471
Celsus, Aulus Cornelius 128
Center for AIDS Prevention Studies
  179
Center for Biologics Evaluation and
  Research 395n, 396
Center for Health Promotion and Disease Prevention 444
Centers for Disease Control and Prevention (CDC)
  adolescents and STDs 403
  Advisory Committee on Immuniza-
    tion Practices 421
  AIDS in older adults 171, 176
  AZT therapy 432
  cervical cancer screening 381n
  chancroid 47n, 315
  chlamydia
    drug treatment 61
    infection 52, 56
    screening 55, 57, 58, 64
  clinical prevention guidelines 305n
  contact information 495
  defined 471
  donovanosis 81n
  Faculty Expansion Program 327
  genital herpes
    medications 320
    pregnancy 140n
  gonorrhea 92
    statistics 29
    symptoms 6

Centers for Disease Control and Prevention (CDC), continued
  health care worker occupational ex-
    posure 456
  hepatitis A 100n
    vaccine 25
  hepatitis B 108n
  hepatitis C 110n
    tests 377
  hepatitis D 121n
  hepatitis E 123n
  HIV 194n
    breastfeeding 435
    infection 150, 152, 156
    testing 392
    treatment, children 188
    women 158
  HIV/AIDS statistics 28
  lymphogranuloma venereum 229n
  maternal infant transmission 184
  National HIV Hotline 5, 38, 188, 497
  occupational exposures 449
  partner notification 22
  PEP registry 455
  PID 254n, 263, 266, 268, 269
  pre-exposure immunization 24
  pregnancy concerns 368
  pubic lice 84n
  resources for STD information 493n
  STD/HIV Prevention Training Cen-
    ters 327
  STDs 323
    guidelines 16, 17, 18, 264, 365
    non-sexual transmission 352
    older adults 40, 42
    pregnancy 427n
    treatment 208, 264, 366
  STD Treatment Guidelines 429
  syphilis 274n, 291
    control 292
    eradication 11
    pregnancy 288n
    statistics 31
  syringe exchange programs 357
  trichomoniasis 294n, 295, 296
  urethra inflammation 246n
  vaccine-preventable STDs 343n
  vaginal infection complications 300
  workplace safety 448

X

Y

Z

Health Reference Series
COMPLETE CATALOG

AIDS Sourcebook, 1st Edition

Basic Information about AIDS and HIV Infection, Featuring Historical and Statistical Data, Current Research, Prevention, and Other Special Topics of Interest for Persons Living with AIDS

Along with Source Listings for Further Assistance

Edited by Karen Bellenir and Peter D. Dresser. 831 pages. 1995. 0-7808-0031-1. $78.

"One strength of this book is its practical emphasis. The intended audience is the lay reader . . . useful as an educational tool for health care providers who work with AIDS patients. Recommended for public libraries as well as hospital or academic libraries that collect consumer materials."
— *Bulletin of the Medical Library Association, Jan '96*

"This is the most comprehensive volume of its kind on an important medical topic. Highly recommended for all libraries."   — *Reference Book Review, '96*

"Very useful reference for all libraries."
— *Choice, Association of College and Research Libraries, Oct '95*

"There is a wealth of information here that can provide much educational assistance. It is a must book for all libraries and should be on the desk of each and every congressional leader. Highly recommended."
— *AIDS Book Review Journal, Aug '95*

"Recommended for most collections."
— *Library Journal, Jul '95*

AIDS Sourcebook, 2nd Edition

Basic Consumer Health Information about Acquired Immune Deficiency Syndrome (AIDS) and Human Immunodeficiency Virus (HIV) Infection, Featuring Updated Statistical Data, Reports on Recent Research and Prevention Initiatives, and Other Special Topics of Interest for Persons Living with AIDS, Including New Antiretroviral Treatment Options, Strategies for Combating Opportunistic Infections, Information about Clinical Trials, and More

Along with a Glossary of Important Terms and Resource Listings for Further Help and Information

Edited by Karen Bellenir. 751 pages. 1999. 0-7808-0225-X. $78.

"Highly recommended."
— *American Reference Books Annual, 2000*

"Excellent sourcebook. This continues to be a highly recommended book. There is no other book that provides as much information as this book provides."
— *AIDS Book Review Journal, Dec-Jan 2000*

"Recommended reference source."
— *Booklist, American Library Association, Dec '99*

"A solid text for college-level health libraries."
— *The Bookwatch, Aug '99*

Cited in *Reference Sources for Small and Medium-Sized Libraries, American Library Association, 1999*

Alcoholism Sourcebook

Basic Consumer Health Information about the Physical and Mental Consequences of Alcohol Abuse, Including Liver Disease, Pancreatitis, Wernicke-Korsakoff Syndrome (Alcoholic Dementia), Fetal Alcohol Syndrome, Heart Disease, Kidney Disorders, Gastrointestinal Problems, and Immune System Compromise and Featuring Facts about Addiction, Detoxification, Alcohol Withdrawal, Recovery, and the Maintenance of Sobriety

Along with a Glossary and Directories of Resources for Further Help and Information

Edited by Karen Bellenir. 635 pages. 2000. 0-7808-0325-6. $78.

SEE ALSO *Drug Abuse Sourcebook, Substance Abuse Sourcebook*

Allergies Sourcebook

Basic Information about Major Forms and Mechanisms of Common Allergic Reactions, Sensitivities, and Intolerances, Including Anaphylaxis, Asthma, Hives and Other Dermatologic Symptoms, Rhinitis, and Sinusitis

Along with Their Usual Triggers Like Animal Fur, Chemicals, Drugs, Dust, Foods, Insects, Latex, Pollen, and Poison Ivy, Oak, and Sumac; Plus Information on Prevention, Identification, and Treatment

Edited by Allan R. Cook. 611 pages. 1997. 0-7808-0036-2. $78.

Alternative Medicine Sourcebook

Basic Consumer Health Information about Alternatives to Conventional Medicine, Including Acupressure, Acupuncture, Aromatherapy, Ayurveda, Bioelectromagnetics, Environmental Medicine, Essence Therapy, Food and Nutrition Therapy, Herbal Therapy, Homeopathy, Imaging, Massage, Naturopathy, Reflexology, Relaxation and Meditation, Sound Therapy, Vitamin and Mineral Therapy, and Yoga, and More

Edited by Allan R. Cook. 737 pages. 1999. 0-7808-0200-4. $78.

"Recommended reference source."
— *Booklist, American Library Association, Feb '00*

■

Alzheimer's, Stroke & 29 Other Neurological Disorders Sourcebook, 1st Edition

Basic Information for the Layperson on 31 Diseases or Disorders Affecting the Brain and Nervous System, First Describing the Illness, Then Listing Symptoms, Diagnostic Methods, and Treatment Options, and Including Statistics on Incidences and Causes

Edited by Frank E. Bair. 579 pages. 1993. 1-55888-748-2. $78.

SEE ALSO Brain Disorders Sourcebook

■

Alzheimer's Disease Sourcebook, 2nd Edition

Basic Consumer Health Information about Alzheimer's Disease, Related Disorders, and Other Dementias, Including Multi-Infarct Dementia, AIDS-Related Dementia, Alcoholic Dementia, Huntington's Disease, Delirium, and Confusional States

Along with Reports Detailing Current Research Efforts in Prevention and Treatment, Long-Term Care Issues, and Listings of Sources for Additional Help and Information

Edited by Karen Bellenir. 524 pages. 1999. 0-7808-0223-3. $78.

Arthritis Sourcebook

Basic Consumer Health Information about Specific Forms of Arthritis and Related Disorders, Including Rheumatoid Arthritis, Osteoarthritis, Gout, Polymyalgia Rheumatica, Psoriatic Arthritis, Spondyloarthropathies, Juvenile Rheumatoid Arthritis, and Juvenile Ankylosing Spondylitis

Along with Information about Medical, Surgical, and Alternative Treatment Options, and Including Strategies for Coping with Pain, Fatigue, and Stress

Edited by Allan R. Cook. 550 pages. 1998. 0-7808-0201-2. $78.

■

Asthma Sourcebook

Basic Consumer Health Information about Asthma, Including Symptoms, Traditional and Nontraditional Remedies, Treatment Advances, Quality-of-Life Aids, Medical Research Updates, and the Role of Allergies, Exercise, Age, the Environment, and Genetics in the Development of Asthma

Along with Statistical Data, a Glossary, and Directories of Support Groups, and Other Resources for Further Information

Edited by Annemarie S. Muth. 628 pages. 2000. 0-7808-0381-7. $78.

■

Back & Neck Disorders Sourcebook

Basic Information about Disorders and Injuries of the Spinal Cord and Vertebrae, Including Facts on Chiropractic Treatment, Surgical Interventions, Paralysis, and Rehabilitation

Along with Advice for Preventing Back Trouble

Edited by Karen Bellenir. 548 pages. 1997. 0-7808-0202-0. $78.

■

Blood & Circulatory Disorders Sourcebook

Basic Information about Blood and Its Components, Anemias, Leukemias, Bleeding Disorders, and Circulatory Disorders, Including Aplastic Anemia, Thalassemia, Sickle-Cell Disease, Hemochromatosis, Hemophilia, Von Willebrand Disease, and Vascular Diseases

Along with a Special Section on Blood Transfusions and Blood Supply Safety, a Glossary, and Source Listings for Further Help and Information

Edited by Karen Bellenir and Linda M. Shin. 554 pages. 1998. 0-7808-0203-9. $78.

"Recommended reference source."
—*Booklist, American Library Association, Feb '99*

"An important reference sourcebook written in simple language for everyday, non-technical users. "
—*Reviewer's Bookwatch, Jan '99*

■

Brain Disorders Sourcebook

Basic Consumer Health Information about Strokes, Epilepsy, Amyotrophic Lateral Sclerosis (ALS/Lou Gehrig's Disease), Parkinson's Disease, Brain Tumors, Cerebral Palsy, Headache, Tourette Syndrome, and More

Along with Statistical Data, Treatment and Rehabilitation Options, Coping Strategies, Reports on Current Research Initiatives, a Glossary, and Resource Listings for Additional Help and Information

Edited by Karen Bellenir. 481 pages. 1999. 0-7808-0229-2. $78.

"Belongs on the shelves of any library with a consumer health collection." —*E-Streams, Mar '00*

"Recommended reference source."
—*Booklist, American Library Association, Oct '99*

SEE ALSO Alzheimer's, Stroke & 29 Other Neurological Disorders Sourcebook, 1st Edition

■

Breast Cancer Sourcebook

Basic Consumer Health Information about Breast Cancer, Including Diagnostic Methods, Treatment Options, Alternative Therapies, Help and Self-Help Information, Related Health Concerns, Statistical and Demographic Data, and Facts for Men with Breast Cancer

Along with Reports on Current Research Initiatives, a Glossary of Related Medical Terms, and a Directory of Sources for Further Help and Information

Edited by Edward J. Prucha and Karen Bellenir. 600 pages. 2001. 0-7808-0244-6. $78.

SEE ALSO Cancer Sourcebook for Women, 1st and 2nd Editions, Women's Health Concerns Sourcebook

■

Burns Sourcebook

Basic Consumer Health Information about Various Types of Burns and Scalds, Including Flame, Heat, Cold, Electrical, Chemical, and Sun Burns

Along with Information on Short-Term and Long-Term Treatments, Tissue Reconstruction, Plastic Surgery, Prevention Suggestions, and First Aid

Edited by Allan R. Cook. 604 pages. 1999. 0-7808-0204-7. $78.

"This key reference guide is an invaluable addition to all health care and public libraries in confronting this ongoing health issue."
—*American Reference Books Annual, 2000*

"This is an exceptional addition to the series and is highly recommended for all consumer health collections, hospital libraries, and academic medical centers." —*E-Streams, Mar '00*

"Recommended reference source."
—*Booklist, American Library Association, Dec '99*

SEE ALSO Skin Disorders Sourcebook

■

Cancer Sourcebook, 1st Edition

Basic Information on Cancer Types, Symptoms, Diagnostic Methods, and Treatments, Including Statistics on Cancer Occurrences Worldwide and the Risks Associated with Known Carcinogens and Activities

Edited by Frank E. Bair. 932 pages. 1990. 1-55888-888-8. $78.

Cited in *Reference Sources for Small and Medium-Sized Libraries, American Library Association, 1999*

"Written in nontechnical language. Useful for patients, their families, medical professionals, and librarians."
—*Guide to Reference Books, 1996*

"Designed with the non-medical professional in mind. Libraries and medical facilities interested in patient education should certainly consider adding the *Cancer Sourcebook* to their holdings. This compact collection of reliable information . . . is an invaluable tool for helping patients and patients' families and friends to take the first steps in coping with the many difficulties of cancer."
—*Medical Reference Services Quarterly, Winter '91*

"Specifically created for the nontechnical reader . . . an important resource for the general reader trying to understand the complexities of cancer."
—*American Reference Books Annual, 1991*

"This publication's nontechnical nature and very comprehensive format make it useful for both the general public and undergraduate students."
—*Choice, Association of College and Research Libraries, Oct '90*

■

New Cancer Sourcebook, 2nd Edition

Basic Information about Major Forms and Stages of Cancer, Featuring Facts about Primary and Secondary Tumors of the Respiratory, Nervous, Lymphatic, Circulatory, Skeletal, and Gastrointestinal Systems, and Specific Organs; Statistical and Demographic Data; Treatment Options; and Strategies for Coping

Edited by Allan R. Cook. 1,313 pages. 1996. 0-7808-0041-9. $78.

"An excellent resource for patients with newly diagnosed cancer and their families. The dialogue is simple, direct, and comprehensive. Highly recommended for patients and families to aid in their understanding of cancer and its treatment."
—*Booklist Health Sciences Supplement, American Library Association, Oct '97*

"The amount of factual and useful information is extensive. The writing is very clear, geared to general readers. Recommended for all levels."
—Choice, Association of College and Research Libraries, Jan '97

Cancer Sourcebook, 3rd Edition

Basic Consumer Health Information about Major Forms and Stages of Cancer, Featuring Facts about Primary and Secondary Tumors of the Respiratory, Nervous, Lymphatic, Circulatory, Skeletal, and Gastrointestinal Systems, and Specific Organs

Along with Statistical and Demographic Data, Treatment Options, Strategies for Coping, a Glossary, and a Directory of Sources for Additional Help and Information

Edited by Edward J. Prucha. 1,069 pages. 2000. 0-7808-0227-6. $78.

Cancer Sourcebook for Women, 1st Edition

Basic Information about Specific Forms of Cancer That Affect Women, Featuring Facts about Breast Cancer, Cervical Cancer, Ovarian Cancer, Cancer of the Uterus and Uterine Sarcoma, Cancer of the Vagina, and Cancer of the Vulva; Statistical and Demographic Data; Treatments, Self-Help Management Suggestions, and Current Research Initiatives

Edited by Allan R. Cook and Peter D. Dresser. 524 pages. 1996. 0-7808-0076-1. $78.

". . . written in easily understandable, non-technical language. Recommended for public libraries or hospital and academic libraries that collect patient education or consumer health materials."
—Medical Reference Services Quarterly, Spring '97

"Would be of value in a consumer health library. . . . written with the health care consumer in mind. Medical jargon is at a minimum, and medical terms are explained in clear, understandable sentences."
—Bulletin of the Medical Library Association, Oct '96

"The availability under one cover of all these pertinent publications, grouped under cohesive headings, makes this certainly a most useful sourcebook."
—Choice, Association of College and Research Libraries, Jun '96

"Presents a comprehensive knowledge base for general readers. Men and women both benefit from the gold mine of information nestled between the two covers of this book. Recommended."
—Academic Library Book Review, Summer '96

"This timely book is highly recommended for consumer health and patient education collections in all libraries."
—Library Journal, Apr '96

SEE ALSO Breast Cancer Sourcebook, Women's Health Concerns Sourcebook

Cancer Sourcebook for Women, 2nd Edition

Basic Consumer Health Information about Specific Forms of Cancer That Affect Women, Including Cervical Cancer, Ovarian Cancer, Endometrial Cancer, Uterine Sarcoma, Vaginal Cancer, Vulvar Cancer, and Gestational Trophoblastic Tumor; and Featuring Statistical Information, Facts about Tests and Treatments, a Glossary of Cancer Terms, and an Extensive List of Additional Resources

Edited by Edward J. Prucha. 600 pages. 2001. 0-7808-0226-8. $78.

SEE ALSO Breast Cancer Sourcebook, Women's Health Concerns Sourcebook

Cardiovascular Diseases & Disorders Sourcebook, 1st Edition

Basic Information about Cardiovascular Diseases and Disorders, Featuring Facts about the Cardiovascular System, Demographic and Statistical Data, Descriptions of Pharmacological and Surgical Interventions, Lifestyle Modifications, and a Special Section Focusing on Heart Disorders in Children

Edited by Karen Bellenir and Peter D. Dresser. 683 pages. 1995. 0-7808-0032-X. $78.

". . . comprehensive format provides an extensive overview on this subject."
—Choice, Association of College and Research Libraries, Jun '96

". . . an easily understood, complete, up-to-date resource. This well executed public health tool will make valuable information available to those that need it most, patients and their families. The typeface, sturdy non-reflective paper, and library binding add a feel of quality found wanting in other publications. Highly recommended for academic and general libraries. "
—Academic Library Book Review, Summer '96

SEE ALSO Healthy Heart Sourcebook for Women, Heart Diseases & Disorders Sourcebook, 2nd Edition

Caregiving Sourcebook

Basic Consumer Health Information for Caregivers, Including a Profile of Caregivers, Caregiving Responsibilities, Tips for Specific Conditions, Care Environments, and the Effects of Caregiving

Along with Legal Issues, Financial Concerns, Future Planning, a Glossary, and a Listing of Additional Resources

Edited by Joyce Brennfleck Shannon. 550 pages. 2001. 0-7808-0331-0. $78.

Colds, Flu & Other Common Ailments Sourcebook

Basic Consumer Health Information about Common Ailments and Injuries, Including Colds, Coughs, the Flu, Sinus Problems, Headaches, Fever, Nausea and Vomiting, Menstrual Cramps, Diarrhea, Constipation, Hemorrhoids, Back Pain, Dandruff, Dry and Itchy Skin, Cuts, Scrapes, Sprains, Bruises, and More

Along with Information about Prevention, Self-Care, Choosing a Doctor, Over-the-Counter Medications, Folk Remedies, and Alternative Therapies, and Including a Glossary of Important Terms and a Directory of Resources for Further Help and Information

Edited by Chad T. Kimball. 600 pages. 2001. 0-7808-0435-X. $78.

Communication Disorders Sourcebook

Basic Information about Deafness and Hearing Loss, Speech and Language Disorders, Voice Disorders, Balance and Vestibular Disorders, and Disorders of Smell, Taste, and Touch

Edited by Linda M. Ross. 533 pages. 1996. 0-7808-0077-X. $78.

"This is skillfully edited and is a welcome resource for the layperson. It should be found in every public and medical library." — *Booklist Health Sciences Supplement, American Library Association, Oct '97*

Congenital Disorders Sourcebook

Basic Information about Disorders Acquired during Gestation, Including Spina Bifida, Hydrocephalus, Cerebral Palsy, Heart Defects, Craniofacial Abnormalities, Fetal Alcohol Syndrome, and More

Along with Current Treatment Options and Statistical Data

Edited by Karen Bellenir. 607 pages. 1997. 0-7808-0205-5. $78.

"Recommended reference source."
— *Booklist, American Library Association, Oct '97*

SEE ALSO Pregnancy & Birth Sourcebook

Consumer Issues in Health Care Sourcebook

Basic Information about Health Care Fundamentals and Related Consumer Issues, Including Exams and Screening Tests, Physician Specialties, Choosing a Doctor, Using Prescription and Over-the-Counter Medications Safely, Avoiding Health Scams, Managing Common Health Risks in the Home, Care Options for Chronically or Terminally Ill Patients, and a List of Resources for Obtaining Help and Further Information

Edited by Karen Bellenir. 618 pages. 1998. 0-7808-0221-7. $78.

"Both public and academic libraries will want to have a copy in their collection for readers who are interested in self-education on health issues."
— *American Reference Books Annual, 2000*

"The editor has researched the literature from government agencies and others, saving readers the time and effort of having to do the research themselves. Recommended for public libraries."
— *Reference and User Services Quarterly, American Library Association, Spring '99*

"Recommended reference source."
— *Booklist, American Library Association, Dec '98*

Contagious & Non-Contagious Infectious Diseases Sourcebook

Basic Information about Contagious Diseases like Measles, Polio, Hepatitis B, and Infectious Mononucleosis, and Non-Contagious Infectious Diseases like Tetanus and Toxic Shock Syndrome, and Diseases Occurring as Secondary Infections Such as Shingles and Reye Syndrome

Along with Vaccination, Prevention, and Treatment Information, and a Section Describing Emerging Infectious Disease Threats

Edited by Karen Bellenir and Peter D. Dresser. 566 pages. 1996. 0-7808-0075-3. $78.

Death & Dying Sourcebook

Basic Consumer Health Information for the Layperson about End-of-Life Care and Related Ethical and Legal Issues, Including Chief Causes of Death, Autopsies, Pain Management for the Terminally Ill, Life Support Systems, Insurance, Euthanasia, Assisted Suicide, Hospice Programs, Living Wills, Funeral Planning, Counseling, Mourning, Organ Donation, and Physician Training

Along with Statistical Data, a Glossary, and Listings of Sources for Further Help and Information

Edited by Annemarie S. Muth. 641 pages. 1999. 0-7808-0230-6. $78.

"This book is a definite must for all those involved in end-of-life care." — *Doody's Review Service, 2000*

Diabetes Sourcebook, 1st Edition

Basic Information about Insulin-Dependent and Non-insulin-Dependent Diabetes Mellitus, Gestational Diabetes, and Diabetic Complications, Symptoms, Treatment, and Research Results, Including Statistics on Prevalence, Morbidity, and Mortality

Along with Source Listings for Further Help and Information

Edited by Karen Bellenir and Peter D. Dresser. 827 pages. 1994. 1-55888-751-2. $78.

". . . very informative and understandable for the layperson without being simplistic. It provides a comprehensive overview for laypersons who want a general understanding of the disease or who want to focus on various aspects of the disease."
— Bulletin of the Medical Library Association, Jan '96

■

Diabetes Sourcebook, 2nd Edition

Basic Consumer Health Information about Type 1 Diabetes (Insulin-Dependent or Juvenile-Onset Diabetes), Type 2 (Noninsulin-Dependent or Adult-Onset Diabetes), Gestational Diabetes, and Related Disorders, Including Diabetes Prevalence Data, Management Issues, the Role of Diet and Exercise in Controlling Diabetes, Insulin and Other Diabetes Medicines, and Complications of Diabetes Such as Eye Diseases, Periodontal Disease, Amputation, and End-Stage Renal Disease

Along with Reports on Current Research Initiatives, a Glossary, and Resource Listings for Further Help and Information

Edited by Karen Bellenir. 688 pages. 1998. 0-7808-0224-1. $78.

"This comprehensive book is an excellent addition for high school, academic, medical, and public libraries. This volume is highly recommended."
—American Reference Books Annual, 2000

"An invaluable reference." — Library Journal, May '00

Selected as one of the 250 "Best Health Sciences Books of 1999." — Doody's Rating Service, Mar-Apr 2000

"Recommended reference source."
—Booklist, American Library Association, Feb '99

". . . provides reliable mainstream medical information . . . belongs on the shelves of any library with a consumer health collection." — E-Streams, Sep '99

"Provides useful information for the general public."
— Healthlines, University of Michigan Health Management Research Center, Sep/Oct '99

■

Diet & Nutrition Sourcebook, 1st Edition

Basic Information about Nutrition, Including the Dietary Guidelines for Americans, the Food Guide Pyramid, and Their Applications in Daily Diet, Nutritional Advice for Specific Age Groups, Current Nutritional Issues and Controversies, the New Food Label and How to Use It to Promote Healthy Eating, and Recent Developments in Nutritional Research

Edited by Dan R. Harris. 662 pages. 1996. 0-7808-0084-2. $78.

"Useful reference as a food and nutrition sourcebook for the general consumer." — Booklist Health Sciences Supplement, American Library Association, Oct '97

"Recommended for public libraries and medical libraries that receive general information requests on nutrition. It is readable and will appeal to those interested in learning more about healthy dietary practices."
— Medical Reference Services Quarterly, Fall '97

"An abundance of medical and social statistics is translated into readable information geared toward the general reader." — Bookwatch, Mar '97

"With dozens of questionable diet books on the market, it is so refreshing to find a reliable and factual reference book. Recommended to aspiring professionals, librarians, and others seeking and giving reliable dietary advice. An excellent compilation." — Choice, Association of College and Research Libraries, Feb '97

SEE ALSO *Digestive Diseases & Disorders Sourcebook, Gastrointestinal Diseases & Disorders Sourcebook*

■

Diet & Nutrition Sourcebook, 2nd Edition

Basic Consumer Health Information about Dietary Guidelines, Recommended Daily Intake Values, Vitamins, Minerals, Fiber, Fat, Weight Control, Dietary Supplements, and Food Additives

Along with Special Sections on Nutrition Needs throughout Life and Nutrition for People with Such Specific Medical Concerns as Allergies, High Blood Cholesterol, Hypertension, Diabetes, Celiac Disease, Seizure Disorders, Phenylketonuria (PKU), Cancer, and Eating Disorders, and Including Reports on Current Nutrition Research and Source Listings for Additional Help and Information

Edited by Karen Bellenir. 650 pages. 1999. 0-7808-0228-4. $78.

"This reference document should be in any public library, but it would be a very good guide for beginning students in the health sciences. If the other books in this publisher's series are as good as this, they should all be in the health sciences collections."
—American Reference Books Annual, 2000

"Recommended reference source."
—Booklist, American Library Association, Dec '99

SEE ALSO *Digestive Diseases & Disorders Sourcebook, Gastrointestinal Diseases & Disorders Sourcebook*

■

Digestive Diseases & Disorders Sourcebook

Basic Consumer Health Information about Diseases and Disorders that Impact the Upper and Lower Digestive System, Including Celiac Disease, Constipation, Crohn's Disease, Cyclic Vomiting Syndrome, Diarrhea, Diverticulosis and Diverticulitis, Gallstones, Heartburn, Hemorrhoids, Hernias, Indigestion (Dyspepsia), Irritable Bowel Syndrome, Lactose Intolerance, Ulcers, and More

Along with Information about Medications and Other Treatments, Tips for Maintaining a Healthy Digestive

Tract, a Glossary, and Directory of Digestive Diseases Organizations

Edited by Karen Bellenir. 335 pages. 1999. 0-7808-0327-2. $48.

"Recommended reference source."
—Booklist, American Library Association, May '00

SEE ALSO Diet & Nutrition Sourcebook, 1st and 2nd Editions, Gastrointestinal Diseases & Disorders Sourcebook

∎

Disabilities Sourcebook

Basic Consumer Health Information about Physical and Psychiatric Disabilities, Including Descriptions of Major Causes of Disability, Assistive and Adaptive Aids, Workplace Issues, and Accessibility Concerns

Along with Information about the Americans with Disabilities Act, a Glossary, and Resources for Additional Help and Information

Edited by Dawn D. Matthews. 616 pages. 2000. 0-7808-0389-2. $78.

"Recommended reference source."
—Booklist, American Library Association, Jul '00

"An involving, invaluable handbook."
—The Bookwatch, May '00

∎

Domestic Violence & Child Abuse Sourcebook

Basic Consumer Health Information about Spousal/Partner, Child, Sibling, Parent, and Elder Abuse, Covering Physical, Emotional, and Sexual Abuse, Teen Dating Violence, and Stalking; Includes Information about Hotlines, Safe Houses, Safety Plans, and Other Resources for Support and Assistance, Community Initiatives, and Reports on Current Directions in Research and Treatment

Along with a Glossary, Sources for Further Reading, and Governmental and Non-Governmental Organizations Contact Information

Edited by Helene Henderson. 1,064 pages. 2000. 0-7808-0235-7. $78.

∎

Drug Abuse Sourcebook

Basic Consumer Health Information about Illicit Substances of Abuse and the Diversion of Prescription Medications, Including Depressants, Hallucinogens, Inhalants, Marijuana, Narcotics, Stimulants, and Anabolic Steroids

Along with Facts about Related Health Risks, Treatment Issues, and Substance Abuse Prevention Programs, a Glossary of Terms, Statistical Data, and Directories of Hotline Services, Self-Help Groups, and Organizations Able to Provide Further Information

Edited by Karen Bellenir. 629 pages. 2000. 0-7808-0242-X. $78.

SEE ALSO Alcoholism Sourcebook, Substance Abuse Sourcebook

∎

Ear, Nose & Throat Disorders Sourcebook

Basic Information about Disorders of the Ears, Nose, Sinus Cavities, Pharynx, and Larynx, Including Ear Infections, Tinnitus, Vestibular Disorders, Allergic and Non-Allergic Rhinitis, Sore Throats, Tonsillitis, and Cancers That Affect the Ears, Nose, Sinuses, and Throat

Along with Reports on Current Research Initiatives, a Glossary of Related Medical Terms, and a Directory of Sources for Further Help and Information

Edited by Karen Bellenir and Linda M. Shin. 576 pages. 1998. 0-7808-0206-3. $78.

"Overall, this sourcebook is helpful for the consumer seeking information on ENT issues. It is recommended for public libraries."
—American Reference Books Annual, 1999

"Recommended reference source."
—Booklist, American Library Association, Dec '98

∎

Endocrine & Metabolic Disorders Sourcebook

Basic Information for the Layperson about Pancreatic and Insulin-Related Disorders Such as Pancreatitis, Diabetes, and Hypoglycemia; Adrenal Gland Disorders Such as Cushing's Syndrome, Addison's Disease, and Congenital Adrenal Hyperplasia; Pituitary Gland Disorders Such as Growth Hormone Deficiency, Acromegaly, and Pituitary Tumors; Thyroid Disorders Such as Hypothyroidism, Graves' Disease, Hashimoto's Disease, and Goiter; Hyperparathyroidism; and Other Diseases and Syndromes of Hormone Imbalance or Metabolic Dysfunction

Along with Reports on Current Research Initiatives

Edited by Linda M. Shin. 574 pages. 1998. 0-7808-0207-1. $78.

"Omnigraphics has produced another needed resource for health information consumers."
—American Reference Books Annual, 2000

"Recommended reference source."
— Booklist, American Library Association, Dec '98

∎

Environmentally Induced Disorders Sourcebook

Basic Information about Diseases and Syndromes Linked to Exposure to Pollutants and Other Substances in Outdoor and Indoor Environments Such as Lead, Asbestos, Formaldehyde, Mercury, Emissions, Noise, and More

Edited by Allan R. Cook. 620 pages. 1997. 0-7808-0083-4. $78.

"Recommended reference source."
— Booklist, American Library Association, Sep '98

"This book will be a useful addition to anyone's library." —*Choice Health Sciences Supplement, Association of College and Research Libraries, May '98*

". . . a good survey of numerous environmentally induced physical disorders . . . a useful addition to anyone's library." —*Doody's Health Sciences Book Reviews, Jan '98*

". . . provide[s] introductory information from the best authorities around. Since this volume covers topics that potentially affect everyone, it will surely be one of the most frequently consulted volumes in the **Health Reference Series**." —*Rettig on Reference, Nov '97*

■

Ethnic Diseases Sourcebook

Basic Consumer Health Information for Ethnic and Racial Minority Groups in the United States, Including General Health Indicators and Behaviors, Ethnic Diseases, Genetic Testing, the Impact of Chronic Diseases, Women's Health, Mental Health Issues, and Preventive Health Care Services

Along with a Glossary and a Listing of Additional Resources

Edited by Joyce Brennfleck Shannon. 600 pages. 2001. 0-7808-0336-1. $78.

■

Family Planning Sourcebook

Basic Consumer Health Information about Planning for Pregancy and Contraception, Including Traditional Methods, Barrier Methods, Hormonal Methods, Permanent Methods, Future Methods, Emergency Contraception, and Birth Control Choices for Women at Each Stage of Life

Along with Statistics, a Glossary, and Sources of Additional Information

Edited by Amy Marcaccio Keyzer. 600 pages. 2001. 0-7808-0379-5. $78.

SEE ALSO *Pregnancy & Birth Sourcebook*

■

Fitness & Exercise Sourcebook, 1st Edition

Basic Information on Fitness and Exercise, Including Fitness Activities for Specific Age Groups, Exercise for People with Specific Medical Conditions, How to Begin a Fitness Program in Running, Walking, Swimming, Cycling, and Other Athletic Activities, and Recent Research in Fitness and Exercise

Edited by Dan R. Harris. 663 pages. 1996. 0-7808-0186-5. $78.

"A good resource for general readers." —*Choice, Association of College and Research Libraries, Nov '97*

"The perennial popularity of the topic . . . make this an appealing selection for public libraries." —*Rettig on Reference, Jun/Jul '97*

Fitness & Exercise Sourcebook, 2nd Edition

Basic Consumer Health Information about the Fundamentals of Fitness and Exercise, Including How to Begin and Maintain a Fitness Program, Fitness as a Lifestyle, the Link between Fitness and Diet, Advice for Specific Groups of People, Exercise as It Relates to Specific Medical Conditions, and Recent Research in Fitness and Exercise

Along with a Glossary of Important Terms and Resources for Additional Help and Information

Edited by Kristen M. Gledhill. 600 pages. 2001. 0-7808-0334-5. $78.

■

Food & Animal Borne Diseases Sourcebook

Basic Information about Diseases That Can Be Spread to Humans through the Ingestion of Contaminated Food or Water or by Contact with Infected Animals and Insects, Such as Botulism, E. Coli, Hepatitis A, Trichinosis, Lyme Disease, and Rabies

Along with Information Regarding Prevention and Treatment Methods, and Including a Special Section for International Travelers Describing Diseases Such as Cholera, Malaria, Travelers' Diarrhea, and Yellow Fever, and Offering Recommendations for Avoiding Illness

Edited by Karen Bellenir and Peter D. Dresser. 535 pages. 1995. 0-7808-0033-8. $78.

"Targeting general readers and providing them with a single, comprehensive source of information on selected topics, this book continues, with the excellent caliber of its predecessors, to catalog topical information on health matters of general interest. Readable and thorough, this valuable resource is highly recommended for all libraries." —*Academic Library Book Review, Summer '96*

"A comprehensive collection of authoritative information." —*Emergency Medical Services, Oct '95*

■

Food Safety Sourcebook

Basic Consumer Health Information about the Safe Handling of Meat, Poultry, Seafood, Eggs, Fruit Juices, and Other Food Items, and Facts about Pesticides, Drinking Water, Food Safety Overseas, and the Onset, Duration, and Symptoms of Foodborne Illnesses, Including Types of Pathogenic Bacteria, Parasitic Protozoa, Worms, Viruses, and Natural Toxins

Along with the Role of the Consumer, the Food Handler, and the Government in Food Safety; a Glossary, and Resources for Additional Help and Information

Edited by Dawn D. Matthews. 339 pages. 1999. 0-7808-0326-4. $48.

"This book takes the complex issues of food safety and foodborne pathogens and presents them in an easily understood manner. [It does] an excellent job of covering a large and often confusing topic." —*American Reference Books Annual, 2000*

■

Forensic Medicine Sourcebook

Basic Consumer Information for the Layperson about Forensic Medicine, Including Crime Scene Investigation, Evidence Collection and Analysis, Expert Testimony, Computer-Aided Criminal Identification, Digital Imaging in the Courtroom, DNA Profiling, Accident Reconstruction, Autopsies, Ballistics, Drugs and Explosives Detection, Latent Fingerprints, Product Tampering, and Questioned Document Examination

Along with Statistical Data, a Glossary of Forensics Terminology, and Listings of Sources for Further Help and Information

Edited by Annemarie S. Muth. 574 pages. 1999. 0-7808-0232-2. $78.

"There are several items that make this book attractive to consumers who are seeking certain forensic data. . . . This is a useful current source for those seeking general forensic medical answers."

—American Reference Books Annual, 2000

"Recommended for public libraries."

—Reference & User Services Quarterly, American Library Association, Spring 2000

"Recommended reference source."

—Booklist, American Library Association, Feb '00

"A wealth of information, useful statistics, references are up-to-date and extremely complete. This wonderful collection of data will help students who are interested in a career in any type of forensic field. It is a great resource for attorneys who need information about types of expert witnesses needed in a particular case. It also offers useful information for fiction and nonfiction writers whose work involves a crime. A fascinating compilation. All levels." —Choice, Association of College and Research Libraries, Jan 2000

■

Gastrointestinal Diseases & Disorders Sourcebook

Basic Information about Gastroesophageal Reflux Disease (Heartburn), Ulcers, Diverticulosis, Irritable Bowel Syndrome, Crohn's Disease, Ulcerative Colitis, Diarrhea, Constipation, Lactose Intolerance, Hemorrhoids, Hepatitis, Cirrhosis, and Other Digestive Problems, Featuring Statistics, Descriptions of Symptoms, and Current Treatment Methods of Interest for Persons Living with Upper and Lower Gastrointestinal Maladies

Edited by Linda M. Ross. 413 pages. 1996. 0-7808-0078-8. $78.

". . . very readable form. The successful editorial work that brought this material together into a useful and understandable reference makes accessible to all readers information that can help them more effectively understand and obtain help for digestive tract problems."

—Choice, Association of College and Research Libraries, Feb '97

SEE ALSO Diet & Nutrition Sourcebook, 1st and 2nd Editions, Digestive Diseases & Disorders Sourcebook

■

Genetic Disorders Sourcebook, 1st Edition

Basic Information about Heritable Diseases and Disorders Such as Down Syndrome, PKU, Hemophilia, Von Willebrand Disease, Gaucher Disease, Tay-Sachs Disease, and Sickle-Cell Disease, Along with Information about Genetic Screening, Gene Therapy, Home Care, and Including Source Listings for Further Help and Information on More Than 300 Disorders

Edited by Karen Bellenir. 642 pages. 1996. 0-7808-0034-6. $78.

"Recommended for undergraduate libraries or libraries that serve the public."

—Science & Technology Libraries, Vol. 18, No. 1, '99

"Provides essential medical information to both the general public and those diagnosed with a serious or fatal genetic disease or disorder."

—Choice, Association of College and Research Libraries, Jan '97

"Geared toward the lay public. It would be well placed in all public libraries and in those hospital and medical libraries in which access to genetic references is limited." —Doody's Health Sciences Book Review, Oct '96

■

Genetic Disorders Sourcebook, 2nd Edition

Basic Consumer Health Information about Hereditary Diseases and Disorders, Including Cystic Fibrosis, Down Syndrome, Hemophilia, Huntington's Disease, Sickle Cell Anemia, and More; Facts about Genes, Gene Research and Therapy, Genetic Screening, Ethics of Gene Testing, Genetic Counseling, and Advice on Coping and Caring

Along with a Glossary of Genetic Terminology and a Resource List for Help, Support, and Further Information

Edited by Kathy Massimini. 650 pages. 2000. 0-7808-0241-1. $78.

■

Head Trauma Sourcebook

Basic Information for the Layperson about Open-Head and Closed-Head Injuries, Treatment Advances, Recovery, and Rehabilitation

Along with Reports on Current Research Initiatives

Edited by Karen Bellenir. 414 pages. 1997. 0-7808-0208-X. $78.

531

Health Insurance Sourcebook

Basic Information about Managed Care Organizations, Traditional Fee-for-Service Insurance, Insurance Portability and Pre-Existing Conditions Clauses, Medicare, Medicaid, Social Security, and Military Health Care

Along with Information about Insurance Fraud

Edited by Wendy Wilcox. 530 pages. 1997. 0-7808-0222-5. $78.

"Particularly useful because it brings much of this information together in one volume. This book will be a handy reference source in the health sciences library, hospital library, college and university library, and medium to large public library."
— *Medical Reference Services Quarterly, Fall '98*

Awarded "Books of the Year Award"
— *American Journal of Nursing, 1997*

"The layout of the book is particularly helpful as it provides easy access to reference material. A most useful addition to the vast amount of information about health insurance. The use of data from U.S. government agencies is most commendable. Useful in a library or learning center for healthcare professional students."
— *Doody's Health Sciences Book Reviews, Nov '97*

Healthy Aging Sourcebook

Basic Consumer Health Information about Maintaining Health through the Aging Process, Including Advice on Nutrition, Exercise, and Sleep, Help in Making Decisions about Midlife Issues and Retirement, and Guidance Concerning Practical and Informed Choices in Health Consumerism

Along with Data Concerning the Theories of Aging, Different Experiences in Aging by Minority Groups, and Facts about Aging Now and Aging in the Future; Featuring a Glossary, a Guide to Consumer Help, Additional Suggested Reading, and Practical Resource Directory

Edited by Jenifer Swanson. 536 pages. 1999. 0-7808-0390-6. $78.

"Recommended reference source."
— *Booklist, American Library Association, Feb '00*

SEE ALSO *Physical & Mental Issues in Aging Sourcebook*

Healthy Heart Sourcebook for Women

Basic Consumer Health Information about Cardiac Issues Specific to Women, Including Facts about Major Risk Factors and Prevention, Treatment and Control Strategies, and Important Dietary Issues

Along with a Special Section Regarding the Pros and Cons of Hormone Replacement Therapy and Its Impact on Heart Health, and Additional Help, Including Recipes, a Glossary, and a Directory of Resources

Edited by Dawn D. Matthews. 336 pages. 2000. 0-7808-0329-9. $48.

SEE ALSO *Cardiovascular Diseases & Disorders Sourcebook, 1st Edition, Heart Diseases & Disorders Sourcebook, 2nd Edition, Women's Health Concerns Sourcebook*

Heart Diseases & Disorders Sourcebook, 2nd Edition

Basic Consumer Health Information about Heart Attacks, Angina, Rhythm Disorders, Heart Failure, Valve Disease, Congenital Heart Disorders, and More, Including Descriptions of Surgical Procedures and Other Interventions, Medications, Cardiac Rehabilitation, Risk Identification, and Prevention Tips

Along with Statistical Data, Reports on Current Research Initiatives, a Glossary of Cardiovascular Terms, and Resource Directory

Edited by Karen Bellenir. 612 pages. 2000. 0-7808-0238-1. $78.

SEE ALSO *Cardiovascular Diseases & Disorders Sourcebook, 1st Edition, Healthy Heart Sourcebook for Women*

Immune System Disorders Sourcebook

Basic Information about Lupus, Multiple Sclerosis, Guillain-Barré Syndrome, Chronic Granulomatous Disease, and More

Along with Statistical and Demographic Data and Reports on Current Research Initiatives

Edited by Allan R. Cook. 608 pages. 1997. 0-7808-0209-8. $78.

Infant & Toddler Health Sourcebook

Basic Consumer Health Information about the Physical and Mental Development of Newborns, Infants, and Toddlers, Including Neonatal Concerns, Nutrition Recommendations, Immunization Schedules, Common Pediatric Disorders, Assessments and Milestones, Safety Tips, and Advice for Parents and Other Caregivers

Along with a Glossary of Terms and Resource Listings for Additional Help

Edited by Jenifer Swanson. 585 pages. 2000. 0-7808-0246-2. $78.

Kidney & Urinary Tract Diseases & Disorders Sourcebook

Basic Information about Kidney Stones, Urinary Incontinence, Bladder Disease, End Stage Renal Disease, Dialysis, and More

Along with Statistical and Demographic Data and Reports on Current Research Initiatives

Edited by Linda M. Ross. 602 pages. 1997. 0-7808-0079-6. $78.

Learning Disabilities Sourcebook

Basic Information about Disorders Such as Dyslexia, Visual and Auditory Processing Deficits, Attention Deficit/Hyperactivity Disorder, and Autism

Along with Statistical and Demographic Data, Reports on Current Research Initiatives, an Explanation of the Assessment Process, and a Special Section for Adults with Learning Disabilities

Edited by Linda M. Shin. 579 pages. 1998. 0-7808-0210-1. $78.

Named "Oustanding Reference Book of 1999."
—*New York Public Library, Feb 2000*

"An excellent candidate for inclusion in a public library reference section. It's a great source of information. Teachers will also find the book useful. Definitely worth reading."
—*Journal of Adolescent & Adult Literacy, Feb 2000*

"Readable . . . provides a solid base of information regarding successful techniques used with individuals who have learning disabilities, as well as practical suggestions for educators and family members. Clear language, concise descriptions, and pertinent information for contacting multiple resources add to the strength of this book as a useful tool."
—*Choice, Association of College and Research Libraries, Feb '99*

"Recommended reference source."
—*Booklist, American Library Association, Sep '98*

"This is a useful resource for libraries and for those who don't have the time to identify and locate the individual publications."
—*Disability Resources Monthly, Sep '98*

■

Liver Disorders Sourcebook

Basic Consumer Health Information about the Liver and How It Works; Liver Diseases, Including Cancer, Cirrhosis, Hepatitis, and Toxic and Drug Related Diseases; Tips for Maintaining a Healthy Liver; Laboratory Tests, Radiology Tests, and Facts about Liver Transplantation

Along with a Section on Support Groups, a Glossary, and Resource Listings

Edited by Joyce Brennfleck Shannon. 591 pages. 2000. 0-7808-0383-3. $78.

"Recommended reference source."
—*Booklist, American Library Association, Jun '00*

■

Medical Tests Sourcebook

Basic Consumer Health Information about Medical Tests, Including Periodic Health Exams, General Screening Tests, Tests You Can Do at Home, Findings of the U.S. Preventive Services Task Force, X-ray and Radiology Tests, Electrical Tests, Tests of Blood and Other Body Fluids and Tissues, Scope Tests, Lung Tests, Genetic Tests, Pregnancy Tests, Newborn Screening Tests, Sexually Transmitted Disease Tests, and Computer Aided Diagnoses

Along with a Section on Paying for Medical Tests, a Glossary, and Resource Listings

Edited by Joyce Brennfleck Shannon. 691 pages. 1999. 0-7808-0243-8. $78.

"A valuable reference guide."
—*American Reference Books Annual, 2000*

"Recommended for hospital and health sciences libraries with consumer health collections."
—*E-Streams, Mar '00*

"This is an overall excellent reference with a wealth of general knowledge that may aid those who are reluctant to get vital tests performed."
—*Today's Librarian, Jan 2000*

■

Men's Health Concerns Sourcebook

Basic Information about Health Issues That Affect Men, Featuring Facts about the Top Causes of Death in Men, Including Heart Disease, Stroke, Cancers, Prostate Disorders, Chronic Obstructive Pulmonary Disease, Pneumonia and Influenza, Human Immunodeficiency Virus and Acquired Immune Deficiency Syndrome, Diabetes Mellitus, Stress, Suicide, Accidents and Homicides; and Facts about Common Concerns for Men, Including Impotence, Contraception, Circumcision, Sleep Disorders, Snoring, Hair Loss, Diet, Nutrition, Exercise, Kidney and Urological Disorders, and Backaches

Edited by Allan R. Cook. 738 pages. 1998. 0-7808-0212-8. $78.

"This comprehensive resource and the series are highly recommended."
—*American Reference Books Annual, 2000*

"Recommended reference source."
—*Booklist, American Library Association, Dec '98*

■

Mental Health Disorders Sourcebook, 1st Edition

Basic Information about Schizophrenia, Depression, Bipolar Disorder, Panic Disorder, Obsessive-Compulsive Disorder, Phobias and Other Anxiety Disorders, Paranoia and Other Personality Disorders, Eating Disorders, and Sleep Disorders

Along with Information about Treatment and Therapies

Edited by Karen Bellenir. 548 pages. 1995. 0-7808-0040-0. $78.

"This is an excellent new book . . . written in easy-to-understand language."
—*Booklist Health Sciences Supplement, American Library Association, Oct '97*

". . . useful for public and academic libraries and consumer health collections."
—*Medical Reference Services Quarterly, Spring '97*

"The great strengths of the book are its readability and its inclusion of places to find more information. Especially recommended."
—*Reference Quarterly, American Library Association, Winter '96*

Mental Health Disorders Sourcebook, 2nd Edition

Basic Consumer Health Information about Anxiety Disorders, Depression and Other Mood Disorders, Eating Disorders, Personality Disorders, Schizophrenia, and More, Including Disease Descriptions, Treatment Options, and Reports on Current Research Initiatives

Along with Statistical Data, Tips for Maintaining Mental Health, a Glossary, and Directory of Sources for Additional Help and Information

Edited by Karen Bellenir. 605 pages. 2000. 0-7808-0240-3. $78.

Mental Retardation Sourcebook

Basic Consumer Health Information about Mental Retardation and Its Causes, Including Down Syndrome, Fetal Alcohol Syndrome, Fragile X Syndrome, Genetic Conditions, Injury, and Environmental Sources

Along with Preventive Strategies, Parenting Issues, Educational Implications, Health Care Needs, Employment and Economic Matters, Legal Issues, a Glossary, and a Resource Listing for Additional Help and Information

Edited by Joyce Brennfleck Shannon. 642 pages. 2000. 0-7808-0377-9. $78.

Obesity Sourcebook

Basic Consumer Health Information about Diseases and Other Problems Associated with Obesity, and Including Facts about Risk Factors, Prevention Issues, and Management Approaches

Along with Statistical and Demographic Data, Information about Special Populations, Research Updates, a Glossary, and Source Listings for Further Help and Information

Edited by Wilma Caldwell and Chad T. Kimball. 376 pages. 2001. 0-7808-0333-7. $48.

Ophthalmic Disorders Sourcebook

Basic Information about Glaucoma, Cataracts, Macular Degeneration, Strabismus, Refractive Disorders, and More

Along with Statistical and Demographic Data and Reports on Current Research Initiatives

Edited by Linda M. Ross. 631 pages. 1996. 0-7808-0081-8. $78.

Oral Health Sourcebook

Basic Information about Diseases and Conditions Affecting Oral Health, Including Cavities, Gum Disease, Dry Mouth, Oral Cancers, Fever Blisters, Canker Sores, Oral Thrush, Bad Breath, Temporomandibular Disorders, and other Craniofacial Syndromes

Along with Statistical Data on the Oral Health of Americans, Oral Hygiene, Emergency First Aid, Information on Treatment Procedures and Methods of Replacing Lost Teeth

Edited by Allan R. Cook. 558 pages. 1997. 0-7808-0082-6. $78.

Osteoporosis Sourcebook

Basic Consumer Health Information about Primary and Secondary Osteoporosis and Juvenile Osteoporosis and Related Conditions, Including Fibrous Dysplasia, Gaucher Disease, Hyperthyroidism, Hypophosphatasia, Myeloma, Osteopetrosis, Osteogenesis Imperfecta, and Paget's Disease

Along with Information about Risk Factors, Treatments, Traditional and Non-traditional Pain Management, a Glossary of Related Terms, and a Directory of Resources

Edited by Allan R. Cook. 600 pages. 2001. 0-7808-0239-X. $78.

SEE ALSO *Women's Health Concerns Sourcebook*

Pain Sourcebook

Basic Information about Specific Forms of Acute and Chronic Pain, Including Headaches, Back Pain, Muscular Pain, Neuralgia, Surgical Pain, and Cancer Pain

Along with Pain Relief Options Such as Analgesics, Narcotics, Nerve Blocks, Transcutaneous Nerve Stimulation, and Alternative Forms of Pain Control, Including Biofeedback, Imaging, Behavior Modification, and Relaxation Techniques

Edited by Allan R. Cook. 667 pages. 1997. 0-7808-0213-6. $78.

"The text is readable, easily understood, and well indexed. This excellent volume belongs in all patient education libraries, consumer health sections of public libraries, and many personal collections."
— American Reference Books Annual, 1999

"A beneficial reference." *— Booklist Health Sciences Supplement, American Library Association, Oct '98*

"The information is basic in terms of scholarship and is appropriate for general readers. Written in journalistic style . . . intended for non-professionals. Quite thorough in its coverage of different pain conditions and summarizes the latest clinical information regarding pain treatment." *— Choice, Association of College and Research Libraries, Jun '98*

"Recommended reference source."
— Booklist, American Library Association, Mar '98

Pediatric Cancer Sourcebook

Basic Consumer Health Information about Leukemias, Brain Tumors, Sarcomas, Lymphomas, and Other Cancers in Infants, Children, and Adolescents, Including Descriptions of Cancers, Treatments, and Coping Strategies

Along with Suggestions for Parents, Caregivers, and Concerned Relatives, a Glossary of Cancer Terms, and Resource Listings

Edited by Edward J. Prucha. 587 pages. 1999. 0-7808-0245-4. $78.

"A valuable addition to all libraries specializing in health services and many public libraries."
— American Reference Books Annual, 2000

"Recommended reference source."
— Booklist, American Library Association, Feb '00

"An excellent source of information. Recommended for public, hospital, and health science libraries with consumer health collections." *— E-Stream, Jun '00*

Physical & Mental Issues in Aging Sourcebook

Basic Consumer Health Information on Physical and Mental Disorders Associated with the Aging Process, Including Concerns about Cardiovascular Disease, Pulmonary Disease, Oral Health, Digestive Disorders, Musculoskeletal and Skin Disorders, Metabolic Changes, Sexual and Reproductive Issues, and Changes in Vision, Hearing, and Other Senses

Along with Data about Longevity and Causes of Death, Information on Acute and Chronic Pain, Descriptions of Mental Concerns, a Glossary of Terms, and Resource Listings for Additional Help

Edited by Jenifer Swanson. 660 pages. 1999. 0-7808-0233-0. $78.

"Recommended for public libraries."
— American Reference Books Annual, 2000

"This is a treasure of health information for the layperson." *— Choice Health Sciences Supplement, Association of College & Research Libraries, May 2000*

"Recommended reference source."
— Booklist, American Library Association, Oct '99

SEE ALSO Healthy Aging Sourcebook

Podiatry Sourcebook

Basic Consumer Health Information about Foot Conditions, Diseases, and Injuries, Including Bunions, Corns, Calluses, Athlete's Foot, Plantar Warts, Hammertoes and Clawtoes, Club Foot, Heel Pain, Gout, and More

Along with Facts about Foot Care, Disease Prevention, Foot Safety, Choosing a Foot Care Specialist, a Glossary of Terms, and Resource Listings for Additional Information

Edited by M. Lisa Weatherford. 600 pages. 2001. 0-7808-0215-2. $78.

Pregnancy & Birth Sourcebook

Basic Information about Planning for Pregnancy, Maternal Health, Fetal Growth and Development, Labor and Delivery, Postpartum and Perinatal Care, Pregnancy in Mothers with Special Concerns, and Disorders of Pregnancy, Including Genetic Counseling, Nutrition and Exercise, Obstetrical Tests, Pregnancy Discomfort, Multiple Births, Cesarean Sections, Medical Testing of Newborns, Breastfeeding, Gestational Diabetes, and Ectopic Pregnancy

Edited by Heather E. Aldred. 737 pages. 1997. 0-7808-0216-0. $78.

"A well-organized handbook. Recommended."
— Choice, Association of College and Research Libraries, Apr '98

"Reecommended reference source."
— Booklist, American Library Association, Mar '98

"Recommended for public libraries."
— American Reference Books Annual, 1998

SEE ALSO Congenital Disorders Sourcebook, Family Planning Sourcebook

Public Health Sourcebook

Basic Information about Government Health Agencies, Including National Health Statistics and Trends, Healthy People 2000 Program Goals and Objectives, the Centers for Disease Control and Prevention, the Food and Drug Administration, and the National Institutes of Health

Along with Full Contact Information for Each Agency

Edited by Wendy Wilcox. 698 pages. 1998. 0-7808-0220-9. $78.

"Recommended reference source."
— *Booklist, American Library Association, Sep '98*

"This consumer guide provides welcome assistance in navigating the maze of federal health agencies and their data on public health concerns."
— *SciTech Book News, Sep '98*

Reconstructive & Cosmetic Surgery Sourcebook

Basic Consumer Health Information on Cosmetic and Reconstructive Plastic Surgery, Including Statistical Information about Different Surgical Procedures, Things to Consider Prior to Surgery, Plastic Surgery Techniques and Tools, Emotional and Psychological Considerations, and Procedure-Specific Information

Along with a Glossary of Terms and a Listing of Resources for Additional Help and Information

Edited by M. Lisa Weatherford. 400 pages. 2001. 0-7808-0214-4. $48.

Rehabilitation Sourcebook

Basic Consumer Health Information about Rehabilitation for People Recovering from Heart Surgery, Spinal Cord Injury, Stroke, Orthopedic Impairments, Amputation, Pulmonary Impairments, Traumatic Injury, and More, Including Physical Therapy, Occupational Therapy, Speech/Language Therapy, Massage Therapy, Dance Therapy, Art Therapy, and Recreational Therapy

Along with Information on Assistive and Adaptive Devices, a Glossary, and Resources for Additional Help and Information

Edited by Dawn D. Matthews. 531 pages. 1999. 0-7808-0236-5. $78.

"Recommended reference source."
— *Booklist, American Library Association, May '00*

Respiratory Diseases & Disorders Sourcebook

Basic Information about Respiratory Diseases and Disorders, Including Asthma, Cystic Fibrosis, Pneumonia, the Common Cold, Influenza, and Others, Featuring Facts about the Respiratory System, Statistical and Demographic Data, Treatments, Self-Help Management Suggestions, and Current Research Initiatives

Edited by Allan R. Cook and Peter D. Dresser. 771 pages. 1995. 0-7808-0037-0. $78.

"Designed for the layperson and for patients and their families coping with respiratory illness. . . . an extensive array of information on diagnosis, treatment, management, and prevention of respiratory illnesses for the general reader." — *Choice, Association of College and Research Libraries, Jun '96*

"A highly recommended text for all collections. It is a comforting reminder of the power of knowledge that good books carry between their covers."
— *Academic Library Book Review, Spring '96*

"A comprehensive collection of authoritative information presented in a nontechnical, humanitarian style for patients, families, and caregivers."
— *Association of Operating Room Nurses, Sep/Oct '95*

Sexually Transmitted Diseases Sourcebook, 1st Edition

Basic Information about Herpes, Chlamydia, Gonorrhea, Hepatitis, Nongonoccocal Urethritis, Pelvic Inflammatory Disease, Syphilis, AIDS, and More

Along with Current Data on Treatments and Preventions

Edited by Linda M. Ross. 550 pages. 1997. 0-7808-0217-9. $78.

Sexually Transmitted Diseases Sourcebook, 2nd Edition

Basic Consumer Health Information about Sexually Transmitted Diseases, Including Information on the Diagnosis and Treatment of Chlamydia, Gonorrhea, Hepatitis, Herpes, HIV, Mononucleosis, Syphilis, and Others

Along with Information on Prevention, Such as Condom Use, Vaccines, and STD Education; And Featuring a Section on Issues Related to Youth and Adolescents, a Glossary, and Resources for Additional Help and Information

Edited by Dawn D. Matthews. 538 pages. 2000. 0-7808-0249-7. $78.

Skin Disorders Sourcebook

Basic Information about Common Skin and Scalp Conditions Caused by Aging, Allergies, Immune Reactions, Sun Exposure, Infectious Organisms, Parasites, Cosmetics, and Skin Traumas, Including Abrasions, Cuts, and Pressure Sores

Along with Information on Prevention and Treatment

Edited by Allan R. Cook. 647 pages. 1997. 0-7808-0080-X. $78.

". . . comprehensive, easily read reference book."
— *Doody's Health Sciences Book Reviews, Oct '97*

SEE ALSO *Burns Sourcebook*

Sleep Disorders Sourcebook

Basic Consumer Health Information about Sleep and Its Disorders, Including Insomnia, Sleepwalking, Sleep Apnea, Restless Leg Syndrome, and Narcolepsy

Along with Data about Shiftwork and Its Effects, Information on the Societal Costs of Sleep Deprivation, Descriptions of Treatment Options, a Glossary of Terms, and Resource Listings for Additional Help

Edited by Jenifer Swanson. 439 pages. 1998. 0-7808-0234-9. $78.

"This text will complement any home or medical library. It is user-friendly and ideal for the adult reader."
—American Reference Books Annual, 2000

"Recommended reference source."
— Booklist, American Library Association, Feb '99

"A useful resource that provides accurate, relevant, and accessible information on sleep to the general public. Health care providers who deal with sleep disorders patients may also find it helpful in being prepared to answer some of the questions patients ask."
—Respiratory Care, Jul '99

Sports Injuries Sourcebook

Basic Consumer Health Information about Common Sports Injuries, Prevention of Injury in Specific Sports, Tips for Training, and Rehabilitation from Injury

Along with Information about Special Concerns for Children, Young Girls in Athletic Training Programs, Senior Athletes, and Women Athletes, and a Directory of Resources for Further Help and Information

Edited by Heather E. Aldred. 624 pages. 1999. 0-7808-0218-7. $78.

"Public libraries and undergraduate academic libraries will find this book useful for its nontechnical language." *—American Reference Books Annual, 2000*

"While this easy-to-read book is recommended for all libraries, it should prove to be especially useful for public, high school, and academic libraries; certainly it should be on the bookshelf of every school gymnasium." *— E-Streams, Mar '00*

Substance Abuse Sourcebook

Basic Health-Related Information about the Abuse of Legal and Illegal Substances Such as Alcohol, Tobacco, Prescription Drugs, Marijuana, Cocaine, and Heroin; and Including Facts about Substance Abuse Prevention Strategies, Intervention Methods, Treatment and Recovery Programs, and a Section Addressing the Special Problems Related to Substance Abuse during Pregnancy

Edited by Karen Bellenir. 573 pages. 1996. 0-7808-0038-9. $78.

"A valuable addition to any health reference section. Highly recommended."
— The Book Report, Mar/Apr '97

". . . a comprehensive collection of substance abuse information that's both highly readable and compact. Families and caregivers of substance abusers will find the information enlightening and helpful, while teachers, social workers and journalists should benefit from the concise format. Recommended."
—Drug Abuse Update, Winter '96/'97

SEE ALSO Alcoholism Sourcebook, Drug Abuse Sourcebook

Traveler's Health Sourcebook

Basic Consumer Health Information for Travelers, Including Physical and Medical Preparations, Transportation Health and Safety, Essential Information about Food and Water, Sun Exposure, Insect and Snake Bites, Camping and Wilderness Medicine, and Travel with Physical or Medical Disabilities

Along with International Travel Tips, Vaccination Recommendations, Geographical Health Issues, Disease Risks, a Glossary, and a Listing of Additional Resources

Edited by Joyce Brennfleck Shannon. 613 pages. 2000. 0-7808-0384-1. $78.

Women's Health Concerns Sourcebook

Basic Information about Health Issues That Affect Women, Featuring Facts about Menstruation and Other Gynecological Concerns, Including Endometriosis, Fibroids, Menopause, and Vaginitis; Reproductive Concerns, Including Birth Control, Infertility, and Abortion; and Facts about Additional Physical, Emotional, and Mental Health Concerns Prevalent among Women Such as Osteoporosis, Urinary Tract Disorders, Eating Disorders, and Depression

Along with Tips for Maintaining a Healthy Lifestyle

Edited by Heather E. Aldred. 567 pages. 1997. 0-7808-0219-5. $78.

"Handy compilation. There is an impressive range of diseases, devices, disorders, procedures, and other physical and emotional issues covered . . . well organized, illustrated, and indexed." *— Choice, Association of College and Research Libraries, Jan '98*

SEE ALSO Breast Cancer Sourcebook, Cancer Sourcebook for Women, 1st and 2nd Editions, Healthy Heart Sourcebook for Women, Osteoporosis Sourcebook

Workplace Health & Safety Sourcebook

Basic Consumer Health Information about Workplace Health and Safety, Including the Effect of Workplace Hazards on the Lungs, Skin, Heart, Ears, Eyes, Brain, Reproductive Organs, Musculoskeletal System, and Other Organs and Body Parts

Along with Information about Occupational Cancer, Personal Protective Equipment, Toxic and Hazardous Chemicals, Child Labor, Stress, and Workplace Violence

Edited by Chad T. Kimball. 626 pages. 2000. 0-7808-0231-4. $78.

Worldwide Health Sourcebook

Basic Information about Global Health Issues, Including Malnutrition, Reproductive Health, Disease Dispersion and Prevention, Emerging Diseases, Risky Health Behaviors, and the Leading Causes of Death

Along with Global Health Concerns for Children, Women, and the Elderly, Mental Health Issues, Research and Technology Advancements, and Economic, Environmental, and Political Health Implications, a Glossary, and a Resource Listing for Additional Help and Information

Edited by Joyce Brennfleck Shannon. 500 pages. 2001. 0-7808-0330-2. $78.

Health Reference Series Cumulative Index 1999

A Comprehensive Index to the Individual Volumes of the Health Reference Series, Including a Subject Index, Name Index, Organization Index, and Publication Index;

Along with a Master List of Acronyms and Abbreviations

Edited by Edward J. Prucha, Anne Holmes, and Robert Rudnick. 990 pages. 2000. 0-7808-0382-5. $78.

116420524